Examination of Intraocular Fluid

Yong Tao • De-Kuang Hwang

Examination of Intraocular Fluid

Springer
PEOPLE'S MEDICAL PUBLISHING HOUSE
PMPH

Yong Tao
Depatment of Ophthalmology
Beijing Chao-Yang Hospital
Beijing, China

De-Kuang Hwang
Department of Ophthalmology
Taipei Veterans General Hospital
Taipei, China

ISBN 978-981-96-2485-0 ISBN 978-981-96-2486-7 (eBook)
https://doi.org/10.1007/978-981-96-2486-7

Jointly published with People's Medical Publishing House, PR of China

This Springer imprint is published by the registered company Springer Nature Singapore Pte Ltd.
The registered company address is: 152 Beach Road, #21-01/04 Gateway East, Singapore 189721, Singapore

Foreword 1

Examination of intraocular fluid is an important tool for advancing ophthalmic diagnosis and treatment in the era of precision medicine. This book provides a detailed and comprehensive summary of the methods, indications, and significance of intraocular fluid testing, which can greatly assist clinical doctors.

Dennis S. C. Lam

C-MER Dennis Lam Eye Center,
C-Mer International Eye Care Group Limited
Hong Kong Hong Kong

International Eye Research Institute of the Chinese
University of Hong Kong (Shenzhen)
Shenzhen China

Foreword 2

I would like to congratulate Professors Tao and Hwang for conceiving and compiling this book on the examination of intraocular fluids. This book is very comprehensive and includes several practical tips that are generally not available elsewhere. It will be helpful not only to clinicians but also to researchers conducting research on human samples.

L V Prasad Eye Institute, Kallam
Anji Reddy Campus, L V Prasad Marg
Hyderabad India

Soumyava Basu

Foreword 3

Prof. DK Hwang and Prof. Yong Tao have published an excellent book on intraocular fluid collection, analysis, and utilization. The content incorporates the latest technologies and is truly remarkable; such a comprehensive book has never been available. I am confident that it will benefit many patients.

Department of Ophthalmology, Faculty of Medicine
Graduate School of Medical Sciences, Kyushu University
Fukuoka Japan

Koh-Hei Sonoda

Foreword 4

In the past, the limited availability of intraocular sample volumes made their use in clinical practice challenging. However, with technological advancements, the testing of intraocular specimens is gradually becoming applicable in clinical practice. Recently, intraocular fluid examination has become increasingly important, especially in diagnosing infectious uveitis. Nowadays, with just a small amount of aqueous humor and vitreous fluid, it is possible to detect and monitor the DNA and RNA of intraocular pathogens, as well as investigate the concentrations of inflammatory cytokines or angiogenesis factors. This capability aids in diagnosing diseases, tracking treatment efficacy, and exploring disease pathophysiology.

The author of this book uses a clear and concise approach to explain the methods for obtaining, testing, and clinically applying intraocular fluids. This provides clinicians with more tools to effectively and quickly treat each patient's unique condition. I highly recommend this book to all ophthalmic clinical practitioners.

Department of Ophthalmology
Kaohsiung Medical University
Kaohsiung Taiwan

Shwu-Jiuan Sheu

Preface

We are going through an era of transformation in the diagnosis and treatment mode of ocular diseases. In the past, patients were accustomed to seeking medical attention in the late stages of severe illness, hereby doctors could make corresponding diagnoses based on typical clinical manifestations. In this case, the prognosis is relatively poor. Nowadays, patients with ocular diseases tend to seek medical attention in the early stage, and the ocular symptoms are often mild or atypical, which makes it difficult for doctors to make a definite judgment in a timely manner. The use of molecular technology to assist ophthalmologists in making early diagnoses has become a trend.

Additionally, many ocular diseases including uveitis are often associated with systemic diseases. Clinically, when dealing with those patients, the most critical task for us is to accurately determine the underlying cause of the disease—whether it is due to infection or autoimmune conditions or other causes. Sometimes, the disease progresses rapidly, requiring ophthalmologist to promptly differentiate the diagnosis to provide timely and effective treatment, thereby preventing blindness of the patients.

With advancements in medical research and innovative techniques, many previously undiagnosable cases of uveitis have now been understand in recent decades. For example, previously idiopathic conditions such as Posner-Schlossman syndrome and Fuchs' heterochromic iridocyclitis are now found to be associated with cytomegalovirus or rubella virus infections. These new insights have significantly reduced the risk of blindness in these patients.

Dr. Hwang and I have been dedicated to studying ocular specimen examination techniques for over a decade. Through continuous experimentation, the clinical importance of analyzing ocular fluid specimens for uveitis has been recognized. This technique has been applied widely in my clinics and successfully cured many patients with complicated ocular diseases, such as uveitis.

This book begins with an explanation of the basic procedures for obtaining ocular specimens, basic protein and cytokine testing, and the latest trends in genetic testing, detailing the principles behind each method. Additionally, it discusses the clinical value of ocular specimen examination for diagnosing and monitoring various types of uveitis. The aim of writing this book is to provide valuable information to clinical practitioners in ophthalmology for treating their patients.

In the era of precision medicine, it is crucial to diagnose the underlying cause of each patient's disease as quickly as possible and provide individualized treatment based on the specific etiology and condition, ensuring the best possible treatment and prognosis for the patient.

Beijing, China Yong Tao

Contents

Introduction of Intraocular Fluids

1

Contents

1.1 Types of Intraocular Fluids

The term "intraocular fluids" encompasses various fluids present within the eyeball, such as aqueous humor, vitreous humor, subretinal fluid, and suprachoroidal effusion.

To ensure optimal functioning of the eye as a visual organ, it is vital for the refractive media to maintain transparency. This necessitates a relatively calm immune environment within the eye. Failure to do so would result in an accumulation of protein components, leading to a reduction in the transparency of the refractive media. The immunological privilege observed in the eye can be attributed to three key factors: (1) the presence of morphological, cellular, and molecular barriers; (2) ocular immune tolerance, also known as anterior chamber-associated immune deviation (ACAID); and (3) the existence of an immunosuppressive environment within the eye.

The aqueous humor is a fluid that is clear in nature. The aqueous humor that circulates throughout the eye serves to provide nourishment to the cornea and lens, facilitate the removal of metabolic waste products, and ultimately drain into the venous blood system [1]. The ophthalmic fluid most frequently employed for detection purposes is the aqueous humor, owing to its ease of extraction. The aqueous humor is responsible for occupying both the anterior and posterior chambers, with

Y. Tao, D.-K. Hwang, *Examination of Intraocular Fluid*,
https://doi.org/10.1007/978-981-96-2486-7_1

a combined volume ranging from 0.15 to 0.3 mL. The primary constituent of the substance is water, comprising around 98.75% of its composition. It exhibits a pH range of 7.5–7.6, a specific gravity of 1.003, a viscosity ranging from 1.025 to 1.100, and a refractive index of 1.336. The aqueous humor is derived from plasma; however, its protein concentration is approximately 0.2 mg/mL, representing a mere fraction of the protein level found in plasma, ranging from 1/400 to 1/300. The composition of aqueous humor differs from plasma due to the presence of the blood-ocular barrier, which includes the blood-aqueous barrier and the blood-retina barrier. The concentrations of albumin, ascorbic acid, and lactic acid in plasma are comparatively higher, whereas the concentrations of globulin, amino acid, and glucose in plasma are relatively lower [2, 3].

The vitreous fluid is contained within the vitreous cavity and encompasses roughly two-thirds of the eyeball's total volume, amounting to approximately 4.5 mL. The primary constituent of the substance is water, comprising around 98% of its composition. In addition, it contains a minor proportion of collagen fibers and hyaluronic acid, each constituting less than 1% of the overall composition. The vitreous body is characterized by its transparency, with a refractive index ranging from 1.3345 to 1.3348 and a density between 1.0053 and 1.0089. The extracellular gel matrix is characterized by a high level of hydration and a near absence of cells. Collagen type 2 is a highly prevalent structural protein found in the vitreous, characterized by a rigid triple helix structure resembling a rod. It plays a crucial role in forming a network that functions as a scaffold within the vitreous. Hyaluronic acid, a disaccharide polymer, possesses a randomly coiled structure while in solution. This structural characteristic enables it to support the collagen network and exert osmotic pressure, so maintaining the proper positioning of the retina. Prior to conducting the examination, it is advisable to employ low-speed centrifugation in order to separate the supernatant for subsequent testing [4]. Furthermore, the composition of 11 chemical constituents, including glucose, inside the vitreous humor undergoes alterations as the postmortem interval increases. This phenomenon can contribute to the forensic determination of the time of death and enhance the precision of estimating the time of death. The levels of glucose, salt, and chlorine in the vitreous humor exhibit a steady decline as the postmortem period increases. Conversely, the concentrations of urea, creatinine, uric acid, potassium, calcium, magnesium, inorganic phosphorus, and trace protein demonstrate a gradual increase with the prolonging of the postmortem interval. A clear and evident linear correlation can be observed between the concentration of potassium ions and the time of death, namely, during a postmortem interval of 72 h [5].

The presence of subretinal fluid is observed in pathological states rather than in normal physiological states. It can occur in a variety of conditions, including exudative retinal detachment and rhegmatogenous retinal detachment [6] caused by intraocular tumors, retinal/choroidal vasculopathy and so forth, and mixed retinal detachment, central serous retinopathy [7], and optic disc pit [8] caused by diabetic retinopathy. The examination of the composition of subretinal fluid can provide valuable insights for determining the underlying cause in certain instances. In the context of proliferative vitreoretinopathy, the subretinal fluid of patients exhibits the presence of neuroretina cells, deep pigment cells, retinal pigment epithelial cells, and macrophages. However, it is noteworthy that lymphocytes are not discernible within this fluid [9]. The presence of collagenase, gelatinase, elastase, and cathepsin G has been observed in the subretinal fluid in cases of retinal detachment. Notably, matrix metalloproteinase-2 (MMP-2) is the primary gelatinase identified in this context [10]. Kowalczuk L et al. [11] took out the subretinal fluid from one patient with refractory central serous retinopathy and compared it with that of two patients with long-standing rhegmatogenous retinal detachment. A total of 128 proteins were identified, with 77 proteins exhibiting downregulation and 51 proteins showing upregulation. Additionally, 76 metabolites were detected, with 43 metabolites displaying downregulation and 33 metabolites demonstrating upregulation. Consequently, these findings indicate differential expression of proteins and metabolites in subretinal fluid under varied conditions.

Suprachoroidal effusion is also found in pathological conditions and has been reported to be associated with several systemic diseases, including systemic lupus erythematosus (SLE) [12–15], leukemia [16], lymphoma [17], IgA nephropathy [18], HIV [19], idiopathic pulmonary arterial hypertension [20], and rhegmatogenous retinal detachment [21]. Iwase T et al. reported the use of 27-gauge needles to drain suprachoroidal effusion during vitrectomy [21]. The analysis of suprachoroidal effusion plays an auxiliary role in the judgment of the etiology and mechanism. For example, Stefater JA et al. analyzed the drainage and composition of suprachoroidal effusion in patients with acute systemic lupus erythematosus and found that the suprachoroidal effusion may be caused by inflammation, rather than secondary to hypoproteinemia or other exudation processes [15]. The results are shown in Table 1.1.

Table 1.1 An examination and comparison of suprachoroidal effusion in individuals diagnosed with acute systemic lupus erythematosus [15]

	Serum	Cerebrospinal fluid (CSF)	Suprachoroidal effusion in the right eye	Suprachoroidal effusion in the left eye
Protein (g/dL)	5.4	2.9	3.4	3.4
LDH (U/L)	235	60	187	154
Suprachoroidal fluid to serum protein ratio		0.54	0.63	0.63
Suprachoroidal fluid to serum LDH ratio		0.26	0.8	0.66
Suprachoroidal fluid LDH/LDH upper-limit-of-normal (the upper limit of normal for LDH is 222 U/L)		0.27	0.84	0.69

1.2 A Guide to the Selection of Items for Intraocular Fluids Examination

The detection of intraocular fluids is a recently developed area of study, and clinicians sometimes experience difficulty while determining the appropriate testing items and situations for intraocular fluid testing.

In addressing this issue, the author proposes the importance of adopting a composed mindset in order to comprehend the examination procedures and principles, in conjunction with the clinical state, with the aim of effectively utilizing this tool. Indeed, the aforementioned phenomenon can be characterized as a cognitive progression, when individuals undergo a period of initial unfamiliarity followed by a gradual acquisition of familiarity.

In a general sense, there are two distinct ways of inspection: "confirmation" and "exclusion." The term "confirmation" pertains to the ability of clinicians to make a comprehensive assessment based on clinical manifestations, conduct specific examinations of intraocular fluids, and validate their clinical judgment. On the other hand, the term "exclusion" refers to scenarios where clinical lesions are in their initial stages, or the clinical manifestations are atypical, or there are inconsistencies in the clinical manifestations, thereby hindering clinicians from making a relatively high probability clinical judgment. Hence, doctors employ a selection of representative examination items with a relatively high probability to assist in the process of narrowing down the diagnosis or investigating the underlying cause (Table 1.2).

It should be noted that in different situations, the items of "exclusion" inspection may vary in different circumstances. For example, when the author encounters atypical situations, the following items are often tested: cytomegalovirus (CMV) and varicella-zoster virus (VZV), the most common exams for intraocular virus infection; Toxocara antibody, the most common exam for intraocular parasite infection; and IL-6 and IL-10, the most common exams for masquerade syndrome. If

Table 1.2 A comparative analysis of inspection modes for the examination of intraocular fluids

Inspection mode	Confirmation	Exclusion
Application	A preliminary judgment can be drawn from the medical history, symptoms, other noninvasive examinations, and other findings	The clinical manifestations are not typical, so that clinicians cannot obtain clinical impressions based on data available
Exam items	Less	More
Pertinence of exams	Strong	Weak
Disadvantages for patients	If the examination results cannot confirm the clinical judgment, the patient faces the risk of continuing to be sampled and delaying the timing of clinical treatment	Additional one-time charges
Benefits for patients	Less initial expenditure	Less probability of repeated exams of intraocular fluids

endophthalmitis is encountered, gene chip, or next-generation sequencing (NGS), G test, GM test, fungal 26S rRNA gene, bacterial 16S rRNA gene, lipopolysaccharide (LPS) experiment, smear, and culture, etc., will be comprehensively carried out to improve the overall inspection efficiency by combined detection.

The selection between "confirmation" and "exclusion" is not determined by a universally standardized approach but rather relies on the clinical expertise of the physician and the observed clinical signs of the disease.

It is anticipated that the usage of "exclusion" will progressively assume a dominant position in the future, owing to many factors. The initial phase of the disease sometimes presents with atypical clinical signs, such as acute retinal necrosis (ARN). In clinic, the prognosis of ARN is often unfavorable, which is due to the frequent occurrence of retinal artery occlusion, extensive retinal necrosis, and even the development of "rag-like changes" in the late stage. If the clinician can confirm the diagnosis of ARN in the early stage, the prognosis of ARN will definitely improve to a large extent. The inevitability of medical advancement lies in the early detection and treatment of diseases. Similarly, alterations in living standards and habits will therefore result in modifications in the clinical presentations of illnesses. In clinical practice, it is commonly observed that a majority of patients diagnosed with syphilitic uveitis do not exhibit symptoms such as chancre and rash. Furthermore, in my experience, patients with tuberculous uveitis usually do not present with low-grade afternoon fever, night sweats, and weight loss, despite that severe systemic tuberculosis patients may be present with those signs.

The advancement of molecular biology technology has led to an accelerated examination process, reduced examination costs, and an expanded scope of microbial species covered by these examinations.

References

1. Pietrowska K, Dmuchowska DA, Krasnicki P, Mariak Z, Kretowski A, Ciborowski M. Analysis of pharmaceuticals and small molecules in aqueous humor. J Pharm Biomed Anal. 2018;159:23–36.
2. Ge J, Wang N. Ophthalmology. People's Medical Publishing House; 2015.
3. Kronfeld PC. The ascorbic acid content of the aqueous of surgically aphakic human eyes. Trans Am Ophthalmol Soc. 1952;50:347–58.
4. Liu X, Tao Y. Use the examination of intraocular fluid well. Chin J Ophthalmol Med (Electronic Edition). 2018;8(05):193–201.
5. Tao T, Xu J, Luo TX, Liao ZG, Pan HF. Contents of vitreous humor of dead body with different postmortem intervals. J Sichuan Univ Med Sci Ed. 2006;37(6):898–900, 927.
6. Fu JL, Shi G, Liu ZX, Su GF, Kang ZC. A systematic review on delayed absorption of subretinal fluid after scleral buckling for rhegmatogenous retinal detachment. J Biol Regul Homeost Agents. 2017;31(3):639–43.
7. Luttrull JK. Low-intensity/high-density subthreshold diode micropulse laser for central serous chorioretinopathy. Retina (Philadelphia, Pa). 2016;36(9):1658–63.
8. Steel DH, Williamson TH, Laidlaw DA, Sharma P, Matthews C, Rees J, Petrou P, Charteris DG, Charles SJ, Patel CK, et al. Extent and location of Intraretinal and subretinal fluid as prognostic factors for the outcome of patients with optic disk pit maculopathy. Retina (Philadelphia, Pa). 2016;36(1):110–8.

9. Xu X, He Z. Cytological study of subretinal fluid. Chin J Ophthalmol. 1997;33(6):450–2.
10. Immonen I, Konttinen YT, Sorsa T, Tommila P, Sirén V. Proteinases in subretinal fluid. Graefe's Arch Clin Exp Ophthalmol = Albrecht von Graefes Archiv fur klinische und experimentelle Ophthalmologie. 1996;234(2):105–9.
11. Kowalczuk L, Matet A, Dor M, Bararpour N, Daruich A, Dirani A, Behar-Cohen F, Thomas A, Turck N. Proteome and Metabolome of subretinal fluid in central serous chorioretinopathy and rhegmatogenous retinal detachment: a pilot case study. Transl Vis Sci Technol. 2018;7(1):3.
12. Han YS, Min Yang C, Lee SH, Shin JH, Moon SW, Kang JH. Secondary angle closure glaucoma by lupus choroidopathy as an initial presentation of systemic lupus erythematosus: a case report. BMC Ophthalmol. 2015;15:148.
13. Wisotsky BJ, Magat-Gordon CB, Puklin JE. Angle-closure glaucoma as an initial presentation of systemic lupus erythematosus. Ophthalmology. 1998;105(7):1170–2.
14. Lavina AM, Agarwal A, Hunyor A, Gass JD. Lupus choroidopathy and choroidal effusions. Retina (Philadelphia, Pa). 2002;22(5):643–7.
15. Stefater JA, Eliott D, Kim LA. Drainage and analysis of suprachoroidal fluid in a patient with acute systemic lupus erythematous. Am J Ophthalmol Case Rep. 2017;5:29–32.
16. Patel AV, Miller JB, Nath R, Shih HA, Yoon MK, Freitag SK, Papaliodis G, Chen TC, Eliott D, Kim IK. Unilateral eye findings: a rare herald of acute leukemia. Ocular Oncol Pathol. 2016;2(3):166–70.
17. Cristol SM, Baumblatt JG, Icasiano E, Grajewski AL, Olivier MM, Parrish RK. Bilateral acute angle-closure associated with systemic lymphoma: a report of 2 cases. J Glaucoma. 2011;20(2):115–7.
18. Pavlin CJ, Easterbrook M, Harasiewicz K, Foster FS. An ultrasound biomicroscopic analysis of angle-closure glaucoma secondary to ciliochoroidal effusion in IgA nephropathy. Am J Ophthalmol. 1993;116(3):341–5.
19. Nash RW, Lindquist TD. Bilateral angle-closure glaucoma associated with uveal effusion: presenting sign of HIV infection. Surv Ophthalmol. 1992;36(4):255–8.
20. Akduman L, Del Priore LV, Kaplan HJ, Meredith T. Uveal effusion syndrome associated with primary pulmonary hypertension and vomiting. Am J Ophthalmol. 1996;121(5):578–80.
21. Iwase T, Ra E, Terasaki H. New technique to drain Suprachoroidal fluid with a 27-gauge needle during Vitrectomy. Retina (Philadelphia, Pa). 2022;42(10):2004–7.

Collection of Intraocular Fluids

2

Contents

2.1 The Safety of Collection of Intraocular Fluids

Anterior chamber puncture refers to the procedure of acquiring or removing aqueous humor as part of the initial medical intervention for managing glaucoma attacks [1]. It is also the prevailing method for collecting intraocular fluids.

Generally speaking, when performed in accordance with correct procedures, it can be considered sufficiently safe. A study conducted by Kitazawa and colleagues, prominent scholars in the field of Japanese ophthalmology, engaged the implementation of anterior chamber puncture in a sample of 301 eyes. The procedure was carried out using a 30-gauge needle, and the decision to perform anterior chamber puncture was based on clinical considerations related to various conditions. These conditions included viral infections such as corneal endothelitis, anterior segment infectious uveitis, cytomegalovirus retinitis, and acute retinal necrosis. Additionally, bacterial infections such as endophthalmitis, as well as malignancies including primary intraocular lymphoma, intraocular metastasis of leukemia, and retinoblastoma, were also considered as indications for anterior chamber puncture. There were no instances of severe sequelae, such as infection, hyphema, lens injury,

Y. Tao, D.-K. Hwang, *Examination of Intraocular Fluid*,
https://doi.org/10.1007/978-981-96-2486-7_2

hypopyon, or extensive fibrous exudation in the anterior chamber [2]. Swiss scholars conducted anterior chamber puncture on a total of 45 eyes. Out of these, one eye experienced a transient exacerbation of anterior chamber inflammation, leading to hospitalization for a duration of 24 h. Fortunately, no long-term consequences were observed in this particular case [3].

To date, the present author has conservatively estimated that the total number of anterior chamber puncture cases exceeds 4000. Notably, no instances of endophthalmitis resulting from anterior chamber puncture have been identified. According to my personal experience, one patient who had undergone bone marrow transplantation and was on long-term oral tacrolimus treatment presented with anterior chamber empyema in the right eye, while the left eye exhibited a clean anterior chamber. Following the administration of anterior chamber puncture to the left eye, the subsequent development of hypopyon was observed in the left eye on the subsequent day. Subsequent verification established that the individual in question experienced an episode of fungemia, resulting in the manifestation of endogenous fungal endophthalmitis in the right eye. It is worth noting that the occurrence of the condition in the left eye was not attributed to the introduction of microorganisms into the anterior chamber via anterior chamber puncture, but rather to a reduction in intraocular pressure (IOP), which facilitated the expedited infiltration of fungi carried by the bloodstream into the ocular region. In the context of stringent operational protocols, the safety profile of anterior chamber puncture remains notably high, even within the ophthalmology clinic rather than operating room [4–8].

Performing an anterior chamber puncture prior to intravitreal medication administration is a very secure surgical technique that effectively mitigates the potential elevation of intraocular pressure resulting from the drug injection into the eye [9]: There have been studies suggesting that the administration of intravitreal medication injections may lead to a significant elevation in intraocular pressure (IOP) [10], and it is speculated that this could potentially result in harm to the optic nerve. The restoration of IOP to its baseline level often occurs within a time frame of 15–30 min [11]. Patients with IOP over 80 mmHg subsequent to intravitreal injection may exhibit no symptoms and remain undiagnosed during clinical assessments immediately following the injection or on the subsequent day. This lack of detection has the potential to result in significant and irreversible damage to the optic nerve [12]. Some scholars performed 230 cases of intravitreal drug injection (0.1 mL), of which 33% ($n = 87$) were combined with anterior chamber paracentesis at the same time, and put forth arguments in favor of the benefits of this procedure [13]. Furthermore, the specimens obtained from anterior chamber puncture prior to intravitreal injection were found to have no theoretical danger of potential drug infiltration into the aqueous humor resulting from posterior chamber spillover into the anterior chamber.

Diagnostic vitrectomy: Diagnostic vitrectomy is a surgical procedure utilized for the purpose of obtaining vitreous and retinal or choroidal specimens in cases of intraocular inflammatory diseases or malignant tumors with unknown etiology and ineffective treatment. This procedure is performed to facilitate a definitive diagnosis through the application of modern molecular biology and laboratory techniques [14]. By carefully selecting acceptable indications and employing skilled surgical methods, the incidence of complications related to diagnostic vitrectomy can be minimized. The main outcomes include temporary low intraocular pressure (IOP) following surgery, development of secondary glaucoma, formation of cataracts, retinal detachment, choroidal hemorrhage, vitreous hemorrhage, endophthalmitis, exacerbation of preexisting inflammatory conditions, proliferative vitreoretinopathy, and some other potential complications [14]. Haruta M et al. reported a case of macular hole after diagnostic vitrectomy for intraocular lymphoma [15].

2.2 The Significance and Value of Collecting Intraocular Fluids

Collecting local tissues or tissue fluids in situ for detection or pathological examination is a widely used method in clinical practice, for example, thoracocentesis to remove pleural effusion [16], lumbar puncture [17], renal biopsy, abdominocentesis, cerebral biopsy [18], amniocentesis, etc. One benefit of this approach is the ability to acquire precise and localized data regarding lesions. Ultimately, the blood test serves as an indicator of the overall systemic state and is not capable of accurately representing the specific local location.

In instances involving lesions, the integrity of the blood-eye barrier is compromised, resulting in the inability of the blood indicator to accurately reflect the intraocular condition. This is mostly due to the relatively small volume of intraocular tissue in relation to the total body volume, resulting in a minimal concentration of the indicator after dilution into the bloodstream. Furthermore, the structure of the eyeball is that of a closed sphere, which presents a challenge for intraocular pathogenic germs to infiltrate the bloodstream. Hence, the analysis of intraocular fluids is necessary due to the presence of the blood-eye barrier, which creates a distinct intraocular milieu. Consequently, relying solely on blood indicators is insufficient to accurately reflect the intraocular circumstances, both in normal and pathological states. The collection of intraocular fluids holds great significance as it allows for the acquisition of localized intraocular pathogenic, immunological, cellular, and molecular pathological data. This information plays a crucial role in aiding the clinical diagnosis and treatment of various disorders.

Serological laboratory techniques are not capable of accurately assessing the intraocular state. Keorochana N et al. [19] collected aqueous humor and serum from 92 patients and found that the proportion of positive serum virus antibodies was 83.3% (HSV), 94.0% (VZV), 98.8% (EBV), and 97.6% (CMV), respectively. Nevertheless, there were no positive results observed in the polymerase chain reaction (PCR) analysis of the nucleic acid of the virus present in the aqueous humor.

The diagnostic vitrectomy procedure has been found to have an overall return rate ranging from 20.0% to 55.3% for cases of unexplained uveitis with unusual clinical symptoms [20–29]. It appears that despite continuous advancements in laboratory technology, there has been minimal alteration in profitability throughout the course of time.

In certain instances, the procedures of diagnostic vitrectomy and therapeutic vitrectomy are indistinguishable and not just employed for the purpose of sampling. Pakdel et al. observed that following diagnostic vitrectomy, the subretinal lymphoma lesions exhibited a reduction in size or resolution [30]. According to the research conducted by Iaccheri B et al., it was observed that vitrectomy exhibited a transient therapeutic impact on intraocular lymphoma [31].

In a broad sense, the primary uses of intraocular fluid testing can be categorized as follows:

Infectious uveitis: Infectious uveitis, including endophthalmitis [32], cytomegalovirus retinitis [33], acute retinal necrosis [34], herpesvirus anterior uveitis [35], ocular toxoplasmosis [36], ocular toxocariasis [37], etc., are the main detection indications for collection of etiological evidence of infection in situ for laboratory diagnosis.

Uveitis with unknown cause [21, 22, 28, 29]: The clinical manifestations can be perplexing. In cases of infectious uveitis, autoimmune uveitis, or masquerade syndrome, when a definitive diagnosis cannot be made based solely on clinical manifestations, additional examinations and blood tests should be conducted. Intraocular fluid samples should be collected and subjected to high-throughput or comprehensive pathogenic microorganism nucleic acid, antibody, and cytokine detection in order to lead to a conclusive diagnosis.

Retinal/choroidal vascular diseases: Different types of retinal/choroidal vascular diseases have different cytokine expression profiles. As biomarkers, they have the advantages of auxiliary diagnosis (such as differentiation of choroidal neovascularization and polypoid choroidal lesions [38]), staging, and typing [39–43]. This type of disease often requires intraocular injection of anti-VEGF drugs/glucocorticoids for treatment. Before injection, collecting aqueous humor for cytokine detection can help accurately determine the intraocular neovascularization/immune status and provide reference for clinical selection of injection types and timing [44–49]. In some cases, retinal/choroidal vascular diseases are vasculitis caused by infectious factors such as tuberculosis [50] and spirochetes [51]. The collection of intraocular fluids for the purpose of pathogenic testing has the potential to offer valuable diagnostic assistance.

Progressive retinal, choroidal, and pigment epithelial lesions with atypical clinical manifestations and unresponsive to treatment by conventional methods [14]: Through the positive results of diagnostic tests, the treatment plans can be adjusted and predictive treatment can be given to manage potential systemic and ocular complications [14, 25].

To meet the demand of precision medicine: one limitation of evaluating the treatment impact purely based on medication-induced clinical manifestations is the potential for delayed response. The evaluation of the treatment's appropriateness and the potential need for altering other medications may require an extended period of time for reflection. By examining the changes of cytokine titers in intraocular fluids after treatment [52], it is possible to evaluate whether drug resistance is present in a short time, and whether the clinical judgment is correct, and to develop a medication plan and treatment timing. For instance, in one my patient with presumed diagnosis of endogenous fungal endophthalmitis, smear of intraocular fluid is negative and culture may take at least several more days. I removed some aqueous humor of measurement of IL-8 and gave intraocular injection of anti-fungi drug. One day later, reduction of aqueous IL-8 was observed, which supported the presumed diagnosis of fungal endophthalmitis, and the subsequent intense anti-fungi treatment can be given more firmly.

Possible future applications: the progressive development of equipment and technology designed for the collection of intraocular fluids has led to potential expansion of indications for clinicians to collect such fluids for the purpose of detection and analysis. This expansion may serve as a means of excluding diseases and providing early warnings in the era of evidence-based medicine. Recent research investigations have indicated an elevation in the levels of IL-36, IL-37, and IL-38 in the aqueous humor of individuals diagnosed with chronic primary angle-closure glaucoma. Furthermore, these elevated levels have been found to be associated with the extent of visual field impairment [53]. Cataract surgery has been found to potentially trigger acute retinal necrosis [54], whereas corneal transplantation has been observed to transfer the cornea from donors with HSV-1 keratitis [55]. If the virus antibody testing is conducted on the discarded aqueous humor, it may facilitate early detection, enabling interventions such as lowering the administration of post-operative glucocorticoid eye drops to mitigate viral reproduction.

2.3 Extraction of Intraocular Fluids

2.3.1 Extraction of Aqueous Humor

The extraction of aqueous humor through anterior chamber puncture necessitates a preliminary slit lamp examination to assess the ocular state. It is imperative to refrain from doing the procedure in cases of active infectious conjunctivitis, blepharitis, lacrimal duct inflammation, and similar conditions. Prior to the extraction of the aqueous humor, it is recommended to provide antibiotic eye drops, such as tobramycin eye drops or levofloxacin eye drops, at a frequency of six times per day for a duration of 3 consecutive days. In the event that the extraction is scheduled on the same day, a temporary administration of the eye drops for a duration of 5 min may be conducted, totally six administrations [56, 57].

2.3.1.1 Extraction of Aqueous Humor in the Outpatient Room

The extraction of aqueous humor in the outpatient treatment room is commonly conducted in office settings in the United States and Canada. This method, known as intravitreal medication injection, is a minimally invasive intraocular intervention [58]; No statistically significant differences were observed among patients who had intravitreal injections in an operating room, a room with adequate space, or an office environment [59]. The author's method for extracting aqueous humor is conducted exclusively within the outpatient treatment room following ultraviolet disinfection. However, some hospitals and departments express apprehension regarding the potential infection risks associated with the outpatient treatment room. At present, there is a lack of unanimity both at the international and domestic levels. Hence, when determining the appropriate setting for extracting the aqueous humor, it is imperative to carefully evaluate the unique circumstances of the entity in question.

Environmental Disinfection

It involves the process of sterilizing the puncture chamber using ultraviolet disinfection for a duration of 40 min. It is important to ensure that doors and windows are closed during the disinfection period.

Ocular Preparation

The conjunctival surface can be effectively anesthetized using oxybuprocaine or tetracaine eye drops. This can be achieved by administering the drops once every 3 min, for a total of three consecutive applications. Following this, the upper and lower eyelids should be disinfected using either alcohol or anisodine. It is important to note that the lid margin and the base of the eyelashes should be cleaned using a cotton swab dipped in a small amount of alcohol or anerdian, while avoiding contact with the conjunctiva (refer to Fig. 2.1). Finally, the conjunctival sac should be rinsed with antibiotic eye drops.

Anterior Chamber Puncture and Fluid Extraction

The patient should be instructed to position their head securely within the slit lamp head frame and firmly affix it to the forehead support, utilizing the slit lamp for assistance. The selection of syringes involves choosing between a 25 G needle, which is equivalent to a 1 mL syringe, and a finer needle tip such as a 31 G or 32 G insulin needle. During the procedure, it is advisable to urge the patient to gently elevate their gaze and access the puncture site through the translucent corneal limbus. It is advisable to situate the needle insertion at the 5 o'clock orientation, as depicted in Fig. 2.2. The needle tip is positioned with its beveled surface facing the surgeon, and it is directed toward the 7 o'clock position. This positioning offers the advantage of reducing the risk of inadvertent lens injury and promoting the formation of a longer corneal tunnel, which is more likely to remain open (Fig. 2.3). Once the needle tip has been introduced into the anterior chamber (Fig. 2.4), it is

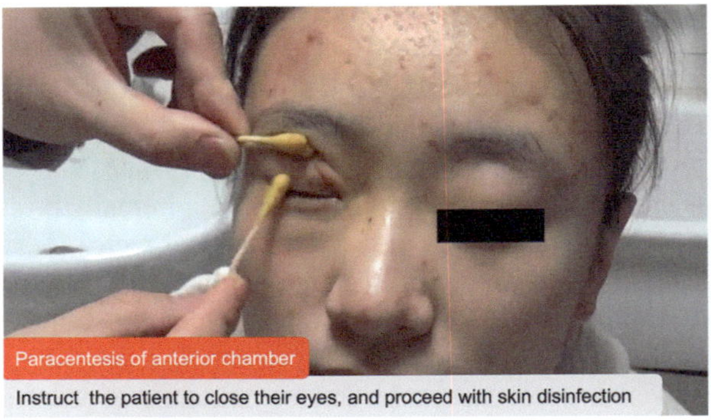

Fig. 2.1 It is recommended to employ anerdian for the purpose of disinfecting the skin Subsequently, delicately invert the edge of the eyelid and proceed to cleanse it utilizing a cotton swab that has been lightly saturated with anerdian

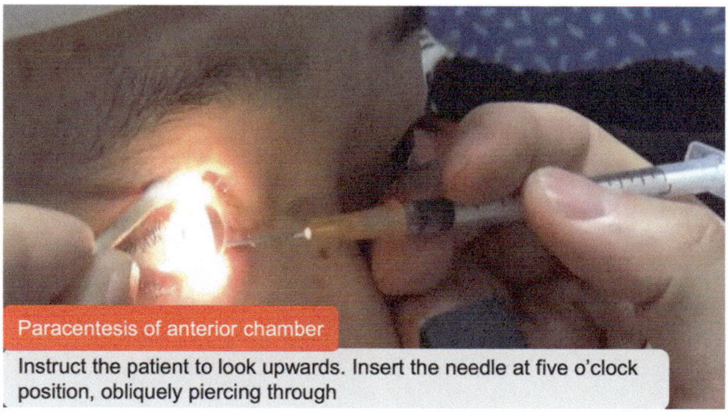

Fig. 2.2 The patient should be directed to stabilize their head by placing it within the slit lamp head frame, ensuring that their forehead is firmly pressed on the frontal support. Next, instruct the patient to direct their gaze in an upward direction and proceed to delicately manipulate the upper eyelid margin by using a cotton swab. The syringe needle is introduced into the anterior chamber through the clear cornea, specifically at the 5 o'clock position. In instances where accessing the anterior chamber proves challenging, one may attempt to facilitate needle rotation by employing a twisting motion including the thumb and index finger

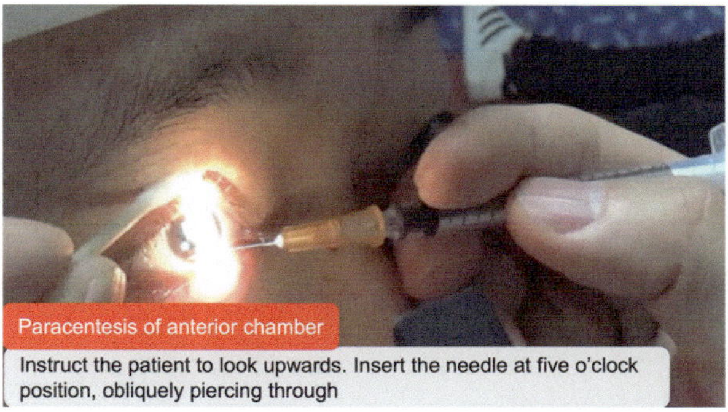

Fig. 2.3 The operator makes an observation of the bevel of the needle in order to ascertain the entry of the syringe needle into the anterior chamber. If the needle is positioned within the layers of the corneal stroma, it is not possible to remove the anterior aqueous humor

advisable to advise the patient to maintain ocular stability. Subsequently, the needle plug should be gradually withdrawn, and the needle tip should be removed after extracting 0.05–0.1 mL of anterior aqueous humor.

Subsequent Processing

Retract the syringe needle in an outward direction. Redeliver antibiotic eye drops to irrigate the conjunctival sac, and provide instructions for the patient to administer antibiotic eye drops at regular intervals of every 30 min until bedtime.

2.3.1.2 Extraction of Aqueous Humor in the Operating Room

it is advisable to adhere to the established protocol for intravitreal medication administration [59]. Prior to extracting the fluid from the anterior chamber, it is recommended to administer antibiotic eye drops, such as tobramycin eye drops or levofloxacin eye drops, six times daily for 3 consecutive days. In the event that the

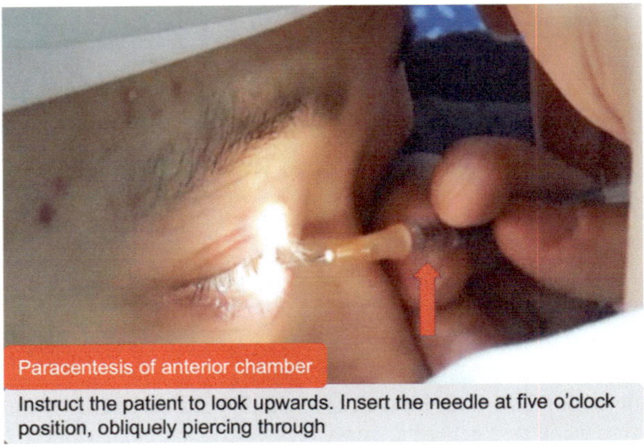

Fig. 2.4 Advise the patient to minimize the frequency of eye closure. The cotton swab should be removed using the operator's left hand, which should then be directed toward the needle plug. Carefully and delicately manipulate the needle plug in an outward direction, subsequently removing approximately 0.1 mL of aqueous humor from the specified location (shown by the red arrow)

procedure is scheduled on the same day, a temporary administration of the eye drops every 5 min, totaling six times, is permissible.

Environmental Disinfection

The implementation of regular environmental disinfection in accordance with the specified guidelines for the ophthalmology operating room is necessary. In cases when numerous procedures have been scheduled in the operating room prior to the anterior chamber puncture procedure, and there has many patients who undergo surgeries before, it is advisable to implement an additional round of disinfection.

Ocular Preparation

Oxybuprocaine or tetracaine is used for eye drops, once every 3 min, for three consecutive times to complete conjunctival surface anesthesia, followed by skin disinfection performed sequentially. It is recommended to use 50 g/L povidone-iodine for skin and conjunctival sac disinfection. Surgical drape, surgical adhesive membrane, and eye speculum to hold the eyelids are performed according to the requirements of ophthalmic surgery.

Anterior Chamber Paracentesis under a Surgical Microscope

Use a 25 G syringe (equivalent to 1 mL syringe) or a finer needle tip (such as a 31 G or 32 G insulin needle). If the surgeon is right-handed, a transparent corneal puncture at 9 o'clock position is recommended with the needle tip oriented toward the 6 o'clock position, because the corneal tunnel is long, easy to close, and it is not easy to damage the lens (Fig. 2.5). If the surgeon is left-handed, it is recommended to perform transparent corneal puncture at 3 o'clock, and the needle tip is toward 6 o'clock position. After entering the anterior chamber, extract 0.05–0.1 mL of anterior aqueous humor, and remove the needle tip. The other hand can close the

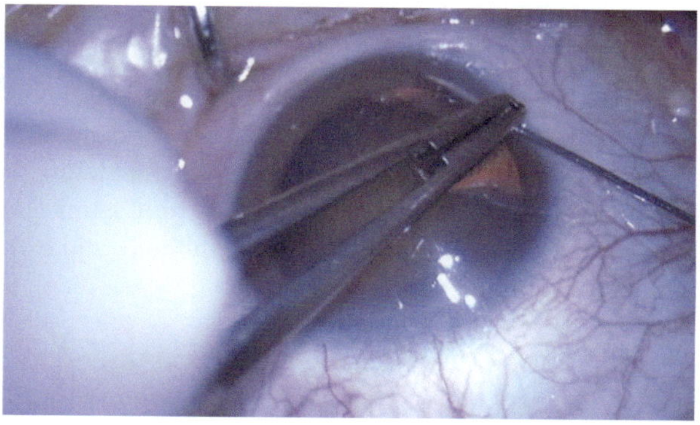

Fig. 2.5 Under the surgical microscope, the needle is inserted from the transparent cornea at 9 o'clock with the needle tip toward the 6 o'clock position to perform anterior chamber puncture drainage. The other hand presses and closes the puncture port with forceps assistance

puncture port for several seconds with the assistance of microforceps or cotton swab, and it is advisable to loosen the puncture port until the operator ensures that there is no further leakage.

Subsequent Treatment

Instruct the patient to continue administering antibiotic eye drops every half an hour until bedtime.

2.3.2 Removal of Vitreous Humor

The utilization of minimally invasive vitrectomy is highly suggested for the extraction of vitreous fluid whenever feasible. In situations when the prerequisites for minimally invasive vitrectomy are not met, the conventional 20 G vitrectomy equipment may be employed for retrieval. Alternatively, in cases where there is evident vitreous liquefaction, direct vitreous aspiration can be accomplished using a syringe.

2.3.2.1 Vitreous Aspiration

Prior to performing a puncture procedure, a regimen of antibiotic eye drops, such as tobramycin eye drops or levofloxacin eye drops, is administered at a frequency of six times each day for a duration of 3 consecutive days. In the event that the puncture procedure is scheduled on the same day as the administration of the eye drops, a temporary adjustment may be made to administer the drops once every 5 min, totaling six administrations.

Environmental Disinfection

Regular environmental disinfection is necessary in accordance with the specified guidelines for maintaining a sterile ophthalmic operating room. In cases where many surgical procedures are scheduled in the operating room prior to vitreous aspiration and there is a significant influx and outflow of individuals, it is advisable to administer an additional round of disinfection.

Ocular Preparation

Oxybuprocaine or tetracaine are administered as ocular drops at intervals of 3 min, repeated three times, to achieve full anesthesia of the conjunctival surface. Subsequently, sequential skin cleaning is conducted. It is advisable to disinfect the skin and conjunctival sac using a solution containing 50 g/L of povidone-iodine. In accordance with the specific demands of ophthalmic surgery, the implementation of a surgical drape, surgical adhesive membrane, and eye speculum for eyelid stabilization is undertaken.

Vitreous Cavity Puncture and Aspiration Under the Surgical Microscope

Instruct the patient to lie flat with eyes looking up, and drop 0.3 mL of 2% lidocaine on the lower conjunctiva.

Select a 23 G (equivalent to a 2 mL syringe) needle, and perform an oblique puncture through the sclera 4.0 mm outside the lower corneal margin (3.5 mm for aphakic eyes) before inserting the needle vertically. After about 1/2 of the needle length enters the vitreous cavity, pull the needle plug outward, and it is time to pull out the needle when 0.3 mL of vitreous fluid is extracted. If the vitreous fluid cannot be smoothly extracted, attempts can be made to rotate the needle direction or to change the angle and position of the needle tip slightly [56, 57]. After extracting 0.3 mL of vitreous humor, press the puncture site with a cotton swab and pull out the needle.

Subsequent Treatment

The patient should be advised to continue administering antibiotic eye drops at intervals of every half hour until they retire for the night.

2.3.2.2 Vitrectomy

Environmental Disinfection

Daily environmental disinfection should be performed in accordance with ophthalmic operating room requirements.

Ocular Preparation

Oxybuprocaine or tetracaine is used for eye drops, once every 3 min, for three consecutive times to complete conjunctival surface anesthesia, followed by skin disinfection. If other surgical procedures are required, such as stripping of membranes, retrobulbar block is recommended. It is recommended to use 50 g/L povidone-iodine for skin and conjunctival sac disinfection. Surgical drape, surgical adhesive membrane, and eye speculum to hold the eyelids are performed according to the requirements of ophthalmic surgery.

Vitrectomy Under an Operating Microscope

The operator should try to choose a minimally invasive vitrectomy surgical system such as 23 G, 25 G, and 27 G. Before puncture, the peripheral fundus should be carefully examined (especially in patients with peripheral anterior proliferation, such as ocular toxocariasis). Avoid obvious sites of proliferation, and perform oblique puncture through the sclera 3.5 mm outside the limbus before inserting the needle vertically, into which a perfusion and vitrectomy cannula are placed respectively. The perfusion is closed before aspiration to ensure that no perfusion fluid enters the vitreous cavity; in the case of ensuring that there is no liquid in the tube of the vitreous body cutter, unscrew the screw cap of the pipeline of the vitreous body cutter, and connect a 2.5 mL syringe needle tube. When the cutting frequency is set at more than 2500 times/min, step on the foot pedal, slowly pull the syringe needle plug outward, and suck out about 0.3–0.5 mL of vitreous humor. Open the perfusion, pull out the cannula after the IOP is restored, and carefully check for leakage. If follow-up cytological examination is required, it is recommended to set the frequency of vitrectomy at 1000 times/min after opening the perfusion, connect a 10 mL syringe needle tube externally, and collect the vitreous cavity washing liquid. The cutting should be directed as far as possible toward the suspicious lesion [57].

Mudhar HS et al. [60] found that inflammatory cells and lymphocytes are more enriched in the vitreous cortex, and only the axis/core vitrectomy is not as effective as the whole vitrectomy to collect cells (7.4–78 times, with an average of 31 times better than axial vitrectomy).

Due to the advancement of minimally invasive surgical equipment and concepts, the minimally invasive diagnostic vitreous surgery has basically reached a widespread level. Prof. Wei summarized the advantages of collecting vitreous fluid specimens for minimally invasive vitrectomy [14] as follows: (1) small surgical injury, the surgical wound is tiny and does not require suturing, the incision heals faster than traditional 20 G vitrectomy, and the patient's postoperative reaction is mild. Due to the long-term and uncontrollable inflammation in some patients considering diagnostic vitrectomy, minimally invasive vitrectomy can reduce postoperative reactions of patients. The ocular surface damage is relatively small, and the postoperative dry eye symptoms are relatively mild; (2) short operation time, suture-free wound can shorten the operation time, especially for the elderly and children with poor physique and patients with high tension and poor cooperation; (3) availability of adequate specimens, through minimally invasive diagnostic vitrectomy, sufficient specimens of vitreous, retina, or choroid can be obtained for laboratory examinations, thereby improving the diagnostic rate.

References

1. Cioboata M, Anghelie A, Chiotan C, Liora R, Serban R, Cornăcel C. Benefits of anterior chamber paracentesis in the management of glaucomatous emergencies. J Med Life. 2014;7 Spec No. 2(Spec Iss 2):5–6.
2. Kitazawa K, Sotozono C, Koizumi N, Nagata K, Inatomi T, Sasaki H, Kinoshita S. Safety of anterior chamber paracentesis using a 30-gauge needle integrated with a specially designed disposable pipette. Br J Ophthalmol. 2017;101(5):548–50.

3. Chronopoulos A, Roquelaure D, Souteyrand G, Seebach JD, Schutz JS, Thumann G. Aqueous humor polymerase chain reaction in uveitis—utility and safety. BMC Ophthalmol. 2016;16(1):189.
4. Zhang EH. Analysis of the application of anterior chamber puncture technique in ophthalmology clinical practice. Diet Health. 2018;005(025):38.
5. Lin WJ. The clinical application of anterior chamber puncture in ophthalmology. Health Horiz. 2019;11:218.
6. Jin SQ. The clinical application of anterior chamber puncture in ophthalmology. China's Rural Health. 2015;14:24.
7. Zhao XM. Application of anterior chamber puncture technique in clinical ophthalmology. Health care Guide. 2019;29:62.
8. Qin SY. Observation on the application of anterior chamber puncture technique in ophthalmology clinical practice. Elect J Clin Med Liter. 2018;97:2.
9. Saxena S, Lai TY, Koizumi H, Farah ME, Ferrara D, Pelayes D, Sato T, Meyer CH, Murray T. Anterior chamber paracentesis during intravitreal injections in observational trials: effectiveness and safety and effects. Int J Retina Vitreous. 2019;5:8.
10. Hollands H, Wong J, Bruen R, Campbell RJ, Sharma S, Gale J. Short-term intraocular pressure changes after intravitreal injection of bevacizumab. Can J Ophthalmol. 2007;42(6):807–11.
11. Gismondi M, Salati C, Salvetat ML, Zeppieri M, Brusini P. Short-term effect of intravitreal injection of Ranibizumab (Lucentis) on intraocular pressure. J Glaucoma. 2009;18(9):658–61.
12. Sharei V, Höhn F, Köhler T, Hattenbach LO, Mirshahi A. Course of intraocular pressure after intravitreal injection of 0.05 mL ranibizumab (Lucentis). Eur J Ophthalmol. 2010;20(1):174–9.
13. Lorenz K, Zwiener I, Mirshahi A. Subconjunctival reflux and need for paracentesis after intravitreal injection of 0.1 ml bevacizumab: comparison between 27-gauge and 30-gauge needle. Graefes Arch Clin Exp Ophthalmol. 2010;248(11):1573–7.
14. Wei WB, Tu Y. Clinical application of diagnostic vitrectomy and prospective microincision techniques. Chi J Ophthalmol. 2010;46(11):1052–6.
15. Haruta M, Taguchi C, Yamakawa R. Macular hole formation after pars plana vitrectomy for primary vitreoretinal lymphoma. Retinal Cases Brief Rep. 2020;14(3):243–6.
16. Schildhouse R, Lai A, Barsuk JH, Mourad M, Chopra V. Safe and effective bedside Thoracentesis: a review of the evidence for practicing clinicians. J Hosp Med. 2017;12(4):266–76.
17. Gorelick PB, Biller J. Lumbar puncture. Technique, indications, and complications. Postgrad Med. 1986;79(8):257–68.
18. Mathon B, Amelot A, Mokhtari K, Bielle F. Increasing the diagnostic yield of stereotactic brain biopsy using intraoperative histological smear. Clin Neurol Neurosurg. 2019;186:105544.
19. Keorochana N, Intaraprasong W, Choontanom R. Herpesviridae prevalence in aqueous humor using PCR. Clinical Ophthalmol (Auckland, NZ). 2018;12:1707–11.
20. Jeroudi A, Yeh S. Diagnostic vitrectomy for infectious uveitis. Int Ophthalmol Clin. 2014;54(2):173–97.
21. Carroll DM, Franklin RM. Vitreous biopsy in uveitis of unknown cause. Retina (Philadelphia, Pa). 1981;1(3):245–51.
22. Priem H, Verbraeken H, de Laey JJ. Diagnostic problems in chronic vitreous inflammation. Graefes Arch Clin Exp Ophthalmol. 1993;231(8):453–6.
23. Palexas GN, Green WR, Goldberg MF, Ding Y. Diagnostic pars plana vitrectomy report of a 21-year retrospective study. Trans Am Ophthalmol Soc. 1995;93:281–308; discussion 308–214.
24. Verbraeken H. Diagnostic vitrectomy and chronic uveitis. Graefes Arch Clin Exp Ophthalmol. 1996;234(Suppl 1):S2–7.
25. Mruthyunjaya P, Jumper JM, McCallum R, Patel DJ, Cox TA, Jaffe GJ. Diagnostic yield of vitrectomy in eyes with suspected posterior segment infection or malignancy. Ophthalmology. 2002;109(6):1123–9.

26. Margolis R, Brasil OF, Lowder CY, Singh RP, Kaiser PK, Smith SD, Perez VL, Sonnie C, Sears JE. Vitrectomy for the diagnosis and management of uveitis of unknown cause. Ophthalmology. 2007;114(10):1893–7.
27. Wittenberg LA, Maberley DA, Ma PE, Wade NK, Gill H, White VA. Contribution of vitreous cytology to final clinical diagnosis fifteen-year review of vitreous cytology specimens from one institution. Ophthalmology. 2008;115(11):1944–50.
28. Oahalou A, Schellekens PA, de Groot-Mijnes JD, Rothova A. Diagnostic pars plana vitrectomy and aqueous analyses in patients with uveitis of unknown cause. Retina (Philadelphia, Pa). 2014;34(1):108–14.
29. Malosse L, Angioi K, Baumann C, Rousseau H, Conart JB. Diagnostic vitrectomy in intraocular inflammations: a retrospective series. J Fr Ophtalmol. 2019;42(6):618–25.
30. Pakdel A, Mammo Z, Hollands H, Forooghian F. Regression of subretinal lymphoma after diagnostic vitrectomy. JAMA Ophthalmol. 2017;135(5):503–5.
31. Iaccheri B, Fiore T, Cerquaglia A, Lupidi M, Cagini C. Transient therapeutic effect of vitrectomy in primary intraocular lymphoma. Int Ophthalmol. 2017;37(6):1333–5.
32. Durand ML. Bacterial and fungal endophthalmitis. Clin Microbiol Rev. 2017;30(3):597–613.
33. Port AD, Orlin A, Kiss S, Patel S, D'Amico DJ, Gupta MP. Cytomegalovirus retinitis: a review. J Ocul Pharmacol Ther. 2017;33(4):224–34.
34. Cochrane TF, Silvestri G, McDowell C, Foot B, McAvoy CE. Acute retinal necrosis in the United Kingdom: results of a prospective surveillance study. Eye (London, England). 2012;26(3):370–377; quiz 378.
35. Neumann R, Barequet D, Rosenblatt A, Amer R, Ben-Arie-Weintrob Y, Hareuveni-Blum T, Vishnevskia-Dai V, Raskin E, Blumenfeld O, Shulman S, et al. Herpetic anterior uveitis—analysis of presumed and PCR proven cases. Ocul Immunol Inflamm. 2019;27(2):211–8.
36. Kijlstra A, Petersen E. Epidemiology, pathophysiology, and the future of ocular toxoplasmosis. Ocul Immunol Inflamm. 2014;22(2):138–47.
37. Molk R. Ocular toxocariasis: a review of the literature. Ann Ophthalmol. 1983;15(3):216–219, 222–217, 230–211.
38. Agrawal R, Balne PK, Wei X, Bijin VA, Lee B, Ghosh A, Narayanan R, Agrawal M, Connolly J. Cytokine profiling in patients with exudative age-related macular degeneration and Polypoidal Choroidal vasculopathy. Invest Ophthalmol Vis Sci. 2019;60(1):376–82.
39. Wu H, Hwang DK, Song X, Tao Y. Association between aqueous cytokines and diabetic retinopathy stage. J Ophthalmol. 2017;2017:9402198.
40. Takeuchi M, Sato T, Sakurai Y, Taguchi M, Harimoto K, Karasawa Y, Ito M. Association between aqueous humor and vitreous fluid levels of Th17 cell-related cytokines in patients with proliferative diabetic retinopathy. PLoS One. 2017;12(5):e0178230.
41. Vujosevic S, Simó R. Local and systemic inflammatory biomarkers of diabetic retinopathy: an integrative approach. Invest Ophthalmol Vis Sci. 2017;58(6):Bio68–bio75.
42. Miao H, Tao Y, Li XX. Inflammatory cytokines in aqueous humor of patients with choroidal neovascularization. Mol Vis. 2012;18:574–80.
43. Jonas JB, Tao Y, Neumaier M, Findeisen P. Monocyte chemoattractant protein 1, intercellular adhesion molecule 1, and vascular cell adhesion molecule 1 in exudative age-related macular degeneration. Arch Ophthalmol (Chicago, Ill : 1960). 2010;128(10):1281–6.
44. Modi A, Sharma K, Sudhakar NP, Yadav NK. Aqueous humor cytokines and therapeutic customization in nonresponding macular edema secondary to retinal vein Occlusion. Retin Case Brief Rep. 2021;15(2):127–30.
45. Matsushima R, Noma H, Yasuda K, Goto H, Shimura M. Role of cytokines in Ranibizumab therapy for macular Edema in patients with central retinal Vein Occlusion. J Ocul Pharmacol Therap. 2019;35(7):407–12.
46. Noma H, Mimura T, Yasuda K, Nakagawa H, Motohashi R, Kotake O, Shimura M. Cytokines and recurrence of macular Edema after Intravitreal Ranibizumab in patients with branch retinal vein occlusion. Ophthalmologica. 2016;236(4):228–34.

47. Felfeli T, Juncal VR, Hillier RJ, Mak MYK, Wong DT, Berger AR, Kohly RP, Kertes PJ, Eng KT, Boyd SR, et al. Aqueous humor cytokines and long-term response to anti-vascular endothelial growth factor therapy in diabetic macular Edema. Am J Ophthalmol. 2019;206:176–83.
48. Di Antonio L, Toto L, Mastropasqua A, Brescia L, Erroi E, Lamolinara A, Di Nicola M, Mastropasqua L. Retinal vascular changes and aqueous humor cytokines changes after aflibercept intravitreal injection in treatment-naïve myopic choroidal neovascularization. Sci Rep. 2018;8(1):15631.
49. Fan X, Gao N, Li J, Lei J, Kang Q. Effects of VEGF levels on anti-VEGF therapy for patients with idiopathic choroidal neovascularization. Mol Cell Biochem. 2018;441(1–2):173–9.
50. Wang TA, Lo KJ, Hwang DK, Chen SJ. Serpiginoid choroiditis associated with presumed ocular tuberculosis. Taiwan J Ophthalmol. 2019;9(2):127–30.
51. Plana-Pla A, Pelegrín-Colás L, Bielsa-Marsol I, Ferrandiz-Foraster C. Secondary syphilis presenting as Oral lesions and posterior Placoid Chorioretinitis in an Immunocompetent patient. Actas Dermo-sifiliogr. 2016;107(9):783–4.
52. Wang B, Tian B, Tao Y, Hou J, Zhao XT, Li XX. Continued decline of aqueous interleukin-8 after multiple intravitreal injections of ganciclovir for cytomegalovirus retinitis. J Ocular Pharmacol Ther. 2014;30(7):587–92.
53. Zhang JL, Song XY, Chen YY, Nguyen THA, Zhang JY, Bao SS, Zhang YY. Novel inflammatory cytokines (IL-36, 37, 38) in the aqueous humor from patients with chronic primary angle closure glaucoma. Int Immunopharmacol. 2019;71:164–8.
54. Mak CY, Sin HP, Ho M, Chan VC, Young AL, Brelen ME. Bilateral acute retinal necrosis after bilateral cataract surgery in an immunocompromised patient: a case report. Int Ophthalmol. 2018;38(3):1329–32.
55. Kaye R, Steger B, Chen JY, Romano V. A serious adverse surgical event: management of suspected HSV-1 keratitis in a donor cornea. Spektrum der Augenheilkunde : Zeitschrift der Osterreichischen Ophthalmologischen Gesellschaft, OOG. 2017;31(1):19–22.
56. Tao Y. Research on examination of intraocular fluid for diagnosis of infectious ocular diseases. Chin J Ophthalmol. 2018;54(7):551–6.
57. Liu X, Tao Y. Use the examination of intraocular fluid well. Chin J Ophthalmol Med (Electr Ed). 2018;8(05):193–201.
58. Xing L, Dorrepaal SJ, Gale J. Survey of intravitreal injection techniques and treatment protocols among retina specialists in Canada. Can J Ophthalmol. 2014;49(3):261–6.
59. Shao Y. Consensus interpretation on the specification of vitreous injection technology by the European society of retinal experts in 2018. Recent Adv Ophthalmol. 2018;38(12):1101–4.
60. Mudhar HS, Sheard R. Diagnostic cellular yield is superior with full pars plana vitrectomy compared with core vitreous biopsy. Eye (Lond). 2013;27(1):50–5.

Preservation and Transportation of Intraocular Fluids

3

Contents

Once the extraction of the intraocular fluid is completed, it is imperative to promptly transfer it into a hermetically sealed sterile receptacle, often a cooled centrifuge tube suitable for cryogenic freezing. In the event that the test laboratory and the ophthalmology operating room are situated in separate units, with a significant distance between them, the issue of specimen transportation arises. It is imperative to give due consideration to the transportation conditions in order to prevent any adverse impact on the test findings.

The circumstances for transportation of specimens are contingent upon the specific characteristics of the substance being evaluated:

1. RNA is a material that is susceptible to rapid degradation. In the event that RNA detection is necessary, it is imperative to promptly store the specimen in a refrigerated container and dispatch it to the laboratory. It is crucial to extract the RNA within a time frame of 48 h [1]. In cases where a prolonged duration is anticipated, it is advisable to promptly combine the sample with an RNA long-acting preservation solution. This solution, comprising a novel combination of tiny molecules, efficiently hinders the activity of RNAase enzymes, thereby mitigating the degradation of RNA molecules.
2. In order to mitigate cellular degradation during transportation, it is advisable for individuals presenting with suspected intraocular lymphoma or those requiring

Y. Tao, D.-K. Hwang, *Examination of Intraocular Fluid*,
https://doi.org/10.1007/978-981-96-2486-7_3

analysis of intraocular fluid cell composition to promptly introduce 2–5 mL of RPMI 1640 cell culture medium subsequent to the removal of vitreous fluid [2].

3. If the substance under examination is DNA and the duration of transportation does not exceed 72 h, it can be carried under ambient conditions. It is advisable to utilize cold chain transportation (maintained below 4 °C) if the duration exceeds 72 h.
4. If the substance that has been detected is a polypeptide or protein, such as an antibody or cytokine, it is advisable to transport it using cold chain methods, maintaining a temperature below 4 °C.
5. After conducting laboratory tests, any residual samples should be retained for subsequent retesting or for the purpose of scientific research. The storage conditions are directly associated with the duration. It is recommended to store protein samples at a temperature of 4 °C in a refrigerator for a duration of 1 week, taking into account the detrimental effects of repeated freeze-thaw cycles. The recommended storage conditions for the sample are as follows: for a storage period of up to 1 month, it can be stored in a freezer set at a temperature of −20 °C. However, for storage periods exceeding 1 month, it is advisable to keep the sample in a refrigerator set at a temperature of −80 °C or in a liquid nitrogen tank.

References

1. Abernathy E, Peairs RR, Chen MH, Icenogle J, Namdari H. Genomic characterization of a persistent rubella virus from a case of Fuch' uveitis syndrome in a 73 year old man. J Clin Virol. 2015;69:104–9.
2. Malinowski SM. The vitreous trap: a simple, surgeon-controlled technique for obtaining undiluted vitreous and subretinal specimens during pars plana vitrectomy. Retina (Philadelphia, Pa). 2010;30(5):828–9.

Items of Examination of Intraocular Fluid

4

Contents

4.1 Cell

Cells serve as the fundamental building blocks that contribute to the structural and functional integrity of living creatures. The cellular components responsible for mediating the inflammatory response are commonly referred to as inflammatory cells. Inflammatory cells encompass a variety of cell types, including lymphocytes,

Y. Tao, D.-K. Hwang, *Examination of Intraocular Fluid*,
https://doi.org/10.1007/978-981-96-2486-7_4

plasma cells, granulocytes (eosinophilic, basophilic, neutral), monocytes, macrophages, mast cells, and others.

Typically, the aqueous humor should not exhibit any cellular presence, whereas the vitreous body of adults is generally devoid of cellular constituents, with the exception of a few cells that may be present in the vitreous cortex [1]. In the context of pathological conditions, such as intraocular inflammation, various forms of cellular infiltration may manifest inside the intraocular fluid. Through cytological examination, it becomes feasible to infer the type of inflammation that is present in the eye. Intraocular cytological examination is generally capable of categorizing intraocular disorders into three main groups: inflammation/infection, hemorrhage, and malignancy [2]. Neutrophils are predominantly detected in instances of fungal and bacterial endophthalmitis. Lymphocytes are predominantly detected in instances of viral uveitis.

Lwamoto et al. analyzed the cells in the aqueous humor using electron microscopy [3]. They found that in two cases of uveitis with hypopyon, neutrophils and monocytes mainly existed in the aqueous humor. In one case of uveitis without hypopyon, neutrophils, eosinophils, suspected monocytes, lymphocytes, and a few cells which belonged to the plasma cell lineage could be detected in the aqueous humor. In other two cases uveitis with hypopyon, lymphocytes predominated in the aqueous humor. Kalogeropoulos CD et al. [4] conducted cytological analysis on the aqueous humor of different types of intraocular diseases and found varied results, which are shown in Table 4.1.

Cytological analysis of the vitreous humor of patients with proliferative vitreoretinopathy showed several types of cells: (1) round, typical retinal pigment epithelial cells; (2) large, partially depigmented cells; (3) large, round, fully depigmented cells (macrophages); (4) small, depigmented cells; and (5) lymphocytes [5].

Stewart J et al. [6] performed cytology analysis of the intraocular fluid sample on a 19-month-old boy with atypical clinical manifestation. Possible diagnosis included persistent hyperplastic primary vitreous and Coats' disease. Numerous cholesterol crystals, rare foamy macrophages, multiple pigmented macrophages, pigmented epithelial cells, and free pigment were shown. Schmorl's stain was positive for melanin. The diagnosis of Coats' disease was supported, and the diagnosis of malignant tumors such as retinoblastoma was hereby excluded.

Table 4.1 Cell types in the aqueous humor of patients with various intraocular diseases

	Phacolytic glaucoma	Phacoanaphylactic endophthalmitis	Infectious endophthalmitis	Ghost-cell glaucoma	Iridocyclitis
Neutrophil	–	++/+++	++++	–	–
Eosinophil	–	+	+	–	+
Histocyte/macrophage	++	+/++	+/++	–	+
Lymphocyte	–	–/+	++	–	+
Ghost cell	–	–	–	++	–

By analyzing T cells in the vitreous humor of ten patients with active ocular toxoplasmosis, Feron EJ et al. found that these T cells did not respond to retinal autoantigens. Compared with the control group, only intraocular T cells in patients with ocular toxoplasmosis respond to *Toxoplasma* antigen [7].

Fujikawa LS et al. [8] performed biopsies on 23 cases of posterior uveitis with poor treatment response. Most patients had T cells (helper T cells) as cell components in the vitreous humor. In patients with Fuchs' syndrome, macrophages were the major cell component, while B cells were the major cell component in phacolytic uveitis.

4.2 DNA

Deoxyribonucleic acid (DNA) is the main genetic material which carries the genetic information necessary for the synthesis of RNA and protein. It is an essential biological macromolecule for the development and normal activity of organisms. DNA is a high-molecular compound, and the basic unit is deoxynucleotide. Each deoxyribonucleotide is composed of three parts, one molecule of nitrogenous base, one molecule of deoxyribose, and one molecule of phosphate. The four nucleobases are adenine (A), thymine (T), cytosine (C) and guanine (G), respectively.

For ophthalmologists, two types of DNA deserve to be tested: (1) DNA of human cells, which are used to detect genetic diseases, polymorphic sites, HLA, etc., and (2) DNA of microorganisms, which are used to identify pathogenic microorganisms in intraocular infections. Most DNA of human cells exists in chromosomes, including 22 pairs of autosomes and 1 pair of allosomes. The exons, which are the coding sequences of proteins, account for only about 1.5% of the total genomic sequence. Mitochondria, an organelle in the cell, also has its own genome. The mitochondrial genome holds significant importance in the context of mitochondrial disorders. For example, Leber's hereditary optic neuropathy is caused by mutations in mitochondrial DNA. The common mutation sites are m. 3460 G > A, m. 11,778 G > A, and m. 14,484 T > C [9, 10]. Gene therapy shed light on the patients with hereditary diseases [11].

The process of identifying pathogenic DNA involves more than just amplifying and identifying specific pieces of a particular bacteria. For example, there are three types of ribosomal RNA in bacteria according to the sedimentation coefficient, namely, 5S, 16S, and 23S rRNA. DNA encoding these three RNAs are 5S, 16S, and 23S rDNA. Primer design aiming at these common DNA can achieve the purpose of broad-spectrum testing. Also, variable regions in DNA sequences which are genus-specific or species-specific enable the identification of different types of bacteria [12, 13]. Similarly, 28 S rDNA of fungi can aid in broad-spectrum detection of suspected fungal endophthalmitis [14].

Separation and purification of DNA are important steps before DNA sequencing. The general principles include keeping the integrity of the primary structure of DNA and excluding contamination by other molecules. In the process of DNA purification, no organic solvents or high concentrations of metal ions should exist in the sample. The contamination of other biological macromolecules and other DNA molecules should be minimized.

4.3 RNA

RNA, also known as ribonucleic acid, is a linear macromolecule composed of ribonucleotides linked together by 3′,5′-phosphodiester linkages. It serves as a carrier of genetic information in biological cells, as well as in certain viruses and viroids. A ribonucleotide is composed of a nitrogenous base, a ribose molecule, and a phosphate molecule. The four primary nitrogenous bases found in RNA are adenine (A), guanine (G), cytosine (C), and uracil (U). It is important to note that uracil (U) substitutes thymine (T) in DNA. RNA is categorized into three main types: ribosomal RNA (rRNA), transfer RNA (tRNA), and messenger RNA (mRNA).

MicroRNAs (miRNAs) are naturally occurring noncoding RNAs found in eukaryotes, typically consisting of 20–25 nucleotides in length. Through the detection of miRNAs in intraocular fluid, it is feasible to ascertain biomarkers for uveitis. According to a newly released review, the following microRNAs have been identified as being linked to uveitis in both people and animals: let-7e, miRNA-1, miR-9-3, miR-20a-5p, miR-23a, mir-29a-3p, miR-140-5p, miR-143, miR-146a, miR-146a-5p, miR-155, miR-182, miR-182-5p, miR-196a2, miR-205, miR-223-3p, and miR-301a [15].

4.4 Antigen

An antigen is a substance that can elicit an immunological response. It typically refers to foreign substances that enter the human body, such as bacteria, viruses, pollen, and so on. The antigen test is highly beneficial for the detection of pathogens. Using cytomegalovirus (CMV) as an illustration, pp65, a matrix phosphoprotein weighing 65KD, serves as an antigenic constituent. This protein is situated within the nucleolus of leukocytes found in peripheral blood. A positive test result for pp65 may occur before the onset of clinical symptoms. A positive test result signifies the presence of an ongoing infection and can be utilized as a marker for assessing the effectiveness of treatment. The antigen test possesses distinctive importance and cannot be entirely substituted by DNA detection. After undergoing allogeneic hematopoietic stem cell transplantation, all patients who tested positive for CMV-pp65 antigen in their peripheral blood showed negative results for CMV-DNA when tested using quantitative polymerase chain reaction (qPCR). However, there were four cases where CMV-DNA was positive by qPCR but CMV-pp65 was negative, and these patients did not develop CMV disease. These findings indicate that the presence of CMV-pp65 antigen in a positive test result is more significant than the detection of CMV-DNA when assessing drug use [16]. The pp65 test is currently considered a standard method for diagnosing active cytomegalovirus (CMV) infection following transplantation [17]. CMV expresses distinct antigens such as pp65, immediate early antigen, and pp67, which is a surface layer protein. Among them, pp67 is the earliest structural antigen that can be detected during active CMV infection [18].

Certain discrete elements within the human body have the potential to transform into antigens. Typically, they are separated from the cells responsible for antibody production and do not induce the formation of autoantibodies. Nevertheless, when these constituents infiltrate the bloodstream as a result of trauma or illness, they can also elicit inflammatory reactions. An instance of ocular damage can result in the rupture of the lens capsule and the overflow of lens protein, ultimately leading to inflammation within the eye. Another instance is autoimmune retinopathy, encompassing paraneoplastic retinopathy (retinopathy associated with malignancy, retinopathy associated with melanoma, and bilateral diffuse uveal melanocyte proliferation) and non-paraneoplastic autoimmune retinopathy. The presence of tumors and other autoantigens triggers the production of autoantibodies by the body, specifically targeting retinal components. This leads to the disruption of normal retinal function [19]. Hence, the immune system identifies the retina, a typical component of the human body, as an antigen and proceeds to assault it.

4.5 Antibody

An antibody is a defensive protein that is generated by the human body in response to the activation of an antigen. Plasma cells, also known as effector B cells, release antibodies to detect and counteract foreign substances like bacteria and viruses. Antibodies identify particular foreign antigens, engage in antigen-antibody interactions, decrease the amount of antigens, and eradicate foreign germs. Often, DNA detection and antigen tests are not feasible due to the absence of viable cells or technical limitations. Antibody detection can be utilized as an alternate test to identify the specific pathogen causing the infection.

Antibodies can be divided into several types according to different ways of classification:

1. According to the object, antibodies can be divided into antitoxin, antibacterial antibody, antiviral antibody, and cytophilic antibody (immunoglobulins (Ig) bind to cells, such as IgE in type 1 hypersensitivity, which can latch on the membrane of the target cell).
2. According to whether there is a visible reaction after binding to the antigen, antibodies can be divided into complete antibodies, which show a visible binding reaction with the participation of the reaction medium, and incomplete antibodies, which show no visible reaction but can inhibit the binding of antigen and its corresponding antibody.
3. According to the source of antibodies, they can be divided into natural antibodies and immune antibodies.
4. According to the physicochemical properties and biological function, antibodies can be divided into IgG, IgA, IgM, IgE, and IgD, respectively. Among them, IgG

is produced by B cells and is the main type of antibody in human serum. The functional structure of IgG is the most clearly studied, with the highest content in serum (75%) and the longest half-life (21–23 days). Therefore, the test of IgG is the mainly used in the examination of intraocular fluid. With a long half-life, the window phase for IgG test is long. The main physiological functions of IgG include neutralizing toxins and viruses, agglutinating and precipitating antigens. Intraocular infection of viruses [20], fungi [21], and parasites [22, 23] can be determined by detection of antibody.

IgM, also known as macroglobulin, has a pentameric structure with the molecular weight of 900 kd. If IgM is pathologically overexpressed in the body, it can cause Waldenström's macroglobulinemia and cause central retinal vein occlusion in both eyes [24]. IgM is the first Ig produced by the humoral immune response, which appears in the early stage of infection. It accounts for 5–10% of the serum Ig, with half-life of 5 days. The increase of IgM level indicates recent infection. In the diagnosis of uveitis, IgM test is relatively few, related to its short window phase [25].

IgA can be divided into serotype and secretory type, accounting for 5–15% of the Ig in serum and with a half-life of 6 days. The secretory type is synthesized by mucosal epithelial cells. The intraocular fluid IgA test is rarely performed due to the lack of mucosal tissue in the eye.

IgD accounts for 1% of the serum Ig content, with a half-life of 3 days. It is rarely used in the examination of intraocular fluid.

IgE content is the lowest in serum (accounting for 0.002% of Ig), with a half-life of 3 days. The level of specific IgE increases during parasitic infection. In parasitic intraocular infections, such as ocular toxocariasis [26], increased IgE level in the intraocular fluid is detected. Comparison between IgE in intraocular fluid and serum IgE can be used in the auxiliary diagnosis.

4.6 Cytokine

Cytokines are a diverse group of proteins, peptides, or glycoproteins that are released by living host cells. They infiltrate other host cells by diffusion, direct cell-to-cell interaction, or transportation through the bloodstream and function at exceedingly low concentrations in bodily fluids. Cytokines are created by cells of different embryonic origins throughout the body and carry information between immune cells, immune cells, and nonimmune cells. These molecules are a specific sort of signals that facilitate and control the processes of immunity, inflammation, and hematopoiesis. Cytokines can be described as the means by which cells communicate with each other. Cytokines, also known by several names based on their proposed function, secreting cell, or target, are widely recognized. For instance, lymphocytes can create cytokines, which are also known as lymphokines. On the other hand, interleukins are produced by a specific type of white blood cell and exert their effects on other white blood cells. Chemokines are a type of cytokines that have the ability to attract and guide cells through a process called chemotaxis.

Cytokines can exert their effects on the cell that produces them (autocrine action), nearby cells (paracrine action), or, in certain instances, distant cells (endocrine action). Cytokines typically work as intercellular signaling molecules that initiate specific biological responses by attaching to receptors on target cells.

Types of cytokines are as follows:

1. Interleukin (IL) is a cytokine produced by lymphocytes, monocytes, or other non-monocytes, which plays an important regulatory role in cell-cell interaction, immune regulation, and hematopoietic and inflammatory processes.
2. Colony-stimulating factor (CSF) stimulates hematopoietic stem cells or hematopoietic cells at different stages of differentiation to form different cell colonies in semisolid medium according to different cytokines. Different CSFs can not only stimulate the proliferation and differentiation of hematopoietic stem and progenitor cells at different developmental stages but also promote the function of mature cells.
3. Interferon (IFN) can be divided into IFN-α, IFN-β, and IFN-γ according to the source and structure of interferon, which are produced by leukocytes, fibroblasts, and activated T cells, respectively. The biological activities of different IFNs are basically the same, and they have antiviral, antitumor, and immune regulation effects.
4. Tumor necrosis factor (TNF) can be divided into TNF-α and TNF-β according to its source and structure, which are produced by monocyte-macrophages and activated T cells, respectively. The alternate name of TNF-β is lymphotoxin (LT). In addition to killing tumor cells, the two types of TNF also participate in immune regulation, the occurrence of fever and inflammation.
5. Transforming growth factor-β (TGF-β) family is a group of polypeptides with hormone-like activity produced by immune cells and nonimmune cells via autocrine or paracrine manner [27]. Their biological functions are highly pleiotropic, and they can regulate the growth, differentiation, and apoptosis of various tissues and cells. Studies have shown that TGF-β can promote the mitosis of osteoblasts, regulate the hematopoietic process, and inhibit the growth of hepatocytes and epithelial cells. But TGF-β can stimulate the growth of human mesothelial cells and prostate cells [28, 29]. In addition, TGF-β has a certain regulatory effect on cell adhesion via activating gene transcription, increasing interstitial protein, and significantly stimulating fibroblasts or cells derived from other mesenchymal tissues, which manifested as increased collagen synthesis. TGF-β also has immunosuppressive effect via inhibiting the proliferation and differentiation of T and B lymphocytes, inhibiting the phagocytosis of macrophages, and inhibiting the synthesis of immunoglobulin.
6. Growth factors (GF) involve epidermal growth factor (EGF), platelet-derived growth factor (PDGF), fibroblast growth factor (FGF), hepatocyte growth factor (HGF), insulin-like growth factor-I (IGF -1), IGF-II, leukemia inhibitory factor (LIF), nerve growth factor (NGF), oncostatin M (OSM), platelet-derived endothelial cell growth factor (PDECGF), transforming growth factor-α (TGF-α), vascular endothelial growth factor (VEGF), etc. FGF, a family of protein factors

that can promote the proliferation of various cells, is secreted by fibroblasts, smooth muscle cells, chondrocytes, and keratinocytes. FGFs that participate in the process of angiogenesis, wound repair, and embryonic development play a role in the nutrition and protection of neurons, promotion of damage repair, and induction of angiogenesis [30]. EGF and its receptors have the effect of promoting proliferation and promoting division of various tissue cells in vivo and in vitro. During the healing and repairing process of ulcer wounds, EGF receptors can be rapidly upregulated. After combining with EGF, they act on cell growth regulator genes, regulate cell glycolysis, promote re-epithelialization of ulcer wounds [31], and accelerate the healing speed of ulcer wounds. Epidermal growth factor can also induce fibroblast proliferation, thicken the stratum corneum, and promote peripheral nerve regeneration [32].

7. Chemokine family (CF) plays an important role in the spread of inflammation and tumor invasion. Genes of chemokine family members have obvious conserved sequences, suggesting that they come from a common ancestral gene. Chemokines are a kind of secreted pro-inflammatory cytokines with a molecular weight of about 8–10KDa. The family is divided into four main types: CXC, CC, C, and CX3C. Chemokines have the following common characteristics: (1) chemokines attract one or more myeloid cells in vitro. (2) Preinflammation cytokines, such as LPS, TNF, and IL-1, can lead to the secretion of most chemokines. (3) Intradermal injection of chemokines can cause inflammatory infiltration. Four factors in the C-X-C subfamily (IL-8, GRO, NAP-2, and ENA-78) can induce neutrophil migration, while members of the C-C subfamily (monocyte chemoattractant protein (MCP)-1, MCP-2, MCP -3, RANTES, MIP-1α, MIP-lβ, etc.) induce the migration of monocytes. T cells can respond to most chemokines. IL-8 has a chemotactic effect on both CD4+ and CD8+ resting T cells. IL-8, GRO, MIP-lα, RANTES, and MCP-1 can induce basophil chemotaxis, release histamine, and promote intracellular calcium flux [33].

Immunocytokines can be divided into type 1 (TNFα, IFN-γ, etc.) that enhances cellular immune responses and type 2 (TGF-β, IL-4, IL-10, IL-13, etc.) that facilitates antibody responses. They can also be classified according to immune response (Table 4.2).

In the following section, several cytokines closely related to the occurrence and development of ocular diseases will be introduced.

4.6.1 VEGF

VEGF is the most potent peptide growth factor found so far to promote angiogenesis [35, 36]. As a member of the large family of angiogenic factors, VEGF is a highly specific mitogen, also known as vascular permeability factor or vascular opsonin. As early as 1939, Ide et al. speculated that there was a "vascular growth stimulating factor" secreted by tumor cells. Senger et al. [37] first identified VEGF

Table 4.2 Classification of cytokines according to immune response [34]

	Family	Members
Acquired immunity	Common γchain receptor ligands	IL-2, IL-4, IL-7, IL-9, IL-15, IL-21
	Common β chain (CD131) receptor ligand	IL-3, IL-5, GM-CSF
	Shared IL-2β chain (CD122)	IL-2, IL-15
	Shared receptors	IL-13 (IL-13R–IL-4R complex) TSLP (TSLPR–IL-7R complex)
Pro-inflammatory signaling	IL-1	IL-1α, IL-1β, IL-1ra, IL-18, IL-33, IL-36α, IL-36β, IL-36γ, IL-36Ra, IL-37, and IL-1Hy2
	IL-6	IL-6, IL-11, IL-31, CNTF, CT-1, LIF, OPN, OSM
	TNFα	TNFα, TNFβ, BAFF, APRIL
	IL-17	IL-17A-F, IL-25 (IL-17E)
	Type I IFN	IFNα, IFNβ, IFNω, IFNκ, Limitin
	Type II IFN	IFNγ
	Type III IFN	IFNλ1 (IL-29), IFNλ2 (IL-28A), IFNλ3 (IL-28B)
Anti-inflammatory signaling	IL-12	IL-12, IL-23, IL-27, IL-35
	IL-10	IL-10, IL-19, IL-20, IL-22, IL-24, IL-26, IL-28, IL-29

as a homodimeric glycoprotein with a relative molecular mass of 4.6×10^4 in highly vascularized tumors. Ferrara et al. [38] isolated and purified bovine pituitary follicular stellate cells from the in vitro culture medium and named them according to their mitotic activity of promoting vascular endothelial cells.

VEGF is widely distributed in human and animal brain, kidney, liver, spleen, lung, bone, eye, and other tissues. Among the ocular tissues, retinal pericytes, pigment epithelial cells, endothelial cells, ganglion cells, amacrine cells, and Müller cells can produce lower levels of VEGF [36].

VEGF has two main biological functions: (1) selectively enhance the mitosis of vascular endothelial cells and lymphatic endothelial cells, promote the proliferation, migration, differentiation and survival of endothelial cells, inhibit the aging and apoptosis of endothelial cells, and then promote the formation of new blood vessels, and (2) increase the permeability of blood vessels, especially venules, support the growth of endothelial cells and provide nutrients for the establishment of new capillary network. By increasing calcium influx, VEGF promotes increased hydraulic conductivity of micro-vessels [39]. Via endothelial cell-derived nitric oxide, VGEF can induce vasodilation in vitro in a dose-dependent manner [40]. Furthermore, studies have found that VEGF is required for normal embryonic angiogenesis. Even the inactivation of a single mouse VEGF allele results in abnormal development and early embryonic death [41, 42]. In addition, VEGF also has pro-inflammatory activity and neuroprotective effect [43, 44].

The VEGF family includes placental growth factor (PLGF), VEGFA, VEGFB, VEGFC, VEGFD, and VEGFE [36, 45]. Usually, VEGF refers to VEGFA [38]. The human VEGFA gene is located on p12–21 of chromosome 6, with a total length of 28 kbp, consisting of eight exons and seven introns [46]. Different exon splicing methods can produce four different isoforms (VEGF121, VEGF165, VEGF189, VEGF206), that is, after the signal sequence is spliced, polypeptides with 121, 165, 189, and 206 amino acids are produced [46]. VEGF165 is the most dominant isoform and lacks residues encoded by exon 6, whereas VEGF121 lacks residues encoded by exons 6 and 7. In addition, there are relatively rare splicing variants such as VEGF145 and VEGF183 [47]. VEGFA is less expressed in normal human and animal tissues, and its expression is often higher in tissues with vigorous metabolism and rich blood supply than in other tissues [36].

Neovascular disease is a common ocular disease. From corneal neovascularization in the anterior segment, rubeosis iridis, and neovascular glaucoma to retinal neovascularization and choroidal neovascularization in the posterior segment, all of these diseases are closely related to the increase of intraocular/local VEGF concentration [48].

4.6.1.1 Formation of Retinal Neovascularization

Retinal neovascularization is not self-limiting. The presence of factors such as a viable retina, low oxygen partial pressure, and venous drainage are prerequisites for neovascularization [36].

Retinal neovascularization is a complex process. First, vasodilation and permeability enhancement appear. The formation of vascular lumen is promoted via the degradation of vascular wall basement membrane, chemotaxis, migration, proliferation of the endothelial cell, and its interaction with pericytes. After binding of VEGF to VEGFR, VEGFR autophosphorylates then activates phosphatidylcholine-specific phospholipase C, hydrolyzes phosphatidylinositol diphosphate, and produces diacylglycerol and inositol triphosphate. Diacylglycerol can activate cell protein kinase C in the cytoplasm and immobilized on the membrane, which induces endothelial cell growth and increases vascular permeability [36, 49].

4.6.1.2 Diabetic Retinopathy

The metabolic disorder characterized by hyperglycemia in diabetic disease leads to the activation of polyol pathway and the formation of nonenzymatic glycation end products. The stimulation of angiotensin II, ischemia, and hypoxia can upregulate VEGF in retinal capillary endothelial cells. The expression of the above-mentioned series of biological effects leads to the occurrence of diabetic microangiopathy. In the early stage, VEGF mainly caused damage to the blood-retinal barrier of retinal venules and superficial capillaries, creating favorable conditions for the formation of retinal neovascularization [50].

By analyzing the specimens of diabetic patients, Witmer et al. [1] found that three VEGFR (1–3) were expressed in the retinal avascular area. VEGFR-1 is expressed in all micro-vessels. The expression of VEGFR-1 is stronger in diabetic patients than in normal controls. Moreover, VEGFR-1 was also found to be expressed in the inner limiting membrane, ganglion cells, inner plexiform layer, inner nuclear layer, and outer plexiform layer. VEGFR-2 was localized in the micro-vessels of the ganglion cell layer and the inner nuclear layer. VEGFR-3 is expressed in micro-vessels of the inner nuclear layer and ganglion cell layer. Similar to VEGFR-2, VEGFR-3 was mainly localized in deep retinal capillaries, accompanied by overexpression and premature appearance of VEGFA and ischemic areas, so it can be considered that VEGFA induces the expression of VEGFR-2 and VEGFR-3 in ischemic areas, leading to the retinal vascular leakage, and finally promoting neovascularization [1, 36].

Previous study found that the concentration of VEGF in the serum of patients with early diabetic microangiopathy was higher than that of other diabetic patients ($P < 0.05$) [51]. The results of our own research also confirmed that the VEGF level in the vitreous ($P < 0.001$) and plasma ($P = 0.03$) of patients with proliferative diabetic retinopathy (PDR) was significantly higher than that in the control group (patients with idiopathic macular hole and epiretinal membrane). Moreover, the expression of VEGF mRNA in the fibrous vascular membrane removed from PDR patients was significantly higher than that in the fibrous membrane removed from patients with epiretinal membrane ($P < 0.01$) [52].

4.6.1.3 Retinal Vein Occlusion

Noma H et al. found that the intraocular VEGF concentration of patients with central retinal vein occlusion was significantly higher than that of the control group without ischemic eye disease (435 pg/mL vs 62.4 pg/mL, $P = 0.0046$) [52]. Their latest research results also showed that the severity of macular edema in patients with central retinal vein occlusion was significantly correlated with the VEGF level in the vitreous humor ($P = 0.008$), but not with the concentration of free VEGFR-2 [53].

We applied retinal photocoagulation on the branch retinal vein of living monkeys, inducing the formation of central retinal vein occlusion (CRVO) and iris neovascularization. After treatment with VEGF RNAi, we found that the formation of iris neovascularization was alleviated compared with the control group, which indirectly suggested that the occurrence of intraocular neovascularization after CRVO was in close relationship with VEGF [54].

Boyd SR et al. found that the concentration of VEGF in aqueous humor in patients with ischemic CRVO was related to the occurrence, persistence and regression of iris neovascularization, the extent of retinal capillary non-perfusion zone, and vascular permeability. Iris neovascularization occurred with the concentration of aqueous VEGF of 849–1569 pg/mL. Conversely, when the concentration of aqueous VEGF was below 550 pg/mL, iris neovascularization completely subsided. Elevated aqueous VEGF level was positively correlated with the elevated aqueous albumin level (a marker of increased vascular permeability) [54].

More direct evidence comes from the histopathological evidence provided by Pe'er J et al. [55], in which ten paraffin specimens of neovascular glaucoma secondary to CRVO were studied. The expression of VEGF mRNA existed in all these ten specimens. Compared with the choroidal melanoma specimens without intraocular neovascularization (control), VEGF expression was upregulated in the inner retinal layer. VEGF mRNA expression was upregulated in the ganglion cell layer in four eyes and was upregulated in the outer retinal layer in two eyes with retinal detachment.

4.6.1.4 Retinopathy of Prematurity

Leske DA et al. [56] used acidosis-induced method to create a rat retinopathy of prematurity (ROP) model and detected the expression of VEGF mRNA during neovascularization by quantitative real-time reverse-transcriptase PCR. The expression of VEGF in the ROP model was closely related to the oxygen concentration in the environment. Stone J et al. [57] used cats as experimental animals to detect the expression of VEGF in the eyes of the ROP model. They found that the expression of VEGF in the inner retinal layer decreased in a high-oxygen environment and increased when returned to the normal environment. VEGF expression was shapely increased with the formation of retinal blood vessels and declined rapidly after vessel formation finished. They also found that compared with the normal developing retina, the retina of the ROP model expressed significantly higher VEGF level. The astrocytes which normally expressing VEGF disappeared, which role was replaced by neurons in the inner layer of the retina.

We analyzed ROP fibrovascular membrane samples obtained from the patients and found that compared with idiopathic epiretinal membrane, the expression of VEGF mRNA in ROP fibrovascular membrane was significantly increased (2.67 ± 0.81, $P < 0.01$). Other studies also found that the intraocular VEGF concentration was 14.77 ± 14.01 ng/mL in stage V ROP and was 44.16 ± 18.72 ng/mL in stage IV ROP, which proved the higher degree of active intraocular neovascularization in stage IV ROP [58].

4.6.1.5 Choroidal Neovascularization

Animal experiments provided strong evidence for the pivotal role of VEGF in the formation of choroidal neovascularization. After 3–5 days of laser exposure, immunohistochemical staining indicated that VGEF was expressed in retinal pigment epithelial cells, choroidal vascular endothelial cells, and inflammatory cells in pigmented rats [59]. In another study, a subretinal injection of adenovirus vector carrying a fragment of rat VEGF164 was performed. After 10 days after injection, the retinal pigment epithelial cells began to overexpress VEGF, and fundus fluorescein angiography indicated vascular leakage. After 80 days of injection, histological examination suggested the neovascularization originating from the choriocapillary layer [60].

The most important evidence came from the specimens of clinical patients. Frank RN et al. conducted histopathological examination on the choroidal neovascular membranes of three patients with age-related macular degeneration (AMD) and found that all of them had positive staining of VEGF. The expressed cells were mainly glial cells, vascular endothelial cells, and retinal pigment epithelial cells [61].

4.6.2 IL-6

IL-6 was first successfully cloned in 1986, which was called B-cell stimulating factor-2 (BSF-2) at that time because of its function of stimulating B cells to produce immunoglobulin. IL-6 has dual affinity for high-affinity receptors and low-affinity receptors of B cells, myeloma plasmacytoma, T cells, liver cells, and hematopoietic stem cell. It plays an important role in the growth and differentiation of these cells [62].

IL-6 is a pro-inflammatory cytokine and plays a key role in various types of uveitis [63, 64]. For example, Murray PI et al. [65] found that in certain types of uveitis, such as Fuchs uveitis syndrome and ocular toxoplasmosis, the level of IL-6 in aqueous humor was significantly increased, but the level of IL-6 in serum did not change. Malecaze F et al. [66] showed that IL-6 plays an important role in uveitis after cataract surgery. In Vogt-Koyanagi Harada disease and sarcoidosis, increased activated T lymphocytes in the aqueous humor further increase IL-6 levels in the aqueous humor and further exacerbating intraocular inflammation, which is independent of T lymphocytes activity in the blood [67, 68].

In addition, in retinal vascular diseases and choroidal diseases, the titer of IL-6 in aqueous humor has also been reported to increase, which indicated the important role of inflammatory factors in the pathogenesis of these diseases. With the progress of DR from no retinal lesion to non-proliferative and proliferative retinopathy, the titer of IL-6 in the aqueous humor increased continuously. Monitoring the aqueous level of IL-6 and VEGF is helpful in the early diagnosis and prognosis evaluation of DR [69–71]. In patients with CRVO and branch retinal vein occlusion (BRVO), the aqueous level of IL-6 increased significantly [72]. After intravitreal injection of ranibizumab, decrease of both aqueous level of IL-6 and VEGF was observed [73], which suggested that anti-VEGF therapy can reduce the degree of intraocular inflammation [74, 75]. In patients with CRVO, the aqueous level of VEGF, soluble intercellular adhesion molecule (sICAM)-1, IL-6 were correlated with the degree of aqueous flare [76]. The aqueous level of IL-6 in patients with chronic central serous chorioretinopathy (CSC) was significantly higher than that in patients with acute CSC (8.09 pg/mL vs 3.16 pg/mL, $P < 0.01$), which indicated that inflammatory factors played a more important role in chronic disease states [77].

4.6.3 IL-8

IL-8 is the first described chemokine which was discovered in 1987 [78]. IL-8 is a small soluble peptide consisting of 99 amino acids with a molecular weight of 8–10 kDa. IL-8 is known as a pro-inflammatory chemokine that induces the accumulation of neutrophils along blood vessel walls. In response to the inflammatory state, sustained, and prolonged presence of IL-8 in the circulation may cause varying degrees of damage. IL-8 has relatively good resistance to temperature, proteolysis, and acidic environments It is not easy to degrade before being transported to the laboratory for testing [79].

IL-8 is confirmed to play an important role in the pathogenesis of uveitis. IL-8 is involved in the pathophysiology of intraocular inflammatory, mainly chemotaxis and degranulation of neutrophils. This process is also considered to be the cause of tissue damage in uveitis [80]. IL-8 was shown to play a role in intraocular inflammation of Behcet's disease and phacoanaphylactic endophthalmitis, in which granulocytes were thought to be the source of IL-8 [81]. Aqueous level of IL-8 was significantly elevated in patients with active uveitis, including HLA-b27-associated uveitis. In patients with Behcet's disease and hypopyon, the mean level of IL-8 in the aqueous humor was significantly higher than in patients without hypopyon [82]. Our previous research found that the level of IL-8 in aqueous humor was related to the degree of recovery of cytomegalovirus retinitis (CMVR), which could be used as a clinical biomarker in judging the drug resistance and the time to stop intraocular injection [83].

In general, IL-8 has at least four different pro-angiogenic properties, which all act through endothelial cells [79]: (1) enhancement of endothelial cell proliferation and capillary formation [84], (2) chemotaxis function of inducing the directional migration of neutrophils, basophils, and T lymphocytes [85], (3) inhibiting the apoptosis of endothelial cells [84]; and (4) protease activation by activating endothelial cells mRNA to promote expression of matrix metalloproteinases (MMPs) MMP-2, 9 and to enhance gelatinase activity [84, 86].

Vitreous IL-8 levels were shown to be associated with the development of proliferative vitreoretinopathy (PVR) [87]. In patients with active PDR, vitreous IL-8 level was significantly elevated [88]. The level of IL-8 in the vitreous humor was also significantly increased after retinal laser photocoagulation [89]. Co-superimposed pro-angiogenic effects of NF-kB protein and IL-8 promoted epiretinal membrane formation during PDR and PVR [90].

4.6.4 IL-10

IL-10, a soluble protein produced by T helper cells (Th), macrophages, monocytes, and B cells, has broad immunosuppressive and immunostimulatory properties [91]. IL-10 has a significant impact on the biological effects of chemokines because IL-10 inhibits the production of chemokines and is a specific chemokine for the differentiation cluster of CD8+ T cells. It inhibits the migratory response of IL-8 to CD4+ T cells (but not CD8+ T cells) [92]. Five novel cytokines (IL-19, IL-20, IL-22, IL-24, and IL-26) have been identified. These cytokines, as well as some cytokines encoded in the viral genome (viral cytokines), form an IL-10-related cytokine family or IL-10 family. They are not only structurally homologous but also similar in receptor subunits and roles [93].

IL-10 may be the cytokine with the strongest inhibitory effect on the secretion of IL-8 and MCP-1 from RPE cells, suggesting that IL-10 has a potential therapeutic effect on ocular inflammatory and proliferative diseases [87]. IL-10 may play an important role in inducing and maintaining antigen-specific T cell anergy, which cannot secrete IL-2, IL-5, IL-10, INF-γ, TNF-α, and GM-CSF [94]. Elevated serum IL-10 levels reduce the risk of developing DR [95].

IL-10 is a regulatory cytokine that suppresses allergic and inflammatory reaction. Mast cells are effector cells of IL-10. Under stimulation, mastocytes release histamine, chemokines, and cytokines as well as trigger allergic inflammatory responses. IL-10 regulates mast cell function by affecting cytokine production [96]. Macrophages synthesize and release a variety of cytokines, including IL-10 [97]. Macrophages control the balance of proinflammatory cytokines IFN-γ and TNF-α and inflammatory suppressors IL-4 and IL-10 during ocular inflammation [98].

The role of IL-10 test in intraocular fluid is to assist in diagnosis of intraocular diffuse large B-cell lymphoma [99], which will be described in detail in Chap. 6.3.1.

The following table (Table 4.3) involves a brief introduction of various interleukins (only covers the main aspects of each interleukin).

4.6.5 FGF

FGF is a large family composed of homologous polypeptides, among which bFGF has been widely studied. Acidic FGF (aFGF) and basic FGF (bFGF) are both heparin-binding factors [105].

FGF plays an important role in the development of PVR [106]. In the first hour after retinal detachment, the infiltration of polymorphonuclear leukocytes begins, releasing growth factors such as FGF, which in turn stimulate the mononuclear cell influx and its differentiation to macrophages. During the next proliferative phase, macrophages stimulate fibroblast proliferation [107]. In the epiretinal membrane samples of patients with PDR and PVR, both mRNA and protein expression of bFGF are present [108]. In animal models of PVR, both aFGF and bFGF mRNA are expressed [109]. Likewise, early clinical studies showed that aFGF was positive in the vitreous and subretinal fluid of all patients with PVR [110].

bFGF can induce angiogenesis via its action on smooth muscle cells and endothelial cells, as well as its role as a chemokine to aid in the proliferation of fibroblasts and epithelial cells [111–113]. In patients with non-PDR, there was a significant correlation between aqueous humor FGF-1 and total retinal blood flow ($r = 0.71$, $P = 0.01$) [114].

The bFGF concentration in the diabetic macular edema group (5.0 ± 10.2 pg/L) was significantly higher than that in the wet AMD group (2.2 ± 7.4 pg/L, $P = 0.002$) and the control group (0.00 pg/L, $P = 0.001$). There was no significant difference between the latter two groups ($P = 0.10$) [115].

4.6.6 MCP-1

MCP-1, also known as CCL2, belongs to the CC chemokine family. During inflammation, MCP-1 and other chemokines are usually expressed in tissues, induced by

Table 4.3 List of secretion sources, targets, and main functions of various interleukins

Cytokine	Sources	Targets	Main functions
IL-1α, IL-1β	Macrophages，many other cells	Macrophages, thymocytes, central nervous system	Costimulation and secretion of cytokines and other acute phase proteins
IL-2	T cells	T cells, B cells, NK cells, and macrophages	Proliferation， enhancement of cytotoxicity, inducing IFNγ secretion, and antibody production
IL-3	T cells，macrophages，eosinophils	Hematopoietic progenitor cells, macrophages, mast cells	Differentiation and survival of lymphoid and bone marrow tissues
IL-4	T cells， macrophages	T cells，B cells，macrophages，monocytes	Proliferation and differentiation of Th2, promotion of IgG and IgE production, inhibition of cell-mediated immunity and Th17 development
IL-5	Th2 cells	Eosinophils，B cells	Proliferation and activation, marker of Th2 effector cells
IL-6	Macrophages，T cells，fibroblasts	B cells，T cells，thymocytes，myeloid cells，osteoclasts	Inflammation and costimulation, induction of proliferation and differentiation, drive Th17 with TGF-β
IL-7	Thymic stromal cells, bone marrow and spleen	B cells，T cells，thymocytes	Maintenance of homeostasis, differentiation and survival
IL-9	Th2 cells	T cells，macrophages，neutrop hils，epithelial cells	Proliferation and promotion of Th2 cytokine secretion
IL-10	Differentiated T helper cells, Tregs, B cells, dendritic cells	Macrophages, T cells, dendritic cells, B cells	Immunosuppression, decrease of MHC class II expression on dendritic cells and antigen presentation cells, downregulating pathogenic Th1, Th2, and Th17 responses
IL-11	Stromal cells	Hematopoietic stem cells, B cells, megakaryocytes	Proliferation

IL-12	Macrophages, dendritic cells, B cells, neutrophils	T cells，NK cells	Differentiation and proliferation promotion of Th1 proliferation and cytotoxicity
IL-13	T cells	B cells，macrophages	Activation of goblet cell in lung and intestine, diffusion and promotion of IgE synthesis, cell-mediated immune regulation
IL-14	T cells	B cells	Promotion of B-cell growth
IL-15	Widely expressed in hematopoietic cells	T cells，NK cells，epithelial cells	Proliferation and survival, secretion of cytokines
IL-16	T cells，eosinophils，macrophages	CD4+ T cells	Recruitment of CD4+ T cells
IL-17a	Th17 cells	Mucosa tissue, epithelium, and endothelium	Maintenance of the protective immunity of the lung, keeping the integrity of tight junction, promotion of the epithelial neutrophil mobilization, cytokine production, and angiogenesis
IL-17b	Bowel and pancreas		
IL-17c	Thymus and spleen		
IL-17d	T cells, smooth muscle cells, epithelial cells		
IL-17f	Th17 cells	Mucosa tissue, epithelium, and endothelium	With function similar to IL-17a but with lower receptor affinity
IL-18	Macrophages	Th1 cells, NK cells, B cells	Proinflammatory effects and induction of IFNγ
IL-19	Monocytes	Keratinocytes	Proinflammatory effects
IL-20	Monocytes	Keratinocytes	Proinflammatory effects
IL-21	Differentiated T helper cells (Th2 and Th17 subsets)	T cells, B cells, NK cells, dendritic cells	Promotion of T cells proliferation, B cells differentiation and cytotoxicity of NK cells
IL-22	Th1 and Th17 cells, NK cells	Fibroblasts, epithelial cells	Proinflammatory and antibacterial effects
IL-23	Macrophages and dendritic cells	T cells	Proinflammatory and promotion of the Th17 proliferation
IL-24	Monocytes, CD4+ T cells	Keratinocytes	Specifical inhibition of the various tumor cells proliferation and inducing tumor cell apoptosis [100]

(continued)

Table 4.3 (continued)

Cytokine	Sources	Targets	Main functions
IL-25 (IL-17e)	Th2 cells, mast cells	Non-B, T, cKit+, FcεR- cells	Promotion of Th2 differentiation and proliferation
IL-26 [101]	Activated T cells, macrophages, NK cells, CD68+ alveolar macrophages	Non-hematopoietic cells, especially epithelial cells, various tissue cells	Proinflammatory effect
IL-27	Activated dendritic cells	T cells	Inducing early Th1 differentiation by stimulating expression of Tbet transcription factor; suppression of Th17 effector responses by inducing STAT-1-dependent blockade of IL-17 production
IL-28b/ IL29 [102] (IFNλ family)	Peripheral blood mononuclear cells (PMBC), dendritic cells, and HeLa cells	Various tissue cells (such as heart, kidney, skin, small intestine, lung, skeletal muscle, liver)	Anti-viral effect, anti-cell proliferation effect and immune regulation
IL-30 [103] (IL-27 subunit p28)	CD4+ T cells and macrophages	NK T cells	Simultaneously antagonizes T helper 1 (Th1) and Th17 responses and may be a novel molecule modulating the tumor and lymph node microenvironment
IL-31	Activated T cells	Bone marrow progenitor cells, lung epithelial cells, keratinocytes	Proinflammatory effect
IL-32	T cells, NK cells, monocytes, endothelial cells, epithelial cells	Vascular endothelial cells	Inflammatory response regulation, cell apoptosis promotion, cell differentiation-inducing, anti-infection [104]
IL-33	Macrophages, dendritic cells	Mast cells, Th2 cells	Costimulation, promotion of Th2 cytokine production
IL-35	Regulatory T cells	Effector T cells	Immunosuppression

pro-inflammatory mediators TNF-α, IL-1, and endotoxin in in vitro cell experiments [116, 117].

MCP-1 stimulates the aggregation and activation of monocytes and macrophages and plays an important role in diabetes-induced retinal inflammation [118, 119]. In addition, MCP-1 increases VEGF production [120] and may also play a role in fibrosis and induction of neovascularization [121].

In patients with diabetic macular edema, after intravitreal injection of anti-inflammatory drugs, the aqueous level of MCP-1 decreased significantly ($P = 0.044$). With the relapse of macular edema, the aqueous level of MCP-1 increased significantly ($P = 0.005$) [122]. MCP-1 was also proved to be associated with recurrence of inflammation after uveitic cataract surgery [123]. In the aqueous humor of patients with wet AMD, the titer of MCP-1 in the aqueous humor increased [124]. The levels of interleukin 6 and MCP-1 were highly correlated with retinal pigment epithelial detachment [125] and also significantly correlated with macular thickness ($r = 0.40$, $P = 0.004$) [126].

4.6.7 TGF-β

TGF-β is a multifunctional cytokine that regulates a diversity of cellular processes such as proliferation, differentiation, migration, ECM plasticity, epithelial-mesenchymal transition, immune function, and apoptosis [127]. Five isoforms (TGF-β1–5) have been identified [128, 129], with different expression and function in different tissues [130, 131]. Although TGF-β is normally involved in the maintenance of tissue homeostasis, it is overexpressed in disease states [132].

Compared with the control group, aqueous level of TGF-β1 and TGF-β2 elevated in patients with non-proliferative DR and with reduced total retinal blood flow [114].

In patients with capsular exfoliation syndrome with/without glaucoma, aqueous levels of TGF-β1, TGF-β2, and TGF-β3 were higher than those in the control group ($P < 0.01$) [133]. An interesting study also found that the aqueous level of TGF-β2 (as a modulator of immunosuppression) in the second cataract-operated eye were significantly higher than those of the first eye ($P = 0.002$) in the same patient [134].

The aqueous level of TGF-β2 in patients with primary open-angle glaucoma was significantly increased, a finding confirmed by many researchers [135–141]. TGF-β increased the secretion of extracellular matrix [142], which was considered to increase resistance to aqueous humor outflow in patients with primary open-angle glaucoma [143–145].

Certain bioactive substances (such as decorin) can be used to inhibit TGF-β, thereby reducing the severity of PV. Injecting high concentrations of TGF-β into the vitreous could accelerate the healing of full-thickness macular holes [146, 147].

4.6.8 TNF-α

TNF-α is a member of the TNF ligand superfamily and is mainly produced by immune cells, including macrophages, T lymphocytes, and natural killer cells [148]. TNF-α helps regulate immune, hematopoietic, and pro-inflammatory activities [149, 150]. In 1975, TNFα was first isolated by Carswell et al. [151].

TNF-α is a well-known key mediator of inflammation, which plays a vital role in the early stages of host resistance to bacterial, viral, and parasitic infections. Usually, inflammation is caused by the release of TNF-α by immune cells, such as macrophages, T lymphocytes, and natural killer cells [152]. In turn, TNFα triggers a series of different cell adhesion molecules, such as selectins, ICAM-1, and vascular cell adhesion molecule (VCAM)-1, to recruit leukocyte accumulation at sites of inflammation through leukocyte adhesion [153]. However, systemic release of high concentrations of TNF-α can lead to vascular decompensation and death [154]. TNF-blocking biologics have been used clinically to treat uveitis and other intraocular autoimmune inflammatory diseases [155, 156].

TNF-α activates macrophages and retinal microglia, leading to the production of reactive oxygen species (ROS) and nitric oxide. TNF-α is pathogenic in DR [157–159] through immune activation of the retinal vasculature as well as chronic low-grade inflammation [160]. Hyperglycemia induces oxidative stress leading to retinal inflammation and neovascularization [161, 162].

TNF-α is also important in the pathogenesis of wet AMD [163, 164]. The mechanisms include macrophage activation, complement activation, and NO/ROS production [165]. TNF-α plays an important role in the pathogenesis of uveitis. Intravitreal injection of TNF-α itself produces uveitis, disrupts the blood-ocular barrier, and promotes neovascularization [166]. A key signaling pathway, IFN-γ (a Th1 cytokine), controls macrophage activation through TNFR1. IFN-γ induces low levels of TNF-α production and trigger autoimmune reaction. After IFN-γ stimulation, macrophages produce NO, which further causes retinal damage [167, 168].

4.6.9 VCAM-1

VCAM-1 is an inducible 90 kDa glycoprotein expressed mainly in endothelial cells [169] and was first identified as an endothelial cell surface glycoprotein in 1989 [170, 171]. VCAM-1 expression is activated by pro-inflammatory cytokines including TNF-α but also by ROS, oxidized LDL, high glucose concentrations, Toll-like receptor agonists [172]. Under highly inflammatory and chronic conditions in certain diseases, VCAM-1 is also expressed on the surface of other cells, including tissue macrophages, dendritic cells, myeloid fibroblasts, myoblasts, oocytes, Kupffer cells, Sertoli cells, and cancer cells [173, 174].

VCAM-1 plays an important role in inflammation via interaction with α4β1 integrin. It is the major regulator of leukocyte adhesion and transendothelial migration. The α4β1 integrin expressed on leukocytes adheres to VCAM-1 on the surface of endothelial cells and activates the signaling pathway in endothelial cells, which helps the migration of leukocytes through endothelial cells [175].

The VCAM-1 level in the vitreous humor of patients with PDR was significantly higher than those of controls ($P = 0.003$) [176]. Interestingly, there was a significant positive correlation between intraocular free VCAM-1 and serum HbA(1)c ($r = 0.590$, $P = 0.007$), suggesting that inadequate metabolism remained an important factor in the development of PDR in diabetes. Risk factors [177].

4.6.10 ICAM-1

ICAM-1 is a membrane-bound glycoprotein that plays an important role in the transportation of leukocytes, the activation of lymphocytes, and various immune functions [178–181]. It is known that ICAM-1 is mainly expressed in leukocyte subsets, endothelial cells, platelets, fibroblasts, epithelial cells, and glial cells [182–187].

Aqueous level of ICAM-1 elevated in patients with diabetic macular edema [188]. Hillier RJ et al. [189] further found that in patients with diabetic macular edema, the aqueous level of ICAM-1 was correlated with the volume of macular edema ($P = 0.002$), which suggested that ICAM-1 in aqueous humor might be the biomarker which could be used to quantitatively.

reflect the severity of diabetic macular edema. Antibodies targeting ICAM-1 attenuated intraocular inflammation in uveitis animal models [190].

4.7 Macro/Micro-Element

The human body contains a total of more than 60 elements, of which more than 20 are essential elements, which are of great significance to maintaining the normal physiological functions of the body. Among them, carbon, hydrogen, oxygen, nitrogen, phosphorus, chlorine, sodium, magnesium, potassium, and calcium are abundant in the human body. Four elements, including carbon, hydrogen, oxygen, and nitrogen, mainly exist in the form of organic matters. Other elements all exist in the form of inorganic salts.

Macro-element refers to any chemical element for which the human body has a daily requirement of greater than about 100 mg. Six elements, including calcium, phosphorus, potassium, sulfur, chlorine, and magnesium, are classified as macro-elements. Micro-elements, also named trace element, refers to elements whose content in the human body is between 0.01% and 0.005% of body weight. Micro-elements essential to the human body include iron, copper, manganese, zinc, cobalt, molybdenum, chromium, nickel, vanadium, fluorine, selenium, iodine, silicon, and tin.

The elemental composition of intraocular fluid was proved to affect the lens transparency. The relationship between the abnormal increase in sodium concentration, or the impaired functional activity of Na-K-ATPase, and the opacification of the human lens cortex has been confirmed [191]. Magnesium deficiency was also confirmed to lead to the development of cataract [192, 193]. In a multi-elemental analysis of the aqueous humor, Flieger J et al. [194] found that the phosphorous level and the ratio of phosphorous/calcium were significant in retinopathy and diabetes, whereas cobalt was significantly higher in AMD. In coexisting hypertension, the levels of tin, titanium, and ruthenium varied in comparison to the controls. In patients with open-angle glaucoma, the aqueous level of zinc was also found to be higher than in control group [195]. In our previous study [196], we found a significantly higher level of phosphorus and copper, and a significantly lower level of potassium and magnesium in the aqueous humor of patients with CMVR. Besides, the aqueous level of copper and selenium was significantly correlated with the concentration of IL-8 in the aqueous humor. Our study indicated that the measurement of trace elements in the aqueous humor might have potential value in the treatment and prognosis evaluation of CMVR.

4.8 Exosome

Exosomes are membrane-bound extracellular vesicles (EVs) that are produced in the endosomal compartment of most eukaryotic cells. It was first discovered in the maturing mammalian reticulocyte (immature red blood cell) by Stahl et al. in 1983 [197] and Johnstone et al. in 1983 [198], and further termed "exosomes" by Johnstone et al. in 1987 [199]. In multicellular organisms, exosomes and other EVs are found in biological fluids including saliva, blood, urine, and cerebrospinal fluid [200]. EVs carry messenger RNA (mRNA), microRNA (miRNA), proteins, and transcription factors from their cell of origin, which make them possible to act as biomarkers in the diagnosis and treatment of disease.

In a study of Dismuke WM et al. in 2015, exosomes were found to be a major constituent of aqueous humor. The authors stated that miRNAs housed within exosomes might function in communication between aqueous humor inflow and outflow tissues [201]. Due to the difficulty of intraocular fluid obtainment and the separation of high-purity aqueous humor exosomes, there are few studies on exosomes in eye diseases, mainly focused on DR, AMD, autoimmune uveitis, glaucoma, and intraocular tumor [202]. In DR, miR-126, secreted by human umbilical cord-derived mesenchymal stem cells, was proved able to alleviate hyperglycemia-induced retinal inflammation by inhibiting the HMGB1 signaling pathway [203]. Other exosomal contents, including IgG, miRNAs, VEGF, CXCL-10, miR-15a, and PPARγ, were also proved to have different biological functions in the pathophysiology of DR [202]. Kang GY et al. [204] identified cytokeratin 8; cytokeratin 14; cathepsin D, Hsp70; myosin-9; and actin, aortic smooth muscle in the aqueous humor, all of them had the potential to diagnose neovascular AMD as novel biomarkers. In brief, exosomes have the potential to act as biomarkers or therapeutic carriers in ocular diseases. However, the functions and mechanisms of exosomes require further investigation.

References

1. Szirmai JA, Balazs EA. Studies on the structure of the vitreous body: III. Cells in the cortical layer. *AMA*. Arch Ophthalmol. 1958;59(1):34–48.
2. Liu K, Klintworth GK, Dodd LG. Cytologic findings in vitreous fluids. Analysis of 74 specimens. Acta Cytol. 1999;43(2):201–6.
3. Iwamoto T, Witmer R. Aqueous humor cytology with the electron microscope. Albrecht Von Graefes Arch Klin Exp Ophthalmol. 1967;174(2):110–26.
4. Kalogeropoulos CD, Malamou-Mitsi VD, Asproudis I, Psilas K. The contribution of aqueous humor cytology in the differential diagnosis of anterior uvea inflammations. Ocul Immunol Inflamm. 2004;12(3):215–25.
5. Baudouin C, Hofman P, Brignole F, Bayle J, Loubière R, Gastaud P. Immunocytology of cellular components in vitreous and subretinal fluid from patients with proliferative vitreoretinopathy. Ophthalmologica. 1991;203(1):38–46.
6. Stewart J, Halliwell T, Gupta RK. Cytodiagnosis of Coats' disease from an ocular aspirate. A case report. Acta Cytologica. 1993;37(5):717–20.
7. Feron EJ, Klaren VN, Wierenga EA, Verjans GM, Kijlstra A. Characterization of toxoplasma gondii-specific T cells recovered from vitreous fluid of patients with ocular toxoplasmosis. Invest Ophthalmol Vis Sci. 2001;42(13):3228–32.
8. Fujikawa LS, Haugen JP. Immunopathology of vitreous and retinochoroidal biopsy in posterior uveitis. Ophthalmology. 1990;97(12):1644–53.
9. Huang LZ, Li TY, Wang B, Li XX. Clinical features and mitochondrial mutation site analysis of Leber hereditary optic neuropathy. Chin J Exp Ophthalmol. 2016;34(10):920–4.
10. Chen XH, Yang M, Wei SH, Xu QG. Clinical features of Leber hereditary optic neuropathy. Ophthalmology (China). 2017;26(05):343–6.
11. Zhang Y, Yuan JJ, Liu HL, Tian Z, Liu SW, Li B. Three cases of Leber's hereditary optic neuropathy with rapid increase in visual acuity after gene therapy. Curr Gene Ther. 2019;19(2):134–8.
12. Mishra D, Satpathy G, Chawla R, Venkatesh P, Ahmed NH, Panda SK. Utility of broad-range 16S rRNA PCR assay versus conventional methods for laboratory diagnosis of bacterial endophthalmitis in a tertiary care hospital. Br J Ophthalmol. 2019;103(1):152–6.
13. Srinivasan R, Karaoz U, Volegova M, MacKichan J, Kato-Maeda M, Miller S, Nadarajan R, Brodie EL, Lynch SV. Use of 16S rRNA gene for identification of a broad range of clinically relevant bacterial pathogens. PLoS One. 2015;10(2):e0117617.
14. Ogawa M, Sugita S, Watanabe K, Shimizu N, Mochizuki M. Novel diagnosis of fungal endophthalmitis by broad-range real-time PCR detection of fungal 28S ribosomal DNA. Graefes Arch Clin Exp Ophthalmol. 2012;250(12):1877–83.
15. Pockar S, Globocnik Petrovic M, Peterlin B, Vidovic Valentincic N. MiRNA as biomarker for uveitis—a systematic review of the literature. Gene. 2019;696:162–75.
16. Zhai WJ, Wei JL, Zhao MF, Wang M, Zhou Z, Liu P, Mu H, Feng SZ, Han MZ. Comparison between CMV quantitative PCR and CMV-pp65 antigen test for detection of CMV infection in allogeneic hematopoietic stem cell transplantation. Zhongguo Shi Yan Xue Ye Xue Za Zhi. 2009;17(6):1522–6.
17. Bergallo M, Costa C, Terlizzi ME, Margio S, Sidoti F, Sinesi F, Cavallo R. Evaluation of two set of primers for detection of immediate early gene UL123 of human cytomegalovirus (HCMV). Mol Biotechnol. 2008;38(1):65–70.
18. Luo CQ, Mo MQ, Mea ZJ. The value of detecting cytomegalovirus (CMV) DNA and its immediate early antigens, pp65 and pp67 in the early diagnosis of CMV infection in kidney transplant recipients. Chin J Histochem Cytochem. 2009;17(6):1522–6.
19. Grewal DS, Fishman GA, Jampol LM. Autoimmune retinopathy and antiretinal antibodies: a review. Retina. 2014;34(5):827–45.
20. Hosogai M, Nakatani Y, Mimura K, Kishi S, Akiyama H. Genetic analysis of varicella-zoster virus in the aqueous humor in uveitis with severe hyphema. BMC Infect Dis. 2017;17(1):427.

21. Malecaze F, Arne JL, Bec P, Séguéla JP, Linas MD, Recco P, Béssières MH. Candida endophthalmitis after heroin abuse. Mycopathologia. 1985;92(2):73–6.
22. Lim SJ, Lee SE, Kim SH, Hong SH, You YS, Kwon OW, Kim HS. Prevalence of toxoplasma gondii and Toxocara canis among patients with uveitis. Ocul Immunol Inflamm. 2015;23(2):111–7.
23. Lim SJ, Lee SE, Kim SH, Hong SH, You YS, Kwon OW, Kim HS. Prevalence of toxoplasma gondii and Toxocara canis among patients with uveitis. Ocul Immunol Inflamm. 2014;22(5):360–6.
24. Chanana B, Gupta N, Azad RV. Case report: bilateral simultaneous central retinal vein occlusion in Waldenström's macroglobulinemia. Optometry. 2009;80(7):350–3.
25. Maslin J, Bigaillon C, Froussard F, Enouf V, Nicand E. Acute bilateral uveitis associated with an active human herpesvirus-6 infection. J Infect. 2007;54(4):e237–40.
26. Wang ZJ, Zhou M, Cao WJ, Ji J, Bi YW, Huang X, Xu GZ. Evaluation of the Goldmann-Witmer coefficient in the immunological diagnosis of ocular toxocariasis. Acta Trop. 2016;158:20–3.
27. Zhu GH, Wang QZ. Research progress on transforming growth factor β and diseases. Chin Med Biotechnol Appl. 2003;02:10–3.
28. XL WU, Wang XY. Research progress of transforming growth factor β. J Nanhua Univ (Med Sci). 2002;02:179–80.
29. Zhang YY, Shi XR. Research progress of transforming growth factor β. Sichuan J Anatomy. 2006;03:30–2.
30. Wang MH, Li HK, Song JY, Zeng XT. Research progress of growth factors in refractory diabetic foot ulcers. J Gannan Med College. 2018;38(06):618–21.
31. Tuyet HL, Nguyen Quynh TT, Vo Hoang Minh H, Thi Bich DN, Do Dinh T, Le Tan D, Van HL LHT, Doan Huu H, Tran Trong TN. The efficacy and safety of epidermal growth factor in treatment of diabetic foot ulcers: the preliminary results. Int Wound J. 2009;6(2):159–66.
32. Tiaka EK, Papanas N, Manolakis AC, Georgiadis GS. Epidermal growth factor in the treatment of diabetic foot ulcers: an update. Perspect Vasc Surg Endovasc Ther. 2012;24(1):37–44.
33. Zhang XH. Advances in chemokine research—chemokine family (1). Foreign Med Immunol. 1995;03:130–133+140.
34. Turner MD, Nedjai B, Hurst T, Pennington DJ. Cytokines and chemokines: At the crossroads of cell signalling and inflammatory disease. Biochim Biophys Acta. 2014;1843(11):2563–82.
35. Ferrara N. Vascular endothelial growth factor. Arterioscler Thromb Vasc Biol. 2009;29(6):789–91.
36. Niu TT, Xu YC. VEGF and intraocular angiogenesis. Adv Ophthalmol. 2008;28(5):394–8.
37. Senger DR, Galli SJ, Dvorak AM, Perruzzi CA, Harvey VS, Dvorak HF. Tumor cells secrete a vascular permeability factor that promotes accumulation of ascites fluid. Science. 1983;219(4587):983–5.
38. Ferrara N, Gerber HP, LeCouter J. The biology of VEGF and its receptors. Nat Med. 2003;9(6):669–76.
39. Bates DO, Curry FE. Vascular endothelial growth factor increases microvascular permeability via a Ca(2+)-dependent pathway. Am J Phys. 1997;273(2 Pt 2):H687–94.
40. Ku DD, Zaleski JK, Liu S, Brock TA. Vascular endothelial growth factor induces EDRF-dependent relaxation in coronary arteries. Am J Phys. 1993;265(2 Pt 2):H586–92.
41. Carmeliet P, Ferreira V, Breier G, Pollefeyt S, Kieckens L, Gertsenstein M, Fahrig M, Vandenhoeck A, Harpal K, Eberhardt C, et al. Abnormal blood vessel development and lethality in embryos lacking a single VEGF allele. Nature. 1996;380(6573):435–9.
42. Ferrara N, Carver-Moore K, Chen H, Dowd M, Lu L, O'Shea KS, Powell-Braxton L, Hillan KJ, Moore MW. Heterozygous embryonic lethality induced by targeted inactivation of the VEGF gene. Nature. 1996;380(6573):439–42.
43. Chen XY, Ye JJ. Basic and clinical research progress of anti-VEGF drugs in the treatment of vascular eye diseases. Ophthalmol Res. 2008;26(9):708–12.
44. Storkebaum E, Lambrechts D, Carmeliet P. VEGF: once regarded as a specific angiogenic factor, now implicated in neuroprotection. BioEssays. 2004;26(9):943–54.

45. Tomanek RJ, Ishii Y, Holifield JS, Sjogren CL, Hansen HK, Mikawa T. VEGF family members regulate myocardial tubulogenesis and coronary artery formation in the embryo. Circ Res. 2006;98(7):947–53.
46. Houck KA, Ferrara N, Winer J, Cachianes G, Li B, Leung DW. The vascular endothelial growth factor family: identification of a fourth molecular species and characterization of alternative splicing of RNA. Mol Endocrinol (Baltimore, Md). 1991;5(12):1806–14.
47. Neufeld G, Cohen T, Gengrinovitch S, Poltorak Z. Vascular endothelial growth factor (VEGF) and its receptors. FASEB J. 1999;13(1):9–22.
48. Siemerink MJ, Augustin AJ, Schlingemann RO. Mechanisms of ocular angiogenesis and its molecular mediators. Dev Ophthalmol. 2010;46:4–20.
49. Distler JH, Hirth A, Kurowska-Stolarska M, Gay RE, Gay S, Distler O. Angiogenic and angiostatic factors in the molecular control of angiogenesis. Quarter J Nuclear Med. 2003;47(3):149–61.
50. D'Amore PA. Mechanisms of retinal and choroidal neovascularization. Invest Ophthalmol Vis Sci. 1994;35(12):3974–9.
51. Ye JH, Ma CH, Zhou BB, Zhong LY, Zhou ZY, Lin XFLY. Changes and significance of vascular endothelial growth factor in early diabetic microangiopathy. J Guangdong Pharm Univ. 2006;02:197–8.
52. Tao Y, Lu Q, Jiang YR, Qian J, Wang JY, Gao L, Jonas JB. Apelin in plasma and vitreous and in fibrovascular retinal membranes of patients with proliferative diabetic retinopathy. Invest Ophthalmol Vis Sci. 2010;51(8):4237–42.
53. Noma H, Funatsu H, Mimura T, Eguchi S, Shimada K. Role of soluble vascular endothelial growth factor receptor-2 in macular oedema with central retinal vein occlusion. Br J Ophthalmol. 2011;95(6):788–92.
54. Yuan MK, Tao Y, Yu WZ, Kai W, Jiang YR. Lentivirus-mediated RNA interference of vascular endothelial growth factor in monkey eyes with iris neovascularization. Mol Vis. 2010;16:1743–53.
55. Pe'er J, Folberg R, Itin A, Gnessin H, Hemo I, Keshet E. Vascular endothelial growth factor upregulation in human central retinal vein occlusion. Ophthalmology. 1998;105(3):412–6.
56. Leske DA, Wu J, Mookadam M, Chen Y, Fautsch MP, Holmes JM, Lanier WL. The relationship of retinal VEGF and retinal IGF-1 mRNA with neovascularization in an acidosis-induced model of retinopathy of prematurity. Curr Eye Res. 2006;31(2):163–9.
57. Stone J, Chan-Ling T, Pe'er J, Itin A, Gnessin H, Keshet E. Roles of vascular endothelial growth factor and astrocyte degeneration in the genesis of retinopathy of prematurity. Invest Ophthalmol Vis Sci. 1996;37(2):290–9.
58. Lashkari K, Hirose T, Yazdany J, McMeel JW, Kazlauskas A, Rahimi N. Vascular endothelial growth factor and hepatocyte growth factor levels are differentially elevated in patients with advanced retinopathy of prematurity. Am J Pathol. 2000;156(4):1337–44.
59. Shen WY, Yu MJ, Barry CJ, Constable IJ, Rakoczy PE. Expression of cell adhesion molecules and vascular endothelial growth factor in experimental choroidal neovascularisation in the rat. Br J Ophthalmol. 1998;82(9):1063–71.
60. Spilsbury K, Garrett KL, Shen WY, Constable IJ, Rakoczy PE. Overexpression of vascular endothelial growth factor (VEGF) in the retinal pigment epithelium leads to the development of choroidal neovascularization. Am J Pathol. 2000;157(1):135–44.
61. Frank RN, Amin RH, Eliott D, Puklin JE, Abrams GW. Basic fibroblast growth factor and vascular endothelial growth factor are present in epiretinal and choroidal neovascular membranes. Am J Ophthalmol. 1996;122(3):393–403.
62. Ghasemi H. Roles of IL-6 in ocular inflammation: a review. Ocul Immunol Inflamm. 2018;26(1):37–50.
63. Zenkel M, Lewczuk P, Jünemann A, Kruse FE, Naumann GO, Schlötzer-Schrehardt U. Proinflammatory cytokines are involved in the initiation of the abnormal matrix process in pseudoexfoliation syndrome/glaucoma. Am J Pathol. 2010;176(6):2868–79.

64. Ohta K, Yamagami S, Taylor AW, Streilein JW. IL-6 antagonizes TGF-beta and abolishes immune privilege in eyes with endotoxin-induced uveitis. Invest Ophthalmol Vis Sci. 2000;41(9):2591–9.
65. Murray PI, Hoekzema R, van Haren MA, de Hon FD, Kijlstra A. Aqueous humor interleukin-6 levels in uveitis. Invest Ophthalmol Vis Sci. 1990;31(5):917–20.
66. Malecaze F, Chollet P, Cavrois E, Vita N, Arné JL, Ferrara P. Role of interleukin 6 in the inflammatory response after cataract surgery. An experimental and clinical study. Arch Ophthalmol. 1991;109(12):1681–3.
67. Norose K, Yano A, Wang XC, Tokushima T, Umihira J, Seki A, Nohara M, Segawa K. Dominance of activated T cells and interleukin-6 in aqueous humor in Vogt-Koyanagi-Harada disease. Invest Ophthalmol Vis Sci. 1994;35(1):33–9.
68. Sakaguchi M, Sugita S, Sagawa K, Itoh K, Mochizuki M. Cytokine production by T cells infiltrating in the eye of uveitis patients. Jpn J Ophthalmol. 1998;42(4):262–8.
69. Cheung CM, Vania M, Ang M, Chee SP, Li J. Comparison of aqueous humor cytokine and chemokine levels in diabetic patients with and without retinopathy. Mol Vis. 2012;18:830–7.
70. Wu H, Hwang DK, Song X, Tao Y. Association between aqueous cytokines and diabetic retinopathy stage. J Ophthalmol. 2017;2017:9402198.
71. Chen H, Zhang X, Liao N, Wen F. Increased levels of IL-6, sIL-6R, and sgp130 in the aqueous humor and serum of patients with diabetic retinopathy. Mol Vis. 2016;22:1005–14.
72. Yi QY, Wang YY, Chen LS, Li WD, Shen Y, Jin Y, Yang J, Wang Y, Yuan J, Cheng L. Implication of inflammatory cytokines in the aqueous humour for management of macular diseases. Acta Ophthalmol. 2020;98(3):e309–15.
73. Matsushima R, Noma H, Yasuda K, Goto H, Shimura M. Role of cytokines in Ranibizumab therapy for macular edema in patients with central retinal vein occlusion. J Ocular Pharmacol Ther. 2019;35(7):407–12.
74. Mashima A, Noma H, Yasuda K, Goto H, Shimura M. Anti-vascular endothelial growth factor agent reduces inflammation in macular edema with central retinal vein occlusion. J Inflamm (Lond). 2019;16:9.
75. Shchuko AG, Zlobin IV, Iureva TN, Ostanin AA, Chernykh ER, Mikhalevich IM. Intraocular cytokines in retinal vein occlusion and its relation to the efficiency of anti-vascular endothelial growth factor therapy. Indian J Ophthalmol. 2015;63(12):905–11.
76. Noma H, Mimura T, Tatsugawa M, Shimada K. Aqueous flare and inflammatory factors in macular edema with central retinal vein occlusion: a case series. BMC Ophthalmol. 2013;13:78.
77. Terao N, Koizumi H, Kojima K, Yamagishi T, Nagata K, Kitazawa K, Yamamoto Y, Yoshii K, Hiraga A, Toda M, et al. Association of Upregulated Angiogenic Cytokines with Choroidal Abnormalities in chronic central serous Chorioretinopathy. Invest Ophthalmol Vis Sci. 2018;59(15):5924–31.
78. Baggiolini M, Dewald B, Moser B. Human chemokines: an update. Annu Rev Immunol. 1997;15:675–705.
79. Ghasemi H, Ghazanfari T, Yaraee R, Faghihzadeh S, Hassan ZM. Roles of IL-8 in ocular inflammations: a review. Ocul Immunol Inflamm. 2011;19(6):401–12.
80. de Boer JH, Hack CE, Verhoeven AJ, Baarsma GS, de Jong PT, Rademakers AJ, de Vries-Knoppert WA, Rothova A, Kijlstra A. Chemoattractant and neutrophil degranulation activities related to interleukin-8 in vitreous fluid in uveitis and vitreoretinal disorders. Invest Ophthalmol Vis Sci. 1993;34(12):3376–85.
81. Sakamoto H, Sakamoto T, Kubota T, Duan H, Koga T, Furue M, Ishibashi T. Interleukin-8 expressed in the granulocytes of the eye in a patient with Behçet's disease complicated by lens-induced endophthalmitis. Jpn J Ophthalmol. 2003;47(6):548–50.
82. El-Asrar AM, Al-Obeidan SS, Kangave D, Geboes K, Opdenakker G, Van Damme J, Struyf S. CXC chemokine expression profiles in aqueous humor of patients with different clinical entities of endogenous uveitis. Immunobiology. 2011;216(9):1004–9.

83. Wang B, Tian B, Tao Y, Hou J, Zhao XT, Li XX. Continued decline of aqueous interleukin-8 after multiple intravitreal injections of ganciclovir for cytomegalovirus retinitis. J Ocular Pharmacol Ther. 2014;30(7):587–92.
84. Li A, Dubey S, Varney ML, Dave BJ, Singh RK. IL-8 directly enhanced endothelial cell survival, proliferation, and matrix metalloproteinases production and regulated angiogenesis. J Immunol (Baltimore, Md: 1950). 2003;170(6):3369–76.
85. Rossi D, Zlotnik A. The biology of chemokines and their receptors. Annu Rev Immunol. 2000;18:217–42.
86. Shono T, Ono M, Izumi H, Jimi SI, Matsushima K, Okamoto T, Kohno K, Kuwano M. Involvement of the transcription factor NF-kappaB in tubular morphogenesis of human microvascular endothelial cells by oxidative stress. Mol Cell Biol. 1996;16(8):4231–9.
87. Aksünger A, Or M, Okur H, Hasanreisoğlu B, Akbatur H. Role of interleukin 8 in the pathogenesis of proliferative vitreoretinopathy. Ophthalmologica. 1997;211(4):223–5.
88. Elner SG, Strieter R, Bian ZM, Kunkel S, Mokhtarzaden L, Johnson M, Lukacs N, Elner VM. Interferon-induced protein 10 and interleukin 8. C-X-C chemokines present in proliferative diabetic retinopathy. Arch Ophthalmol. 1998;116(12):1597–601.
89. Er H, Doganay S, Turkoz Y, Cekmen M, Daglioglu MC, Gunduz A, Evereklioglu C, Isci N. The levels of cytokines and nitric oxide in rabbit vitreous humor after retinal laser photocoagulation. Ophthalmic Surg Lasers. 2000;31(6):479–83.
90. Harada C, Harada T, Mitamura Y, Quah HM, Ohtsuka K, Kotake S, Ohno S, Wada K, Takeuchi S, Tanaka K. Diverse NF-kappaB expression in epiretinal membranes after human diabetic retinopathy and proliferative vitreoretinopathy. Mol Vis. 2004;10:31–6.
91. Mosmann TR. Properties and functions of interleukin-10. Adv Immunol. 1994;56:1–26.
92. Gesser B, Leffers H, Jinquan T, Vestergaard C, Kirstein N, Sindet-Pedersen S, Jensen SL, Thestrup-Pedersen K, Larsen CG. Identification of functional domains on human interleukin 10. Proc Natl Acad Sci USA. 1997;94(26):14620–5.
93. Ghasemi H, Ghazanfari T, Yaraee R, Owlia P, Hassan ZM, Faghihzadeh S. Roles of IL-10 in ocular inflammations: a review. Ocul Immunol Inflamm. 2012;20(6):406–18.
94. Groux H, Bigler M, de Vries JE, Roncarolo MG. Interleukin-10 induces a long-term antigen-specific anergic state in human CD4+ T cells. J Exp Med. 1996;184(1):19–29.
95. Lee JH, Lee W, Kwon OH, Kim JH, Kwon OW, Kim KH, Lim JB. Cytokine profile of peripheral blood in type 2 diabetes mellitus patients with diabetic retinopathy. Ann Clin Lab Sci. 2008;38(4):361–7.
96. Bundoc VG, Keane-Myers A. IL-10 confers protection from mast cell degranulation in a mouse model of allergic conjunctivitis. Exp Eye Res. 2007;85(4):575–9.
97. Cavaillon JM. Cytokines and macrophages. Biomed Pharmacother. 1994;48(10):445–53.
98. McClellan SA, Huang X, Barrett RP, van Rooijen N, Hazlett LD. Macrophages restrict Pseudomonas aeruginosa growth, regulate polymorphonuclear neutrophil influx, and balance pro-and anti-inflammatory cytokines in BALB/c mice. J Immunol (Baltimore, Md: 1950). 2003;170(10):5219–27.
99. Chan CC, Whitcup SM, Solomon D, Nussenblatt RB. Interleukin-10 in the vitreous of patients with primary intraocular lymphoma. Am J Ophthalmol. 1995;120(5):671–3.
100. Zhang Y, Ma QF, Zhang C, Shi YN, Jiang H. Research progress of interleukin-24 genetically engineered protein. Mil Med. 2015;10:797–801.
101. Sun ZH, Wu C. Research progress of interleukin-26 in infectious diseases. Chin J Exp Clin Infect Dis (Elect Ed). 2017;11(2):121–4.
102. Li MC, He SH. Research progress of interleukin-28 and interleukin-29. J Postgrad Med. 2004;17(7):641–3.
103. Li CX, Cui JX, Li JJ, Zhou YY, Guan W. Research progress on the structure and function of IL-30. Shandong Med. 2018;58(41):106–9.
104. Son DJ, Jung YY, Seo YS, Park H, Lee DH, Kim S, Roh YS, Han SB, Yoon DY, Hong JT. Interleukin-32α inhibits endothelial inflammation, vascular smooth muscle cell activation, and atherosclerosis by upregulating timp3 and reck through suppressing microRNA-205 biogenesis. Theranostics. 2017;7(8):2186–203.

105. Rusnati M, Presta M. Interaction of angiogenic basic fibroblast growth factor with endothelial cell heparan sulfate proteoglycans. Biological implications in neovascularization. Int J Clin Lab Res. 1996;26(1):15–23.
106. Ciprian D. The pathogeny of proliferative vitreoretinopathy. Rom J Ophthalmol. 2015;59(2):88–92.
107. Garweg JG, Tappeiner C, Halberstadt M. Pathophysiology of proliferative vitreoretinopathy in retinal detachment. Surv Ophthalmol. 2013;58(4):321–9.
108. Hueber A, Wiedemann P, Esser P, Heimann K. Basic fibroblast growth factor mRNA, bFGF peptide and FGF receptor in epiretinal membranes of intraocular proliferative disorders (PVR and PDR). Int Ophthalmol. 1996;20(6):345–50.
109. Planck SR, Andresevic J, Chen JC, Holmes DL, Rodden W, Westra I, Wu SC, Huang XN, Kay G, Wilson DJ, et al. Expression of growth factor mRNA in rabbit PVR model systems. Curr Eye Res. 1992;11(11):1031–9.
110. Baudouin C, Fredj-Reygrobellet D, Brignole F, Nègre F, Lapalus P, Gastaud P. Growth factors in vitreous and subretinal fluid cells from patients with proliferative vitreoretinopathy. Ophthalmic Res. 1993;25(1):52–9.
111. Arnold F, West DC. Angiogenesis in wound healing. Pharmacol Ther. 1991;52(3):407–22.
112. Krishnamoorthy L, Morris HL, Harding KG. Specific growth factors and the healing of chronic wounds. J Wound Care. 2001;10(5):173–8.
113. Xie JL, Bian HN, Qi SH, Chen HD, Li HD, Xu YB, Li TZ, Liu XS, Liang HZ, Xin BR, et al. Basic fibroblast growth factor (bFGF) alleviates the scar of the rabbit ear model in wound healing. Wound Repair Regen. 2008;16(4):576–81.
114. Khuu LA, Tayyari F, Sivak JM, Flanagan JG, Singer S, Brent MH, Huang D, Tan O, Hudson C. Aqueous humour concentrations of TGF-β, PLGF and FGF-1 and total retinal blood flow in patients with early non-proliferative diabetic retinopathy. Acta Ophthalmol. 2017;95(3):e206–11.
115. Jonas JB, Neumaier M. Vascular endothelial growth factor and basic fibroblast growth factor in exudative age-related macular degeneration and diffuse diabetic macular edema. Ophthalmic Res. 2007;39(3):139–42.
116. Strieter RM, Kunkel SL. The immunopathology of chemotactic cytokines. Adv Exp Med Biol. 1993;351:19–28.
117. Proost P, Wuyts A, Van Damme J. Human monocyte chemotactic proteins-2 and -3: structural and functional comparison with MCP-1. J Leukoc Biol. 1996;59(1):67–74.
118. Behfar S, Hassanshahi G, Nazari A, Khorramdelazad H. A brief look at the role of monocyte chemoattractant protein-1 (CCL2) in the pathophysiology of psoriasis. Cytokine. 2018;110:226–31.
119. Vakilian A, Khorramdelazad H, Heidari P, Sheikh Rezaei Z, Hassanshahi G. CCL2/CCR2 signaling pathway in glioblastoma multiforme. Neurochem Int. 2017;103:1–7.
120. Hong KH, Ryu J, Han KH. Monocyte chemoattractant protein-1-induced angiogenesis is mediated by vascular endothelial growth factor-A. Blood. 2005;105(4):1405–7.
121. Gharaee-Kermani M, Denholm EM, Phan SH. Costimulation of fibroblast collagen and transforming growth factor beta1 gene expression by monocyte chemoattractant protein-1 via specific receptors. J Biol Chem. 1996;271(30):17779–84.
122. Figueras-Roca M, Sala-Puigdollers A, Alforja S, Torras J, Peraza-Nieves J, Zarranz-Ventura J, Adan Civera A, Molins B. Aqueous humour cytokine changes with Intravitreal dexamethasone implant injection for diabetic macular edema. Ocul Immunol Inflamm. 2019;27(8):1203–10.
123. Pei M, Liu X, Zhao C, Gao F, Tao Y, Zhang M. Chemokine and adhesion molecule profiles in aqueous humor of clinically quiescent Uveitic cataracts. Curr Eye Res. 2019;44(2):194–9.
124. Mimura T, Funatsu H, Noma H, Shimura M, Kamei Y, Yoshida M, Kondo A, Watanabe E, Mizota A. Aqueous humor levels of cytokines in patients with age-related macular degeneration. Ophthalmologica. 2019;241(2):81–9.
125. Jonas JB, Tao Y, Neumaier M, Findeisen P. Cytokine concentration in aqueous humour of eyes with exudative age-related macular degeneration. Acta Ophthalmol. 2012;90(5):e381–8.

126. Jonas JB, Tao Y, Neumaier M, Findeisen P. Monocyte chemoattractant protein 1, intercellular adhesion molecule 1, and vascular cell adhesion molecule 1 in exudative age-related macular degeneration. Arch Ophthalmol (Chicago, Ill : 1960). 2010;128(10):1281–6.
127. Shi Y, Massagué J. Mechanisms of TGF-beta signaling from cell membrane to the nucleus. Cell. 2003;113(6):685–700.
128. Liu T. Research progress on β-transforming growth factor and fracture healing (literature review). Sport Sci Res. 2003;02:89–93.
129. Sporn MB, Roberts AB, Wakefield LM, Assoian RK. Transforming growth factor-beta: biological function and chemical structure. Science. 1986;233(4763):532–4.
130. Roberts AB, Sporn MB. Transforming growth factor beta. Adv Cancer Res. 1988;51:107–45.
131. Tandon A, Tovey JC, Sharma A, Gupta R, Mohan RR. Role of transforming growth factor Beta in corneal function, biology and pathology. Curr Mol Med. 2010;10(6):565–78.
132. Wang J, Harris A, Prendes MA, Alshawa L, Gross JC, Wentz SM, Rao AB, Kim NJ, Synder A, Siesky B. Targeting transforming growth factor-β signaling in primary open-angle glaucoma. J Glaucoma. 2017;26(4):390–5.
133. Garweg JG, Zandi S, Gerhardt C, Pfister IB. Isoforms of TGF-β in the aqueous humor of patients with pseudoexfoliation syndrome and a possible association with the long-term stability of the capsular bag after cataract surgery. Graefes Arch Clin Exp Ophthalmol. 2017;255(9):1763–9.
134. Chen Y, Zhang Y, Sun K, Yan H. Higher TGF-β2 level in the aqueous humor of the second eye versus the first eye in the course of sequential cataract surgery. Ocul Immunol Inflamm. 2020;28(3):439–45.
135. Tripathi RC, Li J, Chan WF, Tripathi BJ. Aqueous humor in glaucomatous eyes contains an increased level of TGF-beta 2. Exp Eye Res. 1994;59(6):723–7.
136. Inatani M, Tanihara H, Katsuta H, Honjo M, Kido N, Honda Y. Transforming growth factor-beta 2 levels in aqueous humor of glaucomatous eyes. Graefes Arch Clin Exp Ophthalmol. 2001;239(2):109–13.
137. Picht G, Welge-Luessen U, Grehn F, Lütjen-Drecoll E. Transforming growth factor beta 2 levels in the aqueous humor in different types of glaucoma and the relation to filtering bleb development. Graefes Arch Clin Exp Ophthalmol. 2001;239(3):199–207.
138. Schnaper HW, Hayashida T, Hubchak SC, Poncelet AC. TGF-beta signal transduction and mesangial cell fibrogenesis. Am J Physiol Renal Physiol. 2003;284(2):F243–52.
139. Trivedi RH, Nutaitis M, Vroman D, Crosson CE. Influence of race and age on aqueous humor levels of transforming growth factor-beta 2 in glaucomatous and nonglaucomatous eyes. J Ocul Pharmacol Ther. 2011;27(5):477–80.
140. Ozcan AA, Ozdemir N, Canataroglu A. The aqueous levels of TGF-beta2 in patients with glaucoma. Int Ophthalmol. 2004;25(1):19–22.
141. Yamamoto N, Itonaga K, Marunouchi T, Majima K. Concentration of transforming growth factor beta2 in aqueous humor. Ophthalmic Res. 2005;37(1):29–33.
142. Gamulescu MA, Chen Y, He S, Spee C, Jin M, Ryan SJ, Hinton DR. Transforming growth factor beta2-induced myofibroblastic differentiation of human retinal pigment epithelial cells: regulation by extracellular matrix proteins and hepatocyte growth factor. Exp Eye Res. 2006;83(1):212–22.
143. Lütjen-Drecoll E. Morphological changes in glaucomatous eyes and the role of TGFbeta2 for the pathogenesis of the disease. Exp Eye Res. 2005;81(1):1–4.
144. Tamm ER, Fuchshofer R. What increases outflow resistance in primary open-angle glaucoma? Surv Ophthalmol. 2007;52(Suppl 2):S101–4.
145. Wiederholt M, Thieme H, Stumpff F. The regulation of trabecular meshwork and ciliary muscle contractility. Prog Retin Eye Res. 2000;19(3):271–95.
146. Bai J. Ocular immune diseases and cytokines. J Chongqing Med Univ. 1995;02:145–7.
147. Rosenbaum JT. Cytokines: the good, the bad, and the unknown. Invest Ophthalmol Vis Sci. 1993;34(8):2389–91.
148. Chatzantoni K, Mouzaki A. Anti-TNF-alpha antibody therapies in autoimmune diseases. Curr Top Med Chem. 2006;6(16):1707–14.

149. Kodama S, Davis M, Faustman DL. The therapeutic potential of tumor necrosis factor for autoimmune disease: a mechanistically based hypothesis. Cell Mol Life Sci. 2005;62(16):1850–62.
150. Zhang Y, Harada A, Bluethmann H, Wang JB, Nakao S, Mukaida N, Matsushima K. Tumor necrosis factor (TNF) is a physiologic regulator of hematopoietic progenitor cells: increase of early hematopoietic progenitor cells in TNF receptor p55-deficient mice in vivo and potent inhibition of progenitor cell proliferation by TNF alpha in vitro. Blood. 1995;86(8):2930–7.
151. Carswell EA, Old LJ, Kassel RL, Green S, Fiore N, Williamson B. An endotoxin-induced serum factor that causes necrosis of tumors. Proc Natl Acad Sci USA. 1975;72(9):3666–70.
152. Medzhitov R. Origin and physiological roles of inflammation. Nature. 2008;454(7203):428–35.
153. Pober JS. Endothelial activation: intracellular signaling pathways. Arthritis Res. 2002;4(Suppl 3(Suppl 3)):S109–16.
154. Beutler B, Milsark IW, Cerami AC. Passive immunization against cachectin/tumor necrosis factor protects mice from lethal effect of endotoxin. Science. 1985;229(4716):869–71.
155. Hasegawa E, Takeda A, Yawata N, Sonoda KH. The effectiveness of adalimumab treatment for non-infectious uveitis. Immunol Med. 2019;42(2):79–83.
156. Atienza-Mateo B, Martín-Varillas JL, Calvo-Río V, Demetrio-Pablo R, Beltrán E, Sánchez-Bursón J, Mesquida M, Adan A, Hernández MV, Hernández-Garfella M, et al. Comparative study of infliximab versus Adalimumab in refractory uveitis due to Behçet's disease: National Multicenter Study of 177 cases. Arthritis Rheumatol (Hoboken, NJ). 2019;71(12):2081–9.
157. Gustavsson C, Agardh E, Bengtsson B, Agardh CD. TNF-alpha is an independent serum marker for proliferative retinopathy in type 1 diabetic patients. J Diabetes Complicat. 2008;22(5):309–16.
158. Myśliwiec M, Balcerska A, Zorena K, Myśliwska J, Lipowski P, Raczyńska K. The role of vascular endothelial growth factor, tumor necrosis factor alpha and interleukin-6 in pathogenesis of diabetic retinopathy. Diabetes Res Clin Pract. 2008;79(1):141–6.
159. Zorena K, Myśliwska J, Myśliwiec M, Balcerska A, Hak Ł, Lipowski P, Raczyńska K. Serum TNF-alpha level predicts nonproliferative diabetic retinopathy in children. Mediat Inflamm. 2007;2007:92196.
160. Joussen AM, Poulaki V, Le ML, Koizumi K, Esser C, Janicki H, Schraermeyer U, Kociok N, Fauser S, Kirchhof B, et al. A central role for inflammation in the pathogenesis of diabetic retinopathy. FASEB J. 2004;18(12):1450–2.
161. Ali TK, El-Remessy AB. Diabetic retinopathy: current management and experimental therapeutic targets. Pharmacotherapy. 2009;29(2):182–92.
162. Winkler BS, Boulton ME, Gottsch JD, Sternberg P. Oxidative damage and age-related macular degeneration. Mol Vis. 1999;5:32.
163. Jasielska M, Semkova I, Shi X, Schmidt K, Karagiannis D, Kokkinou D, Mackiewicz J, Kociok N, Joussen AM. Differential role of tumor necrosis factor (TNF)-alpha receptors in the development of choroidal neovascularization. Invest Ophthalmol Vis Sci. 2010;51(8):3874–83.
164. Lichtlen P, Lam TT, Nork TM, Streit T, Urech DM. Relative contribution of VEGF and TNF-alpha in the cynomolgus laser-induced CNV model: comparing the efficacy of bevacizumab, adalimumab, and ESBA105. Invest Ophthalmol Vis Sci. 2010;51(9):4738–45.
165. Xu H, Chen M, Forrester JV. Para-inflammation in the aging retina. Prog Retin Eye Res. 2009;28(5):348–68.
166. Rosenbaum JT, Howes EL Jr, Rubin RM, Samples JR. Ocular inflammatory effects of intravitreally-injected tumor necrosis factor. Am J Pathol. 1988;133(1):47–53.
167. Dick AD, Forrester JV, Liversidge J, Cope AP. The role of tumour necrosis factor (TNF-alpha) in experimental autoimmune uveoretinitis (EAU). Prog Retin Eye Res. 2004;23(6):617–37.
168. Calder CJ, Nicholson LB, Dick AD. A selective role for the TNF p55 receptor in autocrine signaling following IFN-gamma stimulation in experimental autoimmune uveoretinitis. J Immunol (Baltimore, Md : 1950). 2005;175(10):6286–93.
169. Kong DH, Kim YK, Kim MR, Jang JH, Lee S. Emerging roles of vascular cell adhesion Molecule-1 (VCAM-1) in immunological disorders and cancer. Int J Mol Sci. 2018;19(4)

170. Rice GE, Bevilacqua MP. An inducible endothelial cell surface glycoprotein mediates melanoma adhesion. Science. 1989;246(4935):1303–6.
171. Osborn L, Hession C, Tizard R, Vassallo C, Luhowskyj S, Chi-Rosso G, Lobb R. Direct expression cloning of vascular cell adhesion molecule 1, a cytokine-induced endothelial protein that binds to lymphocytes. Cell. 1989;59(6):1203–11.
172. Cook-Mills JM, Marchese ME, Abdala-Valencia H. Vascular cell adhesion molecule-1 expression and signaling during disease: regulation by reactive oxygen species and antioxidants. Antioxid Redox Signal. 2011;15(6):1607–38.
173. Sharma R, Sharma R, Khaket TP, Dutta C, Chakraborty B, Mukherjee TK. Breast cancer metastasis: putative therapeutic role of vascular cell adhesion molecule-1. Cell Oncol (Dordr). 2017;40(3):199–208.
174. van Oosten M, van de Bilt E, de Vries HE, van Berkel TJ, Kuiper J. Vascular adhesion molecule-1 and intercellular adhesion molecule-1 expression on rat liver cells after lipopolysaccharide administration in vivo. Hepatology (Baltimore, Md). 1995;22(5):1538–46.
175. Cerutti C, Ridley AJ. Endothelial cell-cell adhesion and signaling. Exp Cell Res. 2017;358(1):31–8.
176. Hernández C, Carrasco E, García-Arumí J, Maria Segura R, Simó R. Intravitreous levels of hepatocyte growth factor/scatter factor and vascular cell adhesion molecule-1 in the vitreous fluid of diabetic patients with proliferative retinopathy. Diabetes Metab. 2004;30(4):341–6.
177. Adamiec-Mroczek J, Oficjalska-Młyńczak J. Assessment of selected adhesion molecule and proinflammatory cytokine levels in the vitreous body of patients with type 2 diabetes--role of the inflammatory-immune process in the pathogenesis of proliferative diabetic retinopathy. Graefes Arch Clin Exp Ophthalmol. 2008;246(12):1665–70.
178. Liu L, Kubes P. Molecular mechanisms of leukocyte recruitment: organ-specific mechanisms of action. Thromb Haemost. 2003;89(2):213–20.
179. Springer TA. Traffic signals for lymphocyte recirculation and leukocyte emigration: the multistep paradigm. Cell. 1994;76(2):301–14.
180. Steeber DA, Venturi GM, Tedder TF. A new twist to the leukocyte adhesion cascade: intimate cooperation is key. Trends Immunol. 2005;26(1):9–12.
181. Ramos TN, Bullard DC, Barnum SR. ICAM-1: isoforms and phenotypes. J Immunol (Baltimore, Md : 1950). 2014;192(10):4469–74.
182. Lee SJ, Benveniste EN. Adhesion molecule expression and regulation on cells of the central nervous system. J Neuroimmunol. 1999;98(2):77–88.
183. Roebuck KA, Finnegan A. Regulation of intercellular adhesion molecule-1 (CD54) gene expression. J Leukoc Biol. 1999;66(6):876–88.
184. Limb GA, Webster L, Soomro H, Janikoun S, Shilling J. Platelet expression of tumour necrosis factor-alpha (TNF-alpha), TNF receptors and intercellular adhesion molecule-1 (ICAM-1) in patients with proliferative diabetic retinopathy. Clin Exp Immunol. 1999;118(2):213–8.
185. Hubbard AK, Rothlein R. Intercellular adhesion molecule-1 (ICAM-1) expression and cell signaling cascades. Free Radic Biol Med. 2000;28(9):1379–86.
186. Koning GA, Schiffelers RM, Storm G. Endothelial cells at inflammatory sites as target for therapeutic intervention. Endothelium. 2002;9(3):161–71.
187. Tailor A, Cooper D, Granger DN. Platelet-vessel wall interactions in the microcirculation. Microcirculation (New York, NY: 1994). 2005;12(3):275–85.
188. Shimura M, Yasuda K, Motohashi R, Kotake O, Noma H. Aqueous cytokine and growth factor levels indicate response to ranibizumab for diabetic macular oedema. Br J Ophthalmol. 2017;101(11):1518–23.
189. Hillier RJ, Ojaimi E, Wong DT, Mak MY, Berger AR, Kohly RP, Kertes PJ, Forooghian F, Boyd SR, Eng K, et al. Aqueous humor cytokine levels as biomarkers of disease severity in diabetic macular edema. Retina. 2017;37(4):761–9.
190. Whitcup SM, Hikita N, Shirao M, Miyasaka M, Tamatani T, Mochizuki M, Nussenblatt RB, Chan CC. Monoclonal antibodies against CD54 (ICAM-1) and CD11a (LFA-1) prevent and inhibit endotoxin-induced uveitis. Exp Eye Res. 1995;60(6):597–601.

191. El-Sayyad H, Bakr EH, Heba AK, El-Ghawet, El-Desoky TM. Overview of congenital, senile and metabolic cataract. J Ocular Biol. 2015;3:1.
192. Delamere NA, Tamiya S. Expression, regulation and function of Na,K-ATPase in the lens. Prog Retin Eye Res. 2004;23(6):593–615.
193. Zeimer R, Weinreb A, Loewinger E, Kalman ZH, Belkin M. Detection and analysis of metals in the eye by x-ray spectrometry. Med Phys. 1974;1(5):251–6.
194. Flieger J, Dolar-Szczasny J, Rejdak R, Majerek D, Tatarczak-Michalewska M, Proch J, Blicharska E, Flieger W, Baj J, Niedzielski P. The multi-elemental composition of the aqueous humor of patients undergoing cataract surgery, suffering from coexisting diabetes, hypertension, or diabetic retinopathy. Int J Mol Sci. 2021;22(17):9413.
195. Hohberger B, Chaudhri MA, Michalke B, Lucio M, Nowomiejska K, Schlötzer-Schrehardt U, Grieb P, Rejdak R, Jünemann AGM. Levels of aqueous humor trace elements in patients with open-angle glaucoma. J Trace Elem Med Biol. 2018;45:150–5.
196. Zhou Y, Hong F, Wang X, Feng J, Zhu D, Xu Y, Tao Y. Abnormal levels of aqueous humor trace elements in patients with cytomegalovirus retinitis. Eye (Lond). 2019;33(10):1606–12.
197. Harding C, Stahl P. Transferrin recycling in reticulocytes: pH and iron are important determinants of ligand binding and processing. Biochem Biophys Res Commun. 1983;113(2):650–8.
198. Pan BT, Johnstone RM. Fate of the transferrin receptor during maturation of sheep reticulocytes in vitro: selective externalization of the receptor. Cell. 1983;33(3):967–78.
199. Johnstone RM, Adam M, Hammond JR, Orr L, Turbide C. Vesicle formation during reticulocyte maturation. Association of plasma membrane activities with released vesicles (exosomes). J Biol Chem. 1987;262(19):9412–20.
200. Nonaka T, Wong DTW. Saliva Diagnostics. Annu Rev Anal Chem (Palo Alto, Calif). 2022;15(1):107–21.
201. Dismuke WM, Challa P, Navarro I, Stamer WD, Liu Y. Human aqueous humor exosomes. Exp Eye Res. 2015;132:73–7.
202. Liu J, Jiang F, Jiang Y, Wang Y, Li Z, Shi X, Zhu Y, Wang H, Zhang Z. Roles of exosomes in ocular diseases. Int J Nanomedicine. 2020;15:10519–38.
203. Zhang W, Wang Y, Kong Y. Exosomes derived from Mesenchymal stem cells modulate miR-126 to ameliorate hyperglycemia-induced retinal inflammation via targeting HMGB1. Invest Ophthalmol Vis Sci. 2019;60(1):294–303.
204. Kang GY, Bang JY, Choi AJ, Yoon J, Lee WC, Choi S, Yoon S, Kim HC, Baek JH, Park HS, et al. Exosomal proteins in the aqueous humor as novel biomarkers in patients with neovascular age-related macular degeneration. J Proteome Res. 2014;13(2):581–95.

Common Laboratory Testing Methods Used for Examination of Intraocular Fluid

5

Contents

5.1 PCR

Polymerase chain reaction (PCR) is a molecular technique used to exponentially increase the amount of DNA for the purpose of testing and analysis. This method enables the rapid amplification of certain genes or DNA fragments in vitro. PCR technology replicates DNA in a manner similar to its natural process in living organisms and specifically amplifies a targeted section of DNA outside of a living organism. The PCR process is analogous to regular DNA replication and consists of three sequential phases. Initially, the template DNA undergoes denaturation, transitioning from a double-stranded configuration to a single-stranded configuration. Subsequently, the primer is introduced and joined with the template, facilitating the completion of the replication process. Finally, with the presence of DNA polymerase and substrate, complementary DNA is synthesized. The process of repeating these three heat reactions is referred to as a cycle, during which a significant

Y. Tao, D.-K. Hwang, *Examination of Intraocular Fluid*,
https://doi.org/10.1007/978-981-96-2486-7_5

quantity of DNA fragments situated between the two primer sequences can be amplified after 20–40 cycles.

Prior to utilizing PCR for analyzing intraocular fluid, it is necessary to clinically determine the specific type of microorganisms. In the PCR method, primers are intended to specifically target the sequence of a particular bacterium. Viral uveitis, a form of infectious intraocular disease, exhibits distinct clinical characteristics. The viruses responsible for viral uveitis are specifically double-stranded DNA viruses, such as CMV, HSV, and VZV. Therefore, the polymerase chain reaction (PCR) of intraocular fluid primarily focuses on identifying viral species.

The multiplex solid-phase strip PCR assay (strip PCR) is a technique used to amplify DNA. It involves attaching certain primer oligonucleotides to a solid substrate using various ways. Examples of solid supports include agarose beads, polyacrylamide beads, latex beads, magnetic beads, standard glass slides, and silicon wafers. One primary benefit of solid-phase PCR is its facilitation of the separation and purification of PCR products [1].

Nakano S et al. used strip PCR in the nucleic detection of intraocular microorganisms and found it with a similar sensitivity to quantitative PCR [2, 3]. A comparative study was undertaken to assess the testing efficiency of strip PCR, which can detect up to eight pathogens, and loop-mediated isothermal amplification (LAMP), which can detect up to 21 microorganisms, in the analysis of intraocular fluid. The findings were displayed in Table 5.1. We believed that the LAMP had an advantage in terms of its capacity to test a large number of samples, but the strip PCR was advantageous in terms of saving time and samples.

Multiplex PCR is a technology which was improved on the basis of traditional PCR. In the experimental process, multiple pairs of specific primers are added to the same system. Multiple target DNA fragments are amplified based on different DNA templates or different regions of the same template. Microbial identification is performed mainly based on species-or strain-specific DNA change regions. DNA

Table 5.1 Comparison of the characteristics of strip PCR and LAMP

	Strip PCR	LAMP
Sample requirement	13–26 μL	20–50 μL
Sample treatment	None	Required
Through-out	High through-out process, the number of tested samples can be modulated as required	Low through-out process, only one sample can be tested once time
Testing time for one sample	60 min	90 min
Testing time for 12 samples	90–120 min	750 min
Experimental apparatus	Fluorescence PCR instrument	Special instrument
Potential pollution	Several times of sample adding are needed, which add potential pollution	Pollution is prevented by closed space, independent reaction pool

sequence of the primer should have strong specificity; otherwise the primer will bind to other sites and cause nonspecific amplification. Multiplex PCR is improved and developed on the basis of traditional PCR, but not a simple mixture of single PCR. It is often affected by various factors such as reaction conditions and reaction systems in actual operation. Two methods are used in the pathogenic identification using multiplex PCR: one is to conduct multiple detections for a single specific gene of each pathogen and to detect the presence or absence of one or several pathogens at the same time; the other is to perform multiple testing targeting a specific pathogen, which can reduce the occurrence of false positive results.

Multiplex PCR was used to detect multiple pathogenic microorganisms in intraocular fluid: Bispo PJM et al. [4] performed multiplex PCR to HSV-1/2, VZV, CMA, and *Toxoplasma gondii* in intraocular fluid and showed a high sensitivity of this technology. The detection limit was 20 copies for HSV and was 200 copies for the nucleic acid of *Toxoplasma gondii*. At present, there are mainly four centers (two in the United States, one in Japan, and one in India) that use this method for intraocular fluid detection in the world. Generally speaking, the specificity and sensitivity are relatively high [5].

Compared with traditional single-plex PCR, the advantage of this method is undoubtedly more sample-saving. However, if the reaction conditions are not well controlled, the proportion of false positives and false negatives will be higher, and the technical requirements are more complex.

5.2 LAMP

LAMP is a new nucleic acid amplification technology first proposed by Notomi in 2000 [6]. In this technology, four specific primers (including two inner primers and two outer primers) are designed for six regions of the target gene. A BstDNA polymerase with strand displacement properties is used to amplify target sequences efficiently, rapidly, and with high specificity under isothermal conditions. The reaction process includes dumbbell-shaped template synthesis stage, cyclic amplification stage, and finally elongation and recycling stage. The basic principle of this technology is that after the denaturation of the target DNA, the inner and outer primers are extended under the action of BstDNA polymerase, and the extension products of the outer primers replace the extension products of the inner primers to form a dumbbell-shaped DNA, which continue to extend and amplification in the cyclic amplification stage. Finally, a mixture of DNA fragments with stem-loop and polycyclic cauliflower-like structures are formed [7].

The advantages of this technology include the following [8]: (1) fast and efficient. There is no need for prior thermal denaturation of double-stranded DNA, which avoids time loss caused by temperature cycling. (2) High sensitivity. Only a few copies of the template are needed for the amplification of some pathogen, which is several orders of magnitude higher than that of PCR. (3) High specificity. With four specific primers designed for six regions of the target sequence, if any of the six regions does not match the primer, nucleic acid amplification cannot be performed.

(4) Product detection is convenient. During the process of DNA synthesis, LAMP will produce a large amount of pyrophosphate ions, which can combine with magnesium ions to form white magnesium pyrophosphate precipitates. Therefore, the progress of the reaction can be judged according to whether white precipitates are formed in the reaction system. (5) Easy to operate. The LAMP reaction only needs a simple thermostat, and the experiment can be completed in a water bath or a metal bath. No expensive instrument is needed. LAMP has relatively low requirements for sample processing, operating technique, instruments, and equipment, which can also be achieved in the fieldwork [7].

LAMP also has its own disadvantages and limitations [7]: (1) LAMP amplification is the process of strand displacement synthesis, and the length of the target sequence is preferably within 300 base pairs. Thus, long-chain DNA cannot be amplified. (2) Due to the high sensitivity, it is very easy to be contaminated during the experimental process, resulting in false positive results. (3) There are only two types of LAMP reaction results, that is, amplification and non-amplification. It is not easy to identify the occurrence of nonspecific amplification. (4) It is inferior to traditional PCR methods in terms of product recovery, identification, cloning, and single-strand isolation.

Due to these aforementioned limitations, not all microorganisms are suitable for detection by the LAMP method. We conducted research to identify 21 common intraocular pathogens by LAMP. In our experience, LAMP can be used in intraocular infection with unknown origin. But in general, its sensitivity is lower than specific PCR due to the sample size dispersion.

5.3 Metagenomic Next-Generation Sequencing

Metagenomic next-generation sequencing (mNGS) is a technology to sequence millions to billions of DNA molecules parallelly at one time. Three sequencing technologies are currently relative mature, including Roche's 454 sequencing technique, Illumina's Solexa sequencing technique, and ABI's SOLiD sequencing technique [9, 10].

With the rapid development of NGS technology, it has been widely used in chromosomal diseases [11, 12], gene mutations [13, 14], tumor genes [15, 16], and detection of unknown pathogenic microorganisms [17, 18]. NGS has high precision and strong sensitivity. A sequence of 20 base pairs has high specificity. Each sequence larger than 100 base pairs can determine a species, and more than ten million sequences can be tested simultaneously. Theoretically, the throughput of detecting pathogens can reach ten million. Besides, NGS can also be used in pathogen identification, typing, and detection of drug resistance genes and virulence determinant genes. Not only known pathogens but also unknown pathogens can be detected by NGS. The impact of NGS on microbial detection is revolutionary. Researchers rely no longer on isolation and culture. Instead, metagenomics and microbiomics are used to study the interaction between host and microbes [19]. On May 13, 2016, the FDA announced the draft guidances for the diagnosis of NGS infectious diseases, pointing out that NGS can be used for microbial identification and detection of antimicrobial drug resistance and virulence markers. Attention should be paid to the specificity, sensitivity, minimum detection limit, reproducibility, and quality control of clinical NGS product [20]. This is a milestone event marking NGS going out of the laboratory and being applied in the clinic.

In a narrow sense, mNGS takes all bacterial and fungal genome DNA in the ecological environment as the research object. But in a larger sense, this technology studies all biological genetic materials in a specific environment, which determines the life activities of biological groups. It takes all DNA in the ecological environment as the research object, screens useful genes and their products, and studies their functions and the relationship and interaction between them through cloning and heterologous expression.

Four steps are included in mNGS of intraocular fluid: (1) Isolation of biological DNA in a specific environment (intraocular fluid); (2) purification of large molecular weight DNA for cloning; (3) transformation of vectors with metagenomic DNA into model microorganisms to establish the clonal lines; and (4) analysis of the metagenomic library.

mNGS has been clinically used in the pathogenic identification of uveitis. Its advantage is that it can use sequence information to infer the phenotypic behavior of identified pathogens. Doan T et al. showed that for 22% of uveitis in which pathogens could not be found by conventional PCR, mNGS could still help in the pathogenic determination [21]. Previous study of mNGS of intraocular fluids has confirmed its capability of detect bacteria, fungi, and viruses [22]. A recent multicenter study with 488 patients demonstrated that the sensitivity of mNGS utilizing vitreous humor samples was 92.2%, with a total coincidence rate of 81.3%. However, if the aqueous humor was utilized instead, the sensitivity declined to 85.4% and the total coincidence rate dropped to 75.4% [23]. The results of metagenomics study suggested that the disturbance of gut microbes might be related to the pathogenesis of Behcet's disease [24].

5.4 ELISA

Enzyme-linked immunosorbent assay (ELISA) is the most widely used heterogeneous enzyme immunoassay test, not only for the determination of cytokines and antibodies but also for the determination of soluble cytokine receptors or adhesion molecules. Double-antibody sandwich method is the basic principle of ELISA. Two monoclonal antibodies against different epitopes of the same cytokine, or a monoclonal antibody and a polyclonal antibody, are used. One antibody is used for coating as a capture antibody, and the other antibody labels the enzyme as a detection antibody. The high specificity, ease of operation and low cost make this technique easy to be promoted clinically, but its disadvantage is low sensitivity. Another limitation of this technique is that only one to two cytokines or antibodies can be tested with 0.1 mL of intraocular fluid sample, which makes it impossible to perform multiple detection with ELISA.

For antibody detection, the Goldmann-Witmer (GW) coefficient is used to verify the production of antibody in situ. Under normal circumstances, the protein composition in the intraocular fluid is different from that in the blood plasma. The content of immunoglobulin is lower in the intraocular fluid due to the intraocular immune privilege. When the blood-ocular barrier is damaged, the protein components in the serum (including antibody immunoglobulins) can leak into the eye. If the antibody components in the intraocular fluid are tested positive at this time, it will lead to clinical misdiagnosis of the disease. By calculating the GW coefficient, it can help to judge whether the specific antibody in the eye is produced in situ in the eye (intraocular tissue infection pathogen), or a false positive caused by leakage.

The GW coefficient is mainly used in ocular toxoplasmosis, ocular toxocariasis, acute retinal necrosis, viral anterior uveitis caused by CMV, HSV and VZV, and Fuchs syndrome (intraocular infection of rubella virus) [25–34]. Other studies also reported the application of the GW coefficient in the judgment of intraocular infection of EBV [35] and *Coxiella burnetii* [36].

The calculation formula of the GW coefficient is as follows: the GW coefficient = (specific IgG concentration in the intraocular fluid/total IgG concentration in the intraocular fluid)/(specific IgG concentration in serum/total IgG concentration in serum), that is, the ratio of the proportion of a specific IgG in the intraocular fluid to the total IgG in the serum. The higher the ratio, the more it shows that the IgG is produced in situ in the eye; otherwise it may be leaked from the serum. It is generally agreed that if the GW coefficient is between 0.5 and 2, it means that there is no production of intraocular antibody in situ. If the GW coefficient is between 2 and 4, it indicates that there may be suspected intraocular antibody production in situ. If the GW coefficient is more than 4, the production of intraocular antibody in situ is confirmed [37]. In other studies, the cutoff value of 3 was used simply as the threshold [26].

In fact, the cutoff value of the GW coefficient has little effect on the clinical diagnosis of intraocular infection. Mathis T et al. [27] found that if the cutoff value of the GW coefficient was set as 2 (>2 is positive), the specificity was 97.8% for the diagnosis of ocular toxoplasmosis. If the cutoff value was set as 3, the specificity was 100%. The specificity in both cases was high.

It should be noted that the prerequisite for calculating the GW coefficient is that the level of IgG in the intraocular fluid is elevated. The purpose of the GW coefficient calculation is to exclude false positives. In case a specific IgG for one pathogen is negative in the intraocular fluid, it cannot be considered to exist antibody production in situ, even if the calculated GW coefficient is greater than 4.

The Witmer-Desmonts (WD) coefficient has a similar meaning to the GW coefficient, in which total IgG in the formula is replaced by albumin. The calculation formula is specific IgG concentration in the intraocular fluid/total albumin concentration in the intraocular fluid/specific IgG concentration in serum total albumin concentration in serum. In the previous study, the WD coefficient value ≥ 1 was judged as positive [38]. The significance of the WD coefficient is that the total amount of immunoglobulin often changes with the immune status, while the total amount of albumin is relatively constant. For example, in patients with suspected recent viral infections, or with signs of systemic infection such as fever, the serum IgG concentration increases significantly. Therefore, calculation of the WD coefficient is better than the GW coefficient in these cases. However, for patients with abnormal renal function, decreased serum albumin concentration, or even hypoalbuminemia, it is obvious that the WD coefficient is not suitable for calculation.

5.5 CBA

Cytometric bead array (CBA) is one of the suspension array technologies (SAT). SAT is a high throughput, large-scale, and multiplexed screening platform used in molecular biology. SAT has been widely applied to genomic and proteomic research, such as single nucleotide polymorphism (SNP) genotyping, genetic disease screening, gene expression profiling, screening drug discovery, and clinical diagnosis. With the application of CBA, multiple proteins in the intraocular fluid sample can be tested simultaneously. The CBA system uses the flow cytometry with high linear range of fluorescence detection and antibody-coated microspheres to effectively capture the protein to be tested. Each microsphere has a specific fluorescence intensity and can be mixed in a test tube for simultaneous testing. Compared with traditional ELISA and Western blot technologies, this method requires a smaller sample size and has a faster testing speed. In addition, the CBA technique has the advantage of being used for multiplex analysis, where more data can be obtained from a single sample. Especially in the case of small sample volume, multiple cytokine measurement can be performed (up to 30 proteins can be analyzed with sample size of only 25–50 μL), while traditional methods such as ELISA and Western blot can only detect one or two proteins with the same sample volume. According to our experience, the test results of CBA are repeatability. Samples collected for clinical use cannot be accumulated and finally tested once time like samples for scientific research. Clinical samples are often tested separately one by one, which require a high experimental stability. Thus, this technique is more suitable for clinical use.

5.6 Luminex xMAP Technology

Luminex xMAP technology, also known as suspension array technology, is a bead-based multiplexed immunoassay system which can simultaneously detect up to 500 targets in a single sample. In 2001, Luminex technology was certified by the US FDA, becoming the first and only multi-index detection technology for clinical diagnosis approved by the US FDA at that time. This technology is particularly powerful when looking for changes in concentrations of multiple targets under different conditions, for example, tracking the progress of immune responses to a microbial infection and tracking the development of an autoimmune disease. To our experience, the biggest advantage lies in the high throughput: 100 indicators can be tested simultaneously with minimal sample size (as low as 10 μL). However, it is necessary to optimize and match different liquid phase reaction conditions (sample dilution factor, concentration of antibodies, etc.). We conducted batch-to-batch detection and found the repeatability not ideal. In addition, high cost of this assay also limits its application in the clinical examination of intraocular fluid sample.

5.7 Flow Cytometry

Flow cytometry (FCM) is a technique used to detect and measure physical and chemical characteristics of a population of cells or particles [39]. In the experimental process, a sample containing cells or particles is suspended in a fluid and injected into the flow cytometer instrument. The sample is focused to ideally flow one cell at a time through a laser beam, where the light scattered is characteristic to the cells and their components. Cells are often labeled with fluorescent markers so light is absorbed and then emitted in a band of wavelengths. Tens of thousands of cells can be quickly examined and the data gathered are processed by a computer. In clinical practice, FCM can be used for cell counting, cell sorting, determination of cell characteristics and function, identification of microorganisms, biomarker detection, protein engineering detection, diagnosis of blood cancers, and measurement of genome size.

The eye is known as an immune privilege site in which inflammatory cells should not exist in a healthy eye. However, in cases of infectious or noninfectious uveitis, the presence of inflammatory cells in the intraocular fluid could be observed. FCM was reported to be applied in the phenotyping of inflammatory cells in the endotoxin-induced uveitis model [40]. In another study using aqueous and vitreous samples of human uveitis, the author found that T cells (CD3+ CD45++) accounted for the main cellular component in the majority of the samples regardless of the etiology, except for acute bacterial or fungal infections, in which neutrophils predominated in the intraocular fluid [41]. In the diagnosis of ocular sarcoidosis, FCM was also used to calculate the CD4/CD8 ratio. Dave et al. [42] proposed that aqueous humor CD4+/CD8+ ratio > 3.5 measured by FCM was observed to be associated with sarcoid uveitis, with sensitivity of 66.7% and specificity of 95.0%. FCM also act as an important test method in diagnosis of intraocular lymphoma. Tanaka R et al. [43] stated that when two or more of the four tests (atypical cells, IL-10/IL-6 > 1, IgH gene rearrangement, and flow cytometry for B cell clonality) were positive, the sensitivity and specificity values for diagnosis of intraocular lymphoma were 0.929 and 1.00, respectively. FCM permits a comprehensive and quantitative profiling of cell surface markers. Importantly, it can simultaneously analyze several different markers and thereby characterize immunophenotype B-and T-cell subsets [44]. Limitations to FCM include the facts that the laser can only analyze one cell at a time, cells must be in suspension to be analyzed (thereby restricting the analysis of tissue), highly trained operators are required, and cells must be viable to be analyzed [45]. Thus, it is not suitable to perform FCM if samples cannot be processed immediately.

5.8 ICP-MS

Inductively coupled plasma mass spectrometry (ICP-MS) is a type of mass spectrometry that uses an inductively coupled plasma to ionize the sample. It atomizes the sample and creates atomic and small polyatomic ions. It is known and used for its ability to detect metals and several nonmetals in liquid samples at very low concentrations. It can detect different isotopes of the same element, which makes it a versatile tool in isotopic labeling. In clinical work, ICP-MS can be used in suspicion of heavy metal poisoning, metabolic concerns, and even hepatological issues, using samples such as whole blood, urine, plasma, and serum. Like in other body fluids, disturbances in the level of elements in intraocular fluid may also be found in patients with general diseases, which can be detected and analyzed using ICP-MS.

Dolar-Szczasny J et al. [46] performed a study to investigate the change of elemental composition in aqueous humor of patients with dialysis. The elements quantification was established using ICP-MS. Increased levels of manganese and mercury and decreased levels of vanadium and zinc were found. In another study, ICP-MS was used to measure the trace elements in the aqueous humor of patients with primary open-angle glaucoma (POAG) and pseudoexfoliation glaucoma (PEXG). The results showed significantly higher aqueous humor levels of zinc in these two diseases, which indicated its potential role in the pathogenesis of glaucoma [47]. In cases of infectious uveitis such as CMV retinitis, with the application of ICP-MS, the abnormal aqueous levels of trace elements (phosphorus and copper) were also observed [48].

References

1. Tao SC, Zhang ZP, Zhang XE. Progress in PCR technology. Research. 2001;04:26–9.
2. Nakano S, Sugita S, Tomaru Y, Hono A, Nakamuro T, Kubota T, Takase H, Mochizuki M, Takahashi M, Shimizu N. Establishment of multiplex solid-phase strip PCR test for detection of 24 ocular infectious disease pathogens. Invest Ophthalmol Vis Sci. 2017;58(3):1553–9.
3. Nakano S, Tomaru Y, Kubota T, Takase H, Mochizuki M, Shimizu N, Sugita S. Direct strip polymerase chain reaction project G: multiplex solid-phase real-time polymerase chain reaction without DNA extraction: a rapid intraoperative diagnosis using microvolumes. Ophthalmology. 2021;128(5):729–39.
4. Bispo PJM, Davoudi S, Sahm ML, Ren A, Miller J, Romano J, Sobrin L, Gilmore MS. Rapid detection and identification of uveitis pathogens by qualitative multiplex real-time PCR. Invest Ophthalmol Vis Sci. 2018;59(1):582–9.
5. Minkus CL, Bispo PJM, Papaliodis GN, Sobrin L. Real-time multiplex PCR analysis in infectious uveitis. Semin Ophthalmol. 2019;34(4):252–5.
6. Notomi T, Okayama H, Masubuchi H, Yonekawa T, Watanabe K, Amino N, Hase T. Loop-mediated isothermal amplification of DNA. Nucleic Acids Res. 2000;28(12):E63.
7. Wang L, Luo Y, Zhou Q, Lai PA, Bai YD. Research progress of nucleic acid constant temperature amplification technology. Biotechnol Commun. 2011;22(2):296–302.
8. Du FL, Wang TT. Research progress and prospect of loop-mediated isothermal amplification (LAMP) technology. Exp Lab Med. 2018;36(4):1.
9. Mardis ER. Next-generation sequencing platforms. Annu Rev Anal Chem (Palo Alto, Calif). 2013;6:287–303.

10. Wu D, Huang H, Sun LZ. Application of high-throughput sequencing technology in laboratory diagnosis of genetic diseases. Chin J Prenatal Diagnosis (Electr Ed). 2016;8(04):11–6.
11. Fan HC, Blumenfeld YJ, Chitkara U, Hudgins L, Quake SR. Noninvasive diagnosis of fetal aneuploidy by shotgun sequencing DNA from maternal blood. Proc Natl Acad Sci USA. 2008;105(42):16266–71.
12. Sifakis S, Papantoniou N, Kappou D, Antsaklis A. Noninvasive prenatal diagnosis of down syndrome: current knowledge and novel insights. J Perinat Med. 2012;40(4):319–27.
13. Taylor KH, Kramer RS, Davis JW, Guo J, Duff DJ, Xu D, Caldwell CW, Shi H. Ultradeep bisulfite sequencing analysis of DNA methylation patterns in multiple gene promoters by 454 sequencing. Cancer Res. 2007;67(18):8511–8.
14. Wang C, Mitsuya Y, Gharizadeh B, Ronaghi M, Shafer RW. Characterization of mutation spectra with ultra-deep pyrosequencing: application to HIV-1 drug resistance. Genome Res. 2007;17(8):1195–201.
15. Morrissy AS, Morin RD, Delaney A, Zeng T, McDonald H, Jones S, Zhao Y, Hirst M, Marra MA. Next-generation tag sequencing for cancer gene expression profiling. Genome Res. 2009;19(10):1825–35.
16. Tyner JW, Deininger MW, Loriaux MM, Chang BH, Gotlib JR, Willis SG, Erickson H, Kovacsovics T, O'Hare T, Heinrich MC, et al. RNAi screen for rapid therapeutic target identification in leukemia patients. Proc Natl Acad Sci USA. 2009;106(21):8695–700.
17. Hamada H, Sekizuka T, Oba K, Katano H, Kinumaki A, Terai M, Mizutani T, Kuroda M. Comprehensive pathogen detection associated with four recurrent episodes of Kawasaki disease in a patient during a single year using next-generation sequencing. JMM Case Rep. 2016;3(1):e005019.
18. Dyrhovden R, Øvrebø KK, Nordahl MV, Nygaard RM, Ulvestad E, Kommedal Ø. Bacteria and fungi in acute cholecystitis. A prospective study comparing next generation sequencing to culture. J Infect. 2020;80(1):16–23.
19. Aziz N, Zhao Q, Bry L, Driscoll DK, Funke B, Gibson JS, Grody WW, Hegde MR, Hoeltge GA, Leonard DG, et al. College of American Pathologists' laboratory standards for next-generation sequencing clinical tests. Arch Pathol Lab Med. 2015;139(4):481–93.
20. Infectious Disease Next Generation Sequencing Based Diagnostic Devices: Microbial Identification and Detection of Antimicrobial Resistance and Virulence Markers; Draft Guidance for Industry and Food and Drug Administration Staff; Availability. Federal Register / Vol. 81, No. 93 / Friday, May 13, 2016 / Notices.
21. Doan T, Acharya NR, Pinsky BA, Sahoo MK, Chow ED, Banaei N, Budvytiene I, Cevallos V, Zhong L, Zhou Z, et al. Metagenomic DNA sequencing for the diagnosis of intraocular infections. Ophthalmology. 2017;124(8):1247–8.
22. Qian Z, Zhang Y, Wang L, Li Z, Wang H, Kang H, Feng J, Hu X, Tao Y. Application of metagenomic next-generation sequencing in suspected intraocular infections. Eur J Ophthalmol. 2023;33(1):391–7.
23. Qian Z, Xia H, Zhou J, Wang R, Zhu D, Chen L, Kang H, Feng J, Hu X, Wang L, et al. Performance of metagenomic next-generation sequencing of cell-free DNA from vitreous and aqueous humor for diagnoses of intraocular infections. J Infect Dis. 2024;229(1):252–61.
24. Ye Z, Zhang N, Wu C, Zhang X, Wang Q, Huang X, Du L, Cao Q, Tang J, Zhou C, et al. A metagenomic study of the gut microbiome in Behcet's disease. Microbiome. 2018;6(1):135.
25. Baarsma GS, Luyendijk L, Kijlstra A, de Vries J, Peperkamp E, Mertens DA, van Meurs JC. Analysis of local antibody production in the vitreous humor of patients with severe uveitis. Am J Ophthalmol. 1991;112(2):147–50.
26. Dussaix E, Cerqueti PM, Pontet F, Bloch-Michel E. New approaches to the detection of locally produced antiviral antibodies in the aqueous of patients with endogenous uveitis. Ophthalmologica. 1987;194(2–3):145–9.
27. Mathis T, Beccat S, Sève P, Peyron F, Wallon M, Kodjikian L. Comparison of immunoblotting (IgA and IgG) and the Goldmann-Witmer coefficient for diagnosis of ocular toxoplasmosis in immunocompetent patients. Br J Ophthalmol. 2018;102(10):1454–8.

28. de Visser L, Rothova A, de Boer JH, van Loon AM, Kerkhoff FT, Canninga-van Dijk MR, Weersink AY, de Groot-Mijnes JD. Diagnosis of ocular toxocariasis by establishing intraocular antibody production. Am J Ophthalmol. 2008;145(2):369–74.
29. Wang ZJ, Zhou M, Cao WJ, Ji J, Bi YW, Huang X, Xu GZ. Evaluation of the Goldmann-Witmer coefficient in the immunological diagnosis of ocular toxocariasis. Acta Trop. 2016;158:20–3.
30. Takase H, Okada AA, Goto H, Mizuki N, Namba K, Ohguro N, Sonoda KH, Tomita M, Keino H, Kezuka T, et al. Development and validation of new diagnostic criteria for acute retinal necrosis. Jpn J Ophthalmol. 2015;59(1):14–20.
31. Relvas LJM, Antoun J, de Groot-Mijnes JDF, Motulsky E, Ten Dam-Van Loon NH, Makhoul D, Willermain F, Caspers L. Diagnosis of cytomegalovirus anterior uveitis in two European referral centers. Ocul Immunol Inflamm. 2018;26(1):116–21.
32. Wensing B, Mochizuki M, De Boer JH. Clinical characteristics of herpes simplex virus associated anterior uveitis. Ocul Immunol Inflamm. 2018;26(3):333–7.
33. Groen-Hakan F, Babu K, Tugal-Tutkun I, Pathanapithoon K, de Boer JH, Smith JR, de Groot-Mijnes JDF, Rothova A. Challenges of diagnosing viral anterior uveitis. Ocul Immunol Inflamm. 2017;25(5):710–20.
34. Stunf S, Petrovec M, Žigon N, Hawlina M, Kraut A, de Groot-Mijnes JD, Valentinčič NV. High concordance of intraocular antibody synthesis against the rubella virus and Fuchs heterochromic uveitis syndrome in Slovenia. Mol Vis. 2012;18:2909–14.
35. Smit D, Meyer D, Maritz J, de Groot-Mijnes JDF. Polymerase chain reaction and Goldmann-Witmer coefficient to examine the role of Epstein-Barr virus in uveitis. Ocul Immunol Inflamm. 2019;27(1):108–13.
36. Hermans LE, Oosterheert JJ, Kampschreur LM, Ossewaarde-van Norel J, Dekkers J, Rothova A, de Groot-Mijnes JD. Molecular and serological intraocular fluid analysis of Coxiella burnetii-seropositive patients with concurrent idiopathic uveitis. Ocul Immunol Inflamm. 2016;24(1):77–80.
37. Robert-Gangneux F, Binisti P, Antonetti D, Brezin A, Yera H, Dupouy-Camet J. Usefulness of immunoblotting and Goldmann-Witmer coefficient for biological diagnosis of toxoplasmic retinochoroiditis. Euro J Clin Microbiol Infect Dis. 2004;23(1):34–8.
38. Mahalakshmi B, Therese KL, Madhavan HN, Biswas J. Diagnostic value of specific local antibody production and nucleic acid amplification technique-nested polymerase chain reaction (nPCR) in clinically suspected ocular toxoplasmosis. Ocul Immunol Inflamm. 2006;14(2):105–12.
39. Picot J, Guerin CL, Le Van KC, Boulanger CM. Flow cytometry: retrospective, fundamentals and recent instrumentation. Cytotechnology. 2012;64(2):109–30.
40. Chu CJ, Gardner PJ, Copland DA, Liyanage SE, Gonzalez-Cordero A, Kleine Holthaus SM, Luhmann UF, Smith AJ, Ali RR, Dick AD. Multimodal analysis of ocular inflammation using the endotoxin-induced uveitis mouse model. Dis Model Mech. 2016;9(4):473–81.
41. Carreño E, Serrano C, Muñoz N, Romero-Bueno F, Sánchez Pernaute O, Alejandre N. Intraocular leucocyte subpopulations analysis by multiparametric flow cytometry in human uveitis. Br J Ophthalmol. 2021;105(3):322–7.
42. Dave N, Chevour P, Mahendradas P, Venkatesh A, Kawali A, Shetty R, Ghosh A, Sethu S. Increased aqueous humor CD4+/CD8+ lymphocyte ratio in Sarcoid uveitis. Ocul Immunol Inflamm. 2019;27(7):1033–40.
43. Tanaka R, Kaburaki T, Taoka K, Karakawa A, Tsuji H, Nishikawa M, Yatomi Y, Shinozaki-Ushiku A, Ushiku T, Araki F. More accurate diagnosis of Vitreoretinal lymphoma using a combination of diagnostic test results: a prospective observational study. Ocul Immunol Inflamm. 2022;30(6):1354–60.
44. Shumilov E, Mazzeo P, Zinkernagel MS, Legros M, Porret N, Romagna L, Haase D, Lenz G, Novak U, Banz Y, et al. Comprehensive laboratory diagnostic workup for patients with suspected intraocular lymphoma including flow cytometry, molecular genetics and cytopathology. Curr Oncol. 2022;29(2):766–76.
45. Betters DM. Use of flow Cytometry in clinical practice. J Adv Pract Oncol. 2015;6(5):435–40.

46. Dolar-Szczasny J, Flieger J, Kowalska B, Majerek D, Tatarczak-Michalewska M, Zakrocka I, Załuska W, Rejdak R. Hemodialysis effect on the composition of the eye fluid of cataract patients. J Clin Med. 2021;10(23):5485.
47. Hohberger B, Chaudhri MA, Michalke B, Lucio M, Nowomiejska K, Schlötzer-Schrehardt U, Grieb P, Rejdak R, Jünemann AGM. Levels of aqueous humor trace elements in patients with open-angle glaucoma. J Trace Elem Med Biol. 2018;45:150–5.
48. Zhou Y, Hong F, Wang X, Feng J, Zhu D, Xu Y, Tao Y. Abnormal levels of aqueous humor trace elements in patients with cytomegalovirus retinitis. Eye (Lond). 2019;33(10):1606–12.

Approach to Diagnostic Testing

6

Contents

Y. Tao, D.-K. Hwang, *Examination of Intraocular Fluid*,
https://doi.org/10.1007/978-981-96-2486-7_6

6.1 Infectious Uveitis

6.1.1 Cytomegalovirus Anterior Uveitis

6.1.1.1 Brief Introduction

Cytomegalovirus anterior uveitis (CMVAU) can be categorized as a distinct variant of herpetic anterior uveitis (AU) attributable to the common membership of cytomegalovirus (CMV), herpes simplex virus (HSV), and varicella-zoster virus (VZV) in the Herpesviridae family. CMV is classified as a betaherpesvirus owing to its unique linear double-stranded DNA structure. The coexistence of three distinct manifestations of viral anterior uveitis has been extensively described in multiple studies [1–3]. However, a larger body of literature focuses exclusively on the clinical manifestations that differentiate CMVAU from those caused by HSV and VZV [4–13]. For instance, the incidence of secondary glaucoma in patients diagnosed with HSV anterior uveitis (HSV-AU), VZV anterior uveitis (VZV-AU), and CMV anterior uveitis (CMV-AU) was found to be 16%, 9%, and 72%, respectively [14]. Furthermore, the research indicated a significant increase in the presence of small keratic precipitates (KPs), coin-shaped KPs, and diffuse iris atrophy in patients with CMVAU compared to those with HSV-AU and VZV-AU [15].

The detection of CMV IgG antibodies, coupled with the absence of CMV IgM antibodies and antigen in the serum of individuals with CMVAU, suggests that CMVAU is primarily due to the localized reactivation of latent CMV, rather than a widespread infection [16]. Typically found in immunocompetent individuals, CMVAU has been infrequently reported following the use of topical immunosuppressive agents such as tacrolimus or cyclosporin [17, 18], prostaglandin analogues [19], or after cataract surgery [20]. Owing to the mild symptoms and clinical signs in its early stages, diagnoses of CMVAU are often delayed, which can lead to severe functional loss [21].

Elevated intraocular pressure (IOP) is a prominent characteristic of CMVAU. The potential mechanism responsible for the increased IOP observed in anterior viral uveitis may involve the active viral infection within the trabecular meshwork (TM) cells. Furthermore, it has been demonstrated that CMV infection leads to an increase in the production of transforming growth factor (TGF)-β1. This molecule, situated upstream in the signaling pathway, is known for its ability to enhance the resistance of the outflow channel in TM cells [22].

6.1.1.2 Epidemiology

The prevalence of CMVAU has been well-documented globally [3, 20, 23], with a particularly high incidence in the Asian region [20]. In Taiwan, CMV is responsible for 26.5% of HLA-B27 negative anterior uveitis cases in patients with elevated IOP or corneal edema. Additionally, CMV accounts for 64.3% of viral anterior uveitis cases in this demographic [20]. In the southern region of Vietnam, the prevalence of CMV anterior uveitis is reported to be 4% among patients diagnosed with uveitis at two eye hospitals [24]. In Thailand, CMVAU constitutes approximately 33% of viral anterior uveitis cases [25]. In South Korea, 67% of chronic recurrent anterior uveitis cases with elevated IOP are believed to be associated with CMVAU [26]. However, it is important to note that in the United States, CMVAU represents only 2% of viral anterior uveitis cases [27].

The mean age at initial presentation of anterior uveitis is reported to be 57.5 ± 12.6 years [28]. The prevalence of anterior uveitis coupled with elevated IOP varies, ranging from 18% to 34.2% [4, 16, 29–32]. Additionally, CMVAU appears to be more prevalent in males, with a reported rates ranging between 60% and 86% [16, 20, 23, 26, 33, 34].

6.1.1.3 Clinical Manifestation

The primary manifestation of CMVAU often involves unilateral, recurrent episodes of acute or chronic anterior uveitis, typically seen in immunocompetent adults. This condition is commonly accompanied by elevated IOP [34]. Typical ocular characteristics include a mild inflammatory response, characterized by medium-sized floater cells, increased IOP, and either widespread or sector iris atrophy [16, 35]. Although rare, the presence of hypopyon in the anterior chamber and vitreous body opacity may also occur [36]. Additionally, the development of a tonic pupil may be observed in some cases [37].

Glaucoma was diagnosed in 50 to 72% of eyes affected by CMVAU [14, 38]. The IOP at presentation was recorded at an average of 26.01 ± 9.35 mmHg [20]. A strong association was observed between glaucoma and pseudophakic eyes in CMV-positive eyes [20]. Moreover, the mean thickness of the peripapillary retinal nerve fiber layer (pRNFL) was significantly lower in eyes affected by CMVAU compared to their unaffected fellow eyes ($p = 0.012$). Similarly, the mean thickness of the macular ganglion cell-inner plexiform layer (GCIPL) was also significantly lower in the affected eyes compared to normal eyes ($p < 0.001$). These findings suggest the presence of early-stage retinal neural damage in hypertensive CMVAU, even before visual field changes become detectable. Timely and proactive treatment for individuals with glaucoma can potentially mitigate the progression of further damage associated with this condition [39].

Corneal endotheliitis has been reported in approximately 18% of ocular cases [38]. The positive predictive value for CMVAU in cases of corneal endotheliitis characterized by distinct coin-shaped KPs was found to be 90.9% [40]. Among patients with CMVAU, a ring-shaped KP pattern was observed in 53% of the cases, with 76% of these patients exhibiting a decreased number of corneal endothelial cells [41]. The average loss in the number of endothelial cells was reported to be 880.78 ± 882.24 [20]. Additionally, when severe iris depigmentation occurred alongside a decrease in endothelial cell density, the positive and negative predictive values for CMVAU diagnosis rose to 100.0% and 64.9%, respectively [42].

Clinical features of CMVAU may resemble Posner-Schlossman syndrome (50%, see Fig. 6.1), or Fuchs heterochromic iridocyclitis (13%–18%, Fig. 6.2) [43], or present as chronic nonspecific anterior uveitis-like (21%) [38] (see Fig. 6.3a, b). Recently, CMVAU has been categorized into three distinct subtypes: acute relapsing hypertension anterior uveitis, chronic hypertensive anterior uveitis, and recurrent or

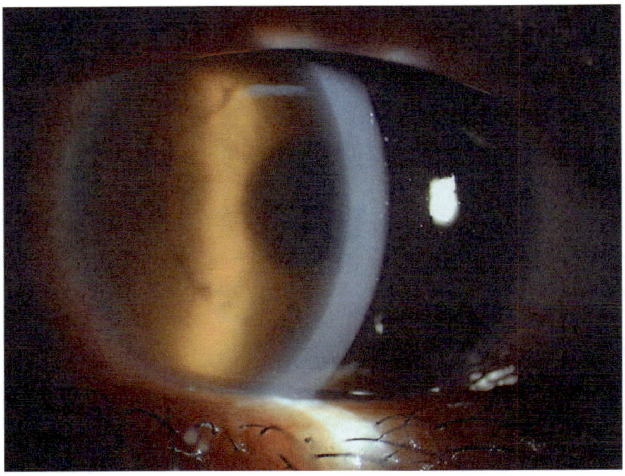

Fig. 6.1 This is a photograph of the anterior segment of the right eye of a 40-year-old female exhibiting changes akin to Posner-Schlossman syndrome. She reported a sensation of swelling in the right eye for 1 day. The intraocular pressure measured 60 mmHg. Observable features include corneal epithelial edema, two medium-sized keratic precipitates located below the pupil area, and a slight reaction in the anterior chamber

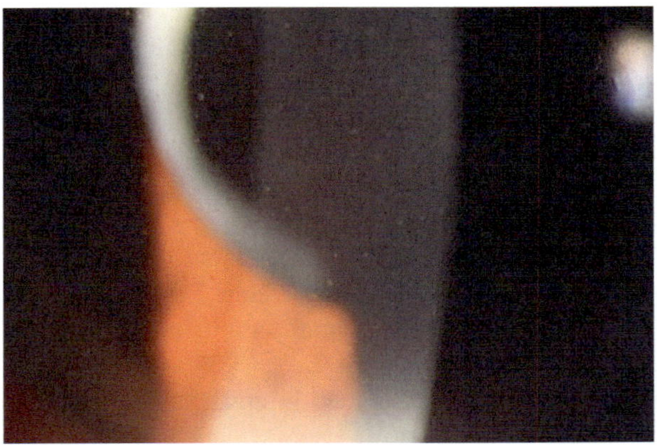

Fig. 6.2 This photograph shows the anterior segment of the right eye of a 43-year-old male displaying changes resembling Fuchs heterochromic iridocyclitis. He reported experiencing blurred vision in his right eye for 2 years. The intraocular pressure was measured at 26 mmHg. Notable observations include small keratic precipitates and a mild reaction in the anterior chamber. Following oral administration of ganciclovir, the intraocular pressure stabilized at 13 to 15 mmHg over the course of year

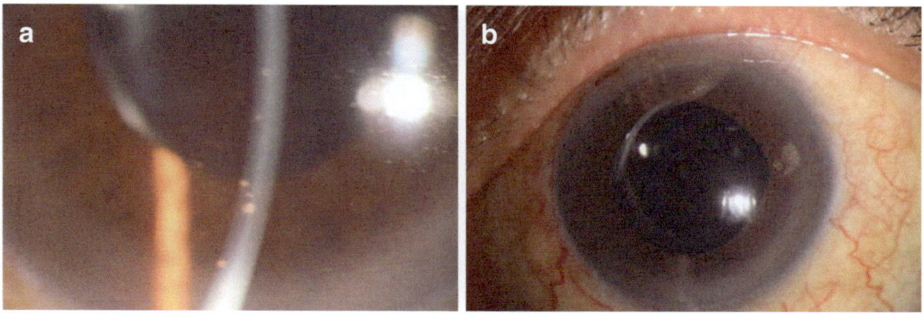

Fig. 6.3 This photograph depicts the anterior segment of the left eye of a 43-year-old male showing changes similar to chronic nonspecific anterior uveitis. He has experienced recurrent episodes of elevated intraocular pressure in his left eye for 2 years. The intraocular pressure was recorded at 38 mmHg. Observable features include a small amount of brown keratic precipitates (**a**), a mild reaction in the anterior chamber, and moth-like changes in the iris (**b**)

chronic iridocyclitis/iritis accompanied by sectoral iris atrophy [4]. Additionally, cataracts have been observed to develop in 69.2% of patients [5].

6.1.1.4 Diagnosis

Typically, the diagnosis of CMVAU is made by combining clinical manifestations with laboratory analysis of intraocular fluids. Given the frequent delays in diagnosing this condition, laboratory evaluation plays a vital role in early detection. In cases suspected of having hypertensive anterior granulomatous uveitis due to CMV, real-time polymerase chain reaction (RT-PCR) and assessment of intraocular antibody production against CMV are performed on aqueous fluid samples [44, 45]. The Goldmann-Witmer coefficient (GWs) is calculated, with a result considered positive if the index exceeds 3.0 [45]. In instances where patients initially test negative for PCR but present significant clinical features, the diagnosis can be confirmed through subsequent positive PCR results (80%) or positive GWc results (20%), accompanied by a repeated aqueous tap [6].

The Classification Criteria for Cytomegalovirus Anterior Uveitis, developed by **THE STANDARDIZATION OF UVEITIS NOMENCLATURE (SUN) WORKING GROUP**, focuses on ensuring on sensitivity in diagnostic criteria and specificity in classification criteria. This classification system includes three distinct components: (1) evidence of anterior uveitis, which encompasses the presence of anterior chamber cells, the condition that if anterior vitreous cells are present, anterior chamber inflammation should also be present, and the absence of evidence of retinitis; (2) evidence of CMV infection in the eye, demonstrated by a positive PCR result for cytomegalovirus on an aqueous specimen; and (3) exclusions criteria, which involve positive serology for syphilis using a treponemal test, evidence of sarcoidosis (either bilateral hilar adenopathy on chest imaging or a tissue biopsy demonstrating noncaseating granulomata), and an aqueous specimen PCR positive for HSV or VZV) [12].

6.1.1.5 Examination of Intraocular Fluids

For CMVAU, the application of real-time PCR on aqueous samples is essential not only for confirming the precise diagnosis [2, 20] but also for tracking the onset of the infection, its clearance, and any potential recurrence [13]. While PCR is renowned for its specificity and accuracy, its diagnostic effectiveness can be further enhanced by incorporating clinical factors and broadening our understanding in this field [46]. Typically, the aqueous tapping procedure is performed in cases of anterior chamber activity, especially in response to spikes in IOP [16], and prior to starting anti-viral and anti-inflammatory treatments [7, 23, 47].

In the current study, 20% of participants yielded negative results upon their initial assessment [11]. For patients' negative taps and persistent or relapsing inflammation, repeated aqueous humor paracentesis for PCR analysis may be indicated [31]. A significant CMV copy count has been identified as a notable risk factor for the development of coin-shaped lesions, recurrent inflammation, decreased endothelial cell densities, and elevated intraocular pressure [48–50]. Furthermore, the concentration of CMV in the aqueous humor was found to be significantly higher in cases with glaucoma ($r = 0.476, p = 0.02$). There is also a strong positive correlation between the delay in performing an aqueous tap after the onset of symptoms and the occurrence of glaucoma ($r = 0.714$, $p < 0.0001$), underscoring the importance of early diagnosis in effectively managing the progression of glaucoma [45]. The average time from the initial onset of uveitis to obtaining a positive result for CMV was approximately 17.4 years, with this duration exceeding 3.6 years in 75% of the cases [31].

Several studies have indicated a higher positive rate for the GWc test, ranging from 67% to 96.2%, compared to real-time PCR, which ranged from 50% to 71.4% [25, 38, 51]. Notably, GWc was the sole positive test in 66.6% of the tested patients [10]. PCR is considered a reliable diagnostic tool for early identification, especially in cases with cellular inflammation in the anterior chamber. In contrast, the GWc test is more suitable for diagnosis at a later stage, when there is a lower level of inflammation in the anterior chamber. When there is a strong clinical suspicion but initial test results are negative, repeating the tap procedure should be considered [10]. Additionally, the presence of endotheliitis has been significantly correlated with the presence of IgG antibodies against CMV in the aqueous humor ($r = 0.418$, $p = 0.047$) [45].

6.1.1.6 Management

Generally, the treatment approaches for CMVAU involve administering systemic antiviral therapy along with the use of topical antiviral and anti-inflammatory eye drops. To manage elevated intraocular pressure (IOP), anti-glaucomatous eye drops or surgical interventions may be employed.

Multiple centers have adopted a similar antiviral regimen for CMVAU, beginning with the administration of systemic ganciclovir intravenously at a dosage of 5 mg/kg/8 h for 10 days. This is followed by oral valganciclovir at 900 mg twice daily for 3 to 6 weeks and then a maintenance dose of 450 mg twice daily for an additional 4 to 6 weeks [7, 47, 51]. Following this regimen, normalization of intraocular pressure, complete remission of corneal edema, and resolution of uveitis have been observed. Valganciclovir, a commonly used antiviral medication [52], and valaciclovir, as a maintenance therapy alternative, have been shown efficacy in this condition [8]. The majority of patients (76.6%) respond to antiviral therapy, but a significant proportion (73.5–75.0%) experience recurrences posttreatment [7, 47, 53]. Oral valganciclovir combined with topical corticosteroids has been noted to reduce the recurrence frequency compared to no prophylactic measures. In cases of CMVAU with uncontrolled IOP, over one-third of patients avoided glaucoma surgery within 2 years by using oral valganciclovir [9]. Biweekly treatment monitoring includes comprehensive blood count, liver enzyme levels, and kidney function assessment [7, 47]. In cases of severe adverse reactions like pancytopenia, therapy discontinuation is advised [51]. Letermovir at a daily dosage of 480 mg is a potential alternative for patients with ongoing inflammation or adverse reactions to valganciclovir [54]. Intraocular injections of ganciclovir (2 mg/0.05 mL) as a loading dose followed by oral valganciclovir (900 mg twice a day), tailed to the severity of the post-injection aqueous inflammation, have been reported to improve or stabilize visual acuity, control the IOP, and manage anterior chamber inflammation [55]. A prophylactic treatment course lasting 3 to 12 months may be considered to prevent recurrences [56]. Recurrences are more common in patients with prior corneal endothelial damage [11].

The use of 0.15% ganciclovir gel is often integrated into the treatment regimen for CMVAU. The recommended protocol is to apply the gel four times daily for a minimum of 3 months. As an alternative, the gel may be applied at least five times a day, with a gradual reduction in frequency based on the degree of inflammation in the anterior chamber, over the same 3-month period [7]. Subsequently, patients are advised to continue with long-term maintenance therapy, applying the gel three to four times daily [6].

The use of topical 0.15% ganciclovir gel has been associated with a significantly lower number of recurrences per year. Posttreatment recurrence rates dropped to 0.76–0.57, compared to the pre-treatment rates of 3.76–2.44 ($P = 0.001$) [6]. Another study highlighted that patients using topical ganciclovir gel experienced statistically fewer episodes of uveitis flare-ups per person-year, with a median of −0.88 episodes/person-years ($p = 0.029$) [28]. Additionally, the early initiation of antiviral treatment seems to correlate with better outcomes regarding the need for glaucoma surgery. In the study, only 8.3% of patients who started treatment early (within 700 days) required glaucoma surgery during the follow-up period [47]. There have also been reports of using ophthalmic 1% valganciclovir ointment, which did not result in clinically evident ocular surface toxicity [57].

Additionally, 0.5% or 2% ganciclovir eye drops have also demonstrated their efficacy and safety in the long-term treatment and prevention of CMVAU [58, 59]. While this topical treatment option is convenient, commercially available ganciclovir eye drops are not widely accessible. Consequently, this treatment is currently recommended primarily in Taiwan.

To manage intraocular inflammation, topical steroids, also known as anti-inflammatory eye drops, were utilized. Typically, the use of these anti-inflammatory medications was gradually reduced as the inflammation subsided [47]. The results of a study with a mean follow-up of 62.1 ± 28.5 months demonstrated that the mean number of uveitis relapses significantly decreased from 0.23 ± 0.17 to 0.03 ± 0.03 ($p < 0.001$) following corticosteroid therapy. This decrease was observed in treatments that combined topical antiviral with or without systemic antiviral therapy [5].

In cases where individuals exhibited IOP levels above 21 mmHg, 80% were found to require an average of 1.97 antiglaucoma drops. Additionally, it was noted that 28.6% of these patients (10 out of 35) needed oral acetazolamide [47]. Surgical intervention for glaucoma is typically advised for patients who experience persistent and uncontrolled IOP over an extended period. A study demonstrated that by the end of a 12-month period following trabectome surgery, the mean IOP could decrease from an initial value of 40 ± 10 mmHg to a normalized level of 13 ± 1 mmHg [60]. It is also recognized that glaucoma surgery not only stabilizes IOP but also has the potential to flush out CMV from the aqueous humor. This can be crucial in preventing the malfunction of corneal endothelial cells and optic nerve damage caused by glaucoma [50].

6.1.2 Herpesvirus Anterior Uveitis

6.1.2.1 Brief Introduction

Herpetic anterior uveitis (HAU) can be caused by either Herpes simplex virus (HSV) or Varicella-zoster virus (VZV) infection, and it is the most common cause of infectious anterior uveitis [61–63]. Inflammation of the anterior chamber occurs in up to 10% of patients with HSV keratitis [62, 64–66] and approximately 50% of immunocompetent patients with herpes zoster ophthalmicus [62, 67]. Risk factors for HSV-related HAU (HSV-AU) reactivation include stress, fever, ultraviolet radiation, menstruation, trauma [63], and YAG peripheral iridotomy [68]. It has been observed that HSV-AU primarily occurs in middle-aged people with a predominance in females [69], whereas HAU caused by VZV (VZV-AU) is more common in patients aged 50 years and older [70]. The recurrence rate of HAU is 0.45 per person-year [71].

6.1.2.2 Epidemiology

HAU accounted for 1% to 10% of all uveitis cases seen at tertiary referral centers [63, 67, 72–76]. It represented 2.8% of all uveitis cases at referral centers in Turkey [77]. In a tertiary military hospital in Thailand, HSV and VZV iridocyclitis accounted for 2.9% of total uveitis cases. Among patients aged 17–60, the rate is 2.4%; for those over 60, it increases to 5.4% [78].

6.1.2.3 Clinical Manifestation

Most patients of HAU are unilaterally involved [79]. They commonly complained of blurred vision accompanied by eye pain, redness, and photophobia [76, 80, 81]. The typical characteristics of HAU include a corneal scar or herpetic dermatitis

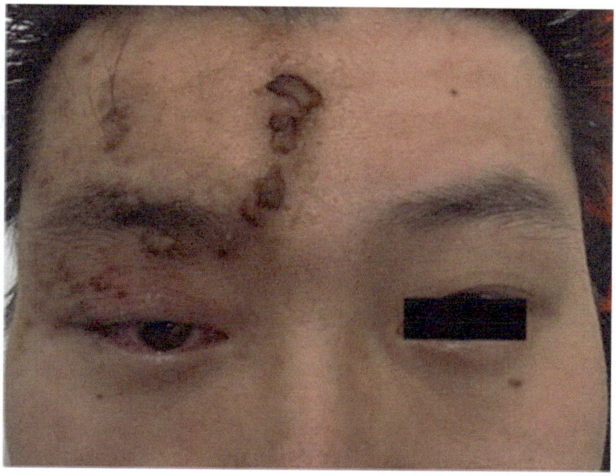

Fig. 6.4 The photograph shows a 26-year-old male who has been suffering from herpetic dermatitis on his right forehead and eyelid for 1 week, accompanied by ocular redness and blurred vision. Varicella-zoster virus DNA is positive (7.52×10^2 copies/mL) in the aqueous humor, confirming the diagnosis of herpetic anterior uveitis

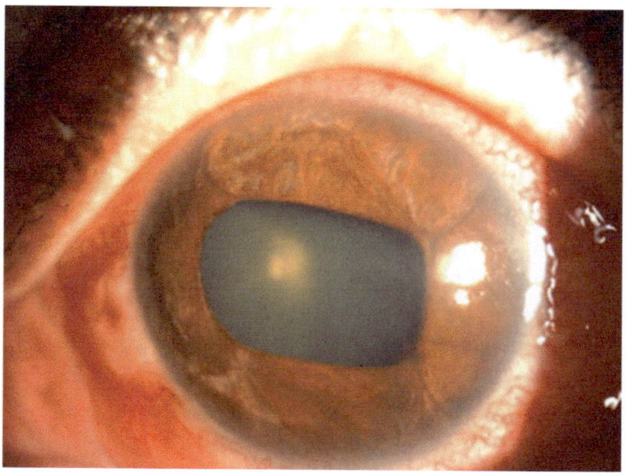

Fig. 6.5 The photograph of the anterior segment shows a 48-year-old female who has experienced recurrent ocular redness and progressively worsening blurred vision in the left eye for 5 months. The intraocular pressure increased to 30 mmHg. The diagnosis of herpesvirus anterior uveitis was confirmed by a positive varicella-zoster virus antibody test (24,225.24 U/mL) in the aqueous humor. Diffuse patchy iris atrophy and pupil deformation are also observable

(Fig. 6.4), keratitis, elevated intraocular pressure (IOP), keratic precipitates (KPs), a distorted pupil (Fig. 6.5), posterior synechiae, loss of accommodation, iridoplegia, and iris atrophy (Fig. 6.6) [69, 71, 79, 82, 83]. Rarely, a hypopyon or hyphema can be observed [84].

Posterior subcapsular cataracts were observed in about 10% of eyes, and decreased corneal sensation was found in 32% of eyes [70, 79]. High intraocular pressure (IOP) is frequently observed and ranges from 46% to 90% in affected eyes [69]. Patients with glaucoma exhibit a greater frequency of IOP peaks during uveitis follow-up compared to individuals without glaucoma [85].

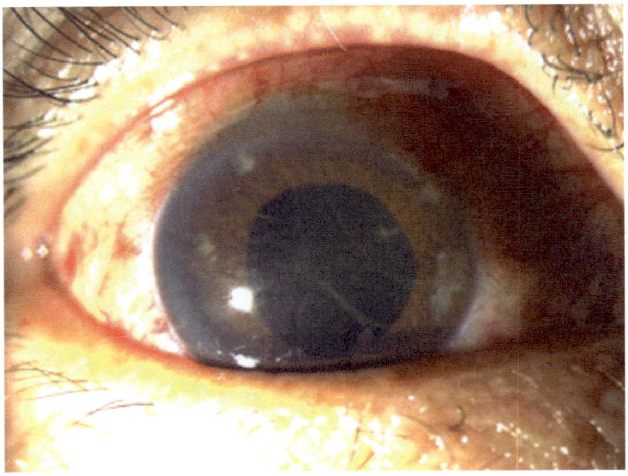

Fig. 6.6 The photograph of the anterior segment depicts a 54-year-old male with recurrent redness and progressively worsening blurred vision in his right eye for 2 years. The intraocular pressure has increased to 50 mmHg. The diagnosis of herpetic anterior uveitis was confirmed by a positive varicella-zoster virus DNA test (1.35×10^8 copies/mL) in the aqueous humor. Multiple areas of patchy iris atrophy are visible

The most common iris features were the sectoral iridoplegia (100%) on biomicroscopy and the disorganization of the iris layers (DIL) (77%) on AS SD-OCT images (anterior segment spectral-domain optical coherence tomography) [86]. Patients with HAU had significantly higher levels of dendritiform inflammatory cells in their subepithelial cornea than patients with Fuchs uveitis syndrome, which can be detected by in vivo confocal microscopy [87]. Corneal edema and opacity can be observed in the late stage due to gradually developing corneal endothelial decompensation (Fig. 6.7). Rarely, herpesvirus anterior uveitis may be complicated by retinal vasculitis apart from necrotizing retinitis [88].

By comparison, eyes affected by HSV-AU exhibited a higher recurrence rate, more corneal involvement, keratic precipitates (KPs), iris atrophy, elevated IOP, and posterior synechiae than those affected by VZV-AU. Conversely, VZV-AU patients exhibited more severe intraocular inflammation, more frequent use of immunomodulatory treatments, and a history of systemic herpetic disease compared to HSV-AU patients [2, 89].

6.1.2.4 Diagnosis

The presumed diagnosis of HAU is usually based on clinical findings [76, 89], such as unilateral involvement, the presence of herpetic dermatitis or dendritic keratitis, which provides the strongest diagnostic support [76], and the presence of KPs, iris atrophy, distorted pupil, and elevated IOP [89]. Although diagnosing anterior herpetic uveitis is usually straightforward in the presence of dermatitis or dendritic keratitis, it can be quite challenging in their absence [61].

However, since new viral pathogens and other etiologies can mimic a similar clinical appearance at onset [90], early misdiagnosis of HAU is common [61].

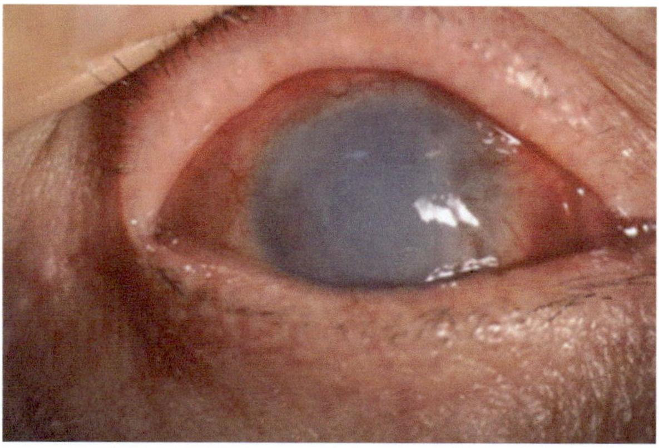

Fig. 6.7 The photograph of the anterior segment features a 67-year-old female who has been experiencing blurred vision and photophobia in her right eye for half a month. The diagnosis of herpetic anterior uveitis was confirmed by positive tests for varicella-zoster virus DNA (4.16×10^5 copies/mL) and antibodies (11,825.25 U/mL) in the aqueous humor. Notable corneal opacity and ciliary conjunctival congestion are also observable

Aqueous humor analysis for PCR and GWC (Goldmann-Witmer coefficient) can be useful in cases of suspected viral uveitis [69]. An anterior chamber (AC) tap is then required to obtain aqueous humor for laboratory diagnosis. The etiology of HAU is confirmed based on positive polymerase chain reaction (PCR) results for the viral genome of HSV or VZV; the production of intraocular antibodies, as determined by a GWC value greater than 3; or both [89]. Seroprevalence of circulating antibodies to HSV is common in the adult population and does not necessarily indicate active herpetic disease, limiting the role of serology in diagnosing HAU [63].

6.1.2.5 Examination of Intraocular Fluids

For confirmation of etiology, isolation of the herpes simplex virus [91, 92] and viral cultures were used in the 1970s, and electron microscopy was employed in the 1980s [93]. However, these procedures pose challenges in terms of complexity and time requirements, while also exhibiting limited sensitivity [76, 81, 94]. In the 1990s, PCR was reported to be used in detecting varicella-zoster virus DNA in iridocyclitis [95].

A more reliable diagnostic approach for herpetic anterior uveitis can be achieved through the utilization of PCR-based analysis on samples of aqueous humor [76]. The positive rate of PCR-based analyses for HSV or VZV DNA in aqueous humor samples can be as high as 100% [96]. However, due to different primer sets used in each laboratory, variations in PCR techniques, and varied clinical criteria for selecting patients with presumed HAU, this rate has ranged from 25% to 100% in various studies [70, 76, 94, 96].

A less widely used method for diagnosing herpetic anterior uveitis is the Goldmann-Witmer coefficient, which measures the intraocular production of antibodies directed against-specific organisms [70, 76]. Notably, the positivity of the

Goldmann-Witmer coefficient seems to vary with the time from the onset of uveitis [76]. Among HAU patients, the proportion of HSV and VZV infections varies between Caucasians and Asians. In a study from the Netherlands involving 24 patients with anterior uveitis and sectoral iris atrophy, most patients were infected by HSV: the Goldmann-Witmer coefficient for HSV >3 was positive in 16 patients, and HSV-DNA was positive in 12 patients, while the coefficient for VZV >3 was positive in 3 patients, and VZV-DNA was positive in 1 patient [70]. However, in a study of Chinese patients with 32 eyes involved, there were 24 eyes with VZV-AU and 8 eyes with HSV-AU [89]. Similarly, a study in Japan found 20 eyes with VZV-AU and 8 eyes with HSV-AU [1].

6.1.2.6 Management

Currently, the therapy options for people with HAU include oral antiviral medications and topical corticosteroids.

Long-term oral acyclovir use appears to remain effective in decreasing the number of ocular herpes simplex virus recurrences beyond 12 months (78% vs. 36%) and in prolonging recurrence-free survival ($P = 0.001$) [97]. A daily maintenance dose of acyclovir for longer than 6 months, or even for a minimum of 2 years after the first uveitis attack, is suggested [98]. Patients with adverse outcomes due to HSV-AU were typically not receiving oral antiviral prophylaxis [99].

In HAU patients experiencing uveitis attacks, topical steroids are typically initiated and tapered very cautiously to prevent severe rebound attacks [98]. By contrast, most topical antiviral agents fail to reach therapeutic levels in the aqueous humor [61, 100]. Additionally, prolonged use of topical antivirals can be toxic to both the corneal and conjunctival epithelium, resulting in either allergic blepharoconjunctivitis or corneal epitheliopathy in 5% to 10% of patients [65, 66]. Low-temperature treatment has been reported to be used in the management of iridocyclitis and herpetic infections of the cornea [101, 102]. Each episode of HAU can last from 1 week to several months [76, 80, 81].

6.1.3 Cytomegalovirus Retinitis

6.1.3.1 Brief Introduction

Cytomegalovirus (CMV) belongs to the *Herpesviridae* family, a double-stranded DNA virus that is widely prevalent in nature. In developed areas, the population infection rate for CMV ranges from 27.4% to 50.4% [103–105], while this proportion can exceed 90% in densely populated developing countries [106, 107]. CMV is transmitted through body fluids, such as saliva, tears, cervical secretions, urine, semen, feces, blood, or milk excreted by infected individuals. It becomes a source of infection and can be transmitted via droplets. Infection can also occur through organ donations from individuals infected with CMV.

CMV enters the body and spreads through the bloodstream to the eyes, infecting retinal tissue cells, mainly vascular endothelial cells. In immunocompetent individuals, the replication of CMV is suppressed, forming a symbiotic steady-state balance. However, this balance is disrupted in immunocompromised individuals, leading to retinal vasculitis caused by CMV, which results in retinal dysfunction.

CMV retinitis (CMVR) has been reported to be significantly associated with a CD4+ cell count below 50 cells/μL [108]. The occurrence of CMVR correlates well with the level of CD4+ T lymphocytes, with occurrences of 16.8%, 5.4%, and 1.4% in patients with CD4+ T lymphocyte counts of less than 50, 50 to 99, and 100 to 199 cells/μL, respectively [109].

CMVR is primarily reported in patients with human immunodeficiency virus (HIV) infection and acquired immunodeficiency syndrome (AIDS) [110], as well as in those with systemic malignancies following systemic immunosuppressive therapies [111–113]. It also affects those treated with long-term systemic corticosteroids or immunomodulatory therapy for rheumatoid or autoimmune disorders [114, 115]. Additionally, CMVR may occur after local immunosuppressive therapies, such as intravitreal dexamethasone implants [116–118] and intravitreal triamcinolone injections [119, 120].

6.1.3.2 Epidemiology

Before the advent of highly active antiretroviral therapy (HAART), 20.2% to 37% of AIDS patients were reported to be affected by CMVR [108, 110, 121–123]. However, with the widespread development of HAART (commonly known as cocktail therapy), the proportion of CMVR in AIDS patients decreased remarkably to about 9.0% [108, 124, 125]. On the other hand, the incidence of CMVR in patients with acute leukemia, malignant lymphoma, and organ transplantation using immunosuppressive drugs has been reported to be 3% [126].

6.1.3.3 Clinical Manifestation

Patients with CMVR generally exhibit a mild reaction in the anterior segment. Gray or white dusty, medium-sized, fatty keratic precipitates (mainly in the inferior area of the cornea, Fig. 6.8) along with a few floating cells in the anterior chamber and

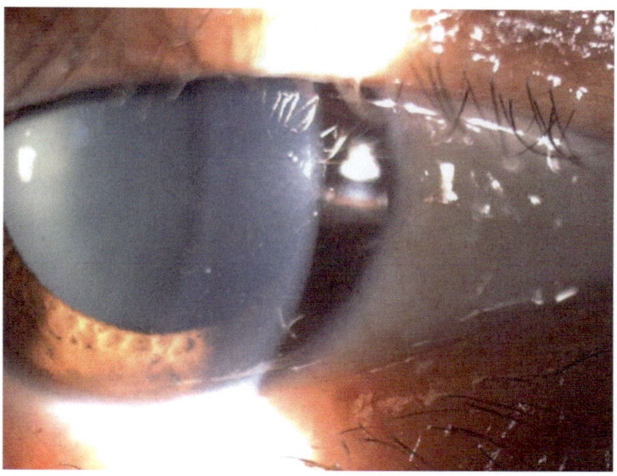

Fig. 6.8 The photograph of the anterior segment of a patient diagnosed with CMVR following allogeneic hematopoietic stem cell transplantation for leukemia. Gray or white dusty, medium-sized, fatty keratic precipitates in the inferior area of the cornea can be observed

slight anterior chamber flare can be observed. Vitreous opacity is generally mild, but vitreous floating cells can be detected with careful examination.

The fundus manifestations of CMVR are characteristic, primarily presenting as typical necrotizing retinitis. The most common type of CMVR lesions, resembling "cheese and ketchup" (retinal hemorrhage and exudate with fuzzy boundaries), appears as wedge-shaped areas of whitening with variable small dot-like lesions (granular type) and associated hemorrhage (brush-fire) (Fig. 6.9a). In fundus fluorescein angiography (FA), areas of hemorrhage and active retinitis may exhibit hypofluorescence with stippled hyperfluorescence (Fig. 6.9b).

White sheathing of retinal veins and even frost-like branching changes can be observed if extensive retinal vessels are involved (Fig. 6.10). Retinal fibrotic scars, retinal atrophy, RPE depigmentation or proliferation (Fig. 6.11), and subretinal crystallization (commonly seen in children, Fig. 6.12) can be observed in the chronic form of CMVR.

In infants younger than 1 year with CMVR, the disease tends to manifest in the macula, whereas in adults, it tends to manifest in the periphery of the retina [127].

The initial visual acuity, type, zone, and extent of CMVR did not differ significantly between patients with HIV infection and patients with immunocompromised conditions from various causes. However, intraocular inflammation is more frequently associated with active retinitis in non-HIV patients, while immune recovery uveitis is more prevalent in HIV patients [128].

Recurrence occurred in 33.3% of cases at a mean time of 6.4 ± 3.3 weeks after discontinuation of anti-CMV therapy. The retinal detachment rate was 21.7% per eye-year, and the mortality rate was 11.7% per person-year [129].

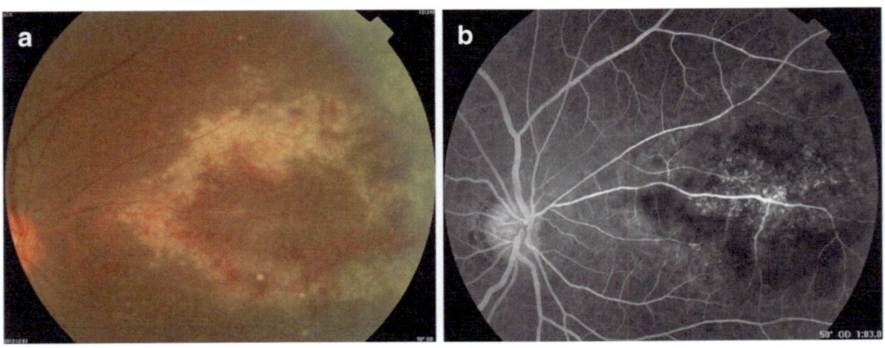

Fig. 6.9 The photographs (**a**) and fluorescein angiography (**b**) of the fundus of the right eye of a patient with AIDS (acquired immunodeficiency syndrome) diagnosed with CMVR, confirmed by positive CMV DNA in the aqueous humor. The nasal area of the retina exhibits a mixture of grayish-yellow granular retinal necrosis and retinal hemorrhage with unclear boundaries, resembling a "cheese + ketchup" appearance (**a**). The fundus fluorescein angiography displays a circular hypofluorescence with stippled hyperfluorescence (**b**)

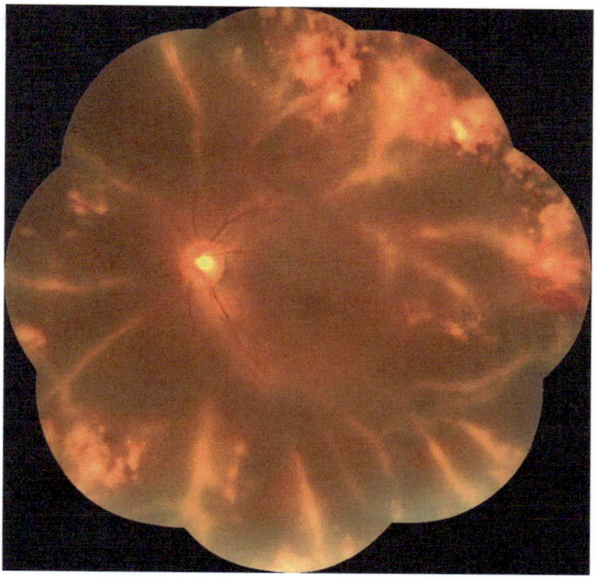

Fig. 6.10 Fundus photography of the left eye of a patient with cytomegalovirus retinitis, showing frost-like branching changes of retinal veins

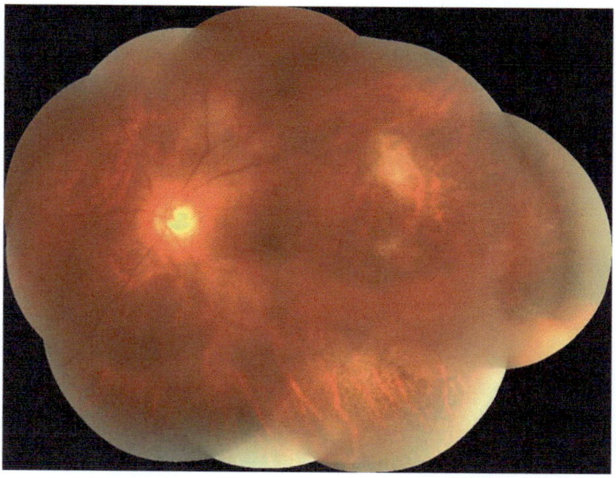

Fig. 6.11 Fundus photography of the left eye of a patient with CMVR who underwent repeated intravitreal injections of ganciclovir. Fibrous scar formation (near the upper temporal vascular arch), retinal neuroepithelial atrophy, and retinal pigment epithelium depigmentation in the peripheral area are observable

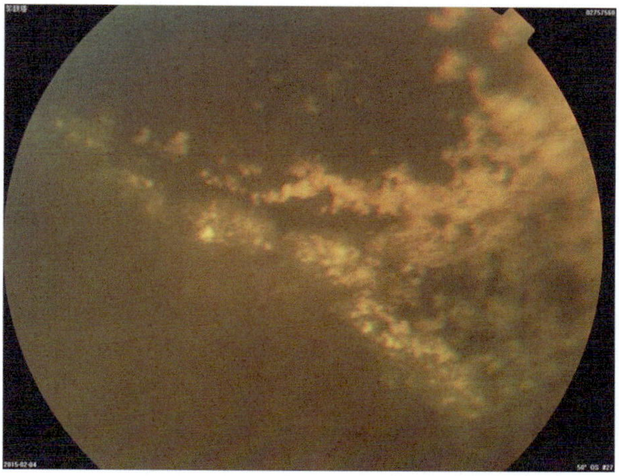

Fig. 6.12 Fundus photography of a child with chronic cytomegalovirus retinitis after allogeneic hematopoietic stem cell transplantation due to leukemia. Subretinal crystallization is observable

6.1.3.4 Diagnosis

The diagnosis of CMVR is predominantly clinical and relies on the observation of characteristic retinitis during dilated funduscopic examination, based on the classic appearance of lesions. Confirmation of CMVR diagnosis can be achieved by obtaining an aqueous or vitreous sample, in which CMV may be detected by PCR.

The diagnosis of CMVR in children is challenging due to the absence of external ocular signs or the inability to express visual symptoms [130], and artificial intelligence has shed light on routine CMVR screening in children in the inpatient ward [131].

A classification criteria for CMVR has been proposed by the Standardization of Uveitis Nomenclature (SUN) working group as follows [132] (requires #1 and #2 and either #3 or #4):

1. Necrotizing retinitis with indistinct borders due to numerous small (<50 μm) satellites.
2. Immune compromise:
3. Systemic (e.g., AIDS, organ transplant, chemotherapy)
4. Ocular (e.g., intraocular corticosteroids or chemotherapy)
5. Characteristic clinical picture ([a or b or c] AND d)
   (a) Wedge-shaped area of retinitis OR
   (b) Hemorrhagic appearance of the retinitis OR
   (c) Granular appearance of the retinitis AND
   (d) Absent to mild vitritis
6. Evidence of intraocular infection with cytomegalovirus
   (a) Positive PCR for cytomegalovirus from either the aqueous or vitreous specimen.

Exclusions:

1. Positive serology for syphilis using a treponemal test.
2. Intraocular specimen PCR-positive for infection by herpes simplex virus, varicella-zoster virus, or Toxoplasma gondii (unless there is immune compromise, morphologic evidence for >1 infection, the characteristic picture of cytomegalovirus retinitis, and the intraocular fluid specimen also has a positive PCR result for cytomegalovirus).

6.1.3.5 Examination of Intraocular Fluids

CMVR diagnosis could be confirmed by laboratory examination of cytomegalovirus DNA in the intraocular fluid sample. Detection of CMV genome by PCR in the aqueous humor could be used as a specific and highly predictive method for confirming this infection in the retina, as well as aiding in the differentiation of immune recovery uveitis. In HIV-infected patients with ambiguous ocular changes, the detection of varicella-zoster virus (VZV), herpes simplex virus (HSV), and *Toxoplasma gondii* DNA together with CMV in the aqueous is suggested to further make an etiological diagnosis of retinitis of unclear origin and to exclude the presence of combined infection or contribute to differentiation diagnosis. Furthermore, it also provides accurate markers to differentiate active and inactive CMV retinitis (aqueous or vitreous PCR, $P < 0.001$). Positive rates of aqueous CMV-DNA were 0 in AIDS patients with microvascular retinopathy (MVR) but not CMVR.

The positive rate of CMV detection in the aqueous humor of clinically diagnosed CMVR is 89% [129], and the specificity of either aqueous or vitreous is equally 93% [133]. Given the belief that examination of intraocular fluids should simplify the diagnosis without the need for invasive posterior diagnostic procedures in complicated patients and should be performed in adults for definitive prompt diagnosis, a wider application of the aqueous PCR method is advocated [134].

Local anti-CMV antibody secretion in the eye helps confirm the presumed diagnosis of CMVR in 50% of the investigated AIDS patients [135]. However, antibody production against CMV does not show an increase in the Goldmann-Witmer coefficient [136]. The application of a PCR assay detecting CMV DNA is a more sensitive method for confirming a diagnosis in indistinct cases than analysis of locally produced antibodies using the Goldmann-Witmer coefficient [137].

Interleukin-8 (IL-8) concentration in the aqueous demonstrates a strong correlation with CMV DNA burden, indicative of a Th1 and monocyte-macrophage-mediated response, and decreases longitudinally over the course of treatment [138–140]. Moreover, IL-8 declines continuously after multiple intravitreal injections of antiviral drugs, showing a remarkable declining trend. Therefore, IL-8 may be regarded as a reliable quantitative laboratory indicator of the recovery of CMVR [139]. Additionally, the aqueous levels of trace elements (phosphorus and copper) were found to be abnormal in CMVR patients [141].

6.1.3.6 Management

Ganciclovir is widely utilized as the primary pharmacological intervention for the management of CMVR. The standard intravenous dose regimen for therapy typically involves the administration of ganciclovir. During the induction phase, patients are given a dosage of 5 mg/kg twice daily for a duration of 14 to 21 days. Subsequently, during the maintenance phase, patients receive a daily dosage of 5 mg/kg of ganciclovir [110]. Foscarnet also provides a useful alternative therapy for patients with CMV isolates that have become resistant to ganciclovir. The intravenous dosing regimen of foscarnet for therapy is as follows: during the induction phase, foscarnet is given at 90 mg/kg twice daily for 14 days, and during the maintenance phase, it is administered at 120 mg/kg/day [110]. Present recommendations for cessation of maintenance therapy involve the presence of a consistent increase in CD4+ cells above 100 cells/μL (with a minimum rise of 50 cells/μL), as well as relapse-free periods lasting between 3 and 6 months [142–146].

However, the widely used systemic antiviral medication, ganciclovir, has been found to be frequently associated with neutropenia. Consequently, the dosage of ganciclovir needs to be reduced in cases of renal failure, neutropenia, or thrombocytopenia. These conditions are commonly observed in patients with severe systemic morbidity, particularly myelosuppression [147, 148]. Additional drawbacks of intravenous administration of antiviral drugs include reduced bioavailability inside ocular tissues, necessitating the need for extended treatment duration [130, 149]. Consequently, the administration of antiviral medicines via intravitreal injections has emerged as a prominent approach in current therapeutic practices.

The documented dosage range for intravitreal injections of ganciclovir (IVG) spans from 200 μg to 6 mg, as reported in studies [150–156]. The most commonly used intravitreal dosages are 2 mg/0.1 mL for ganciclovir and 2.4 mg/0.1 mL for foscarnet [134, 157]. The interval between successive injections is typically 1 week [148].

The initial efficacy of treating CMVR after four consecutive weekly intravitreal injections does not exhibit a statistically significant variance when compared to the administration of ganciclovir alone or in combination with foscarnet. The administration of ganciclovir alone through continuous injection has been found to be an effective treatment for immunosuppressed patients who have recently developed CMVR [155]. Intravitreal injection was stopped when the aqueous CMV DNA became undetectable ($<1.0 \times 10^3$ copies/mL in the aqueous humor) or aqueous IL-8 level <30 pg/mL and scar tissue formation could be observed [111, 140, 158]. It is regarded that incorporating aqueous humor IL-8 level into the criteria of CMVR treatment decision can safely and effectively reduce the number of intravitreal injections needed and can be used as important indicators to assess treatment endpoint [111].

6.1.4 Acute Retinal Necrosis

6.1.4.1 Brief Introduction

Acute retinal necrosis (ARN) is a sight-threatening form of uveitis. Varicella-zoster virus (VZV) and herpes simplex virus (HSV) I and II are primarily implicated, with cytomegalovirus (CMV) and Epstein Barr virus (EBV) being less common causes of the disease [135, 159–166]. Histology reveals profound acute necrosis of the retina, retinal arteritis, and eosinophilic intranuclear inclusions in retinal cells [160]. Although ARN typically occurs in immunocompetent individuals, it has been observed in an adult with a history of HSV encephalitis treated with a dexamethasone intravitreal implant (Ozurdex®) [167]. Documented cases have linked ARN to natalizumab administration [168, 169], herpes zoster vaccination [170], and complications with encephalitis [171–173]. For HSV-2-induced retinitis, a history of neonatal herpes, triggering events such as neurosurgery, periocular trauma, high-dose corticosteroids, and chorioretinal scars suggest reactivation of the HSV-2 infection [174].

6.1.4.2 Epidemiology

The incidence of ARN in the United Kingdom is approximately one case per 1.6 to 2.0 million people per year [175, 176]. Among ARN cases caused by HSV, 23.9% had histories of prior encephalitis [177].

6.1.4.3 Clinical Manifestation

Some patients with VZV-related ARN had a history of skin shingles or cold sores before the onset of ARN, while many other patients exhibited no obvious systemic symptoms. Symptoms include eye redness, periorbital pain, photophobia, gradual vision decline, or seeing dark shadows fluttering in front of the eyes. In the acute stage, it often involves anterior segment inflammation. Ocular examinations reveal anterior segment inflammation, gray and white fatty keratic precipitates (KPs) (Fig. 6.13), anterior chamber flare, floating cells in the anterior chamber, posterior pupil synechiae, etc. Vitreous inflammatory cell infiltration (Fig. 6.14), occlusive retinal arteritis (Fig. 6.15), and yellow and white necrosis in the peripheral retina are also noted. Optical coherence tomography angiography may show decreased vascular density in the superficial and deep plexuses [178]. In the late stage, proliferative vitreoretinopathy, full-thickness necrotizing retinitis, and retinal detachment may develop.

Involvement of the second eye occurs in about one-third of patients, typically within 6 weeks [179], and some reports indicate that the contralateral eye may be affected even decades after the initial onset [180]. These reports suggest that inflammation and retinal necrosis tend to be less severe in the later-affected eye, resulting in fewer instances of retinal detachment and better visual outcomes [181].

Vision-threatening complications of ARN include retinal detachment, macular edema, ischemia, and optic neuropathy [182]. The retinal detachment rate is 37% for HSV-ARN and 46% for VZV-ARN; it is 52% in immunocompetent patients and 39% in immunocompromised patients [183]. Most often, retinal detachment in ARN is rhegmatogenous, occurring due to breaks and holes formed after retinal necrosis, while exudative retinal detachment should be particularly monitored in children with ARN [184].

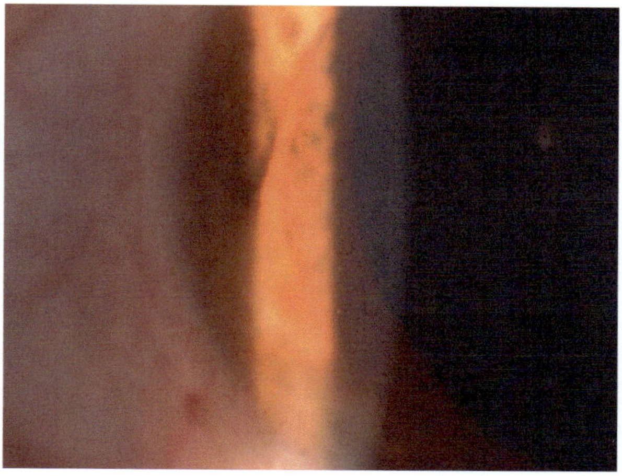

Fig. 6.13 The photograph shows the anterior segment of the right eye of a 48-year-old male presenting with red eye and blurred vision for half a month. The diagnosis of acute retinal necrosis was confirmed by clinical examination and a positive laboratory test for varicella-zoster virus DNA in the aqueous humor. Medium-sized fatty keratic precipitates are observable

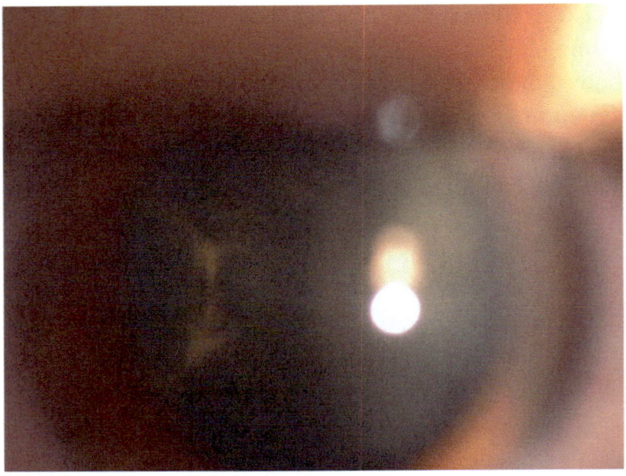

Fig. 6.14 This photograph pertains to the same patient as Fig. 6.13. Anterior vitreous opacity and inflammatory cell infiltration are evident

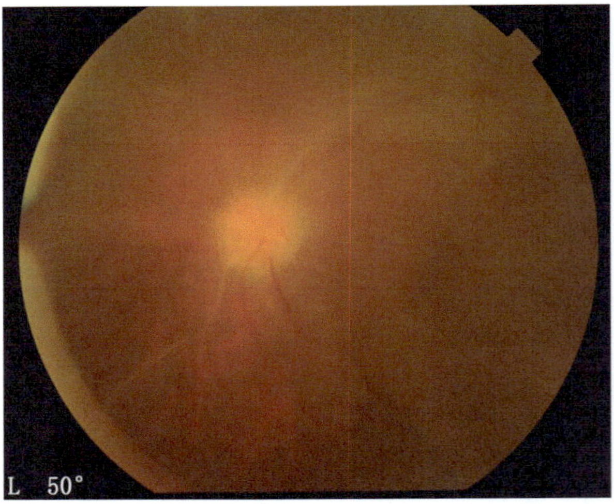

Fig. 6.15 The photograph reveals the posterior segment of the left eye of a 66-year-old male who has experienced blurred vision for 3 weeks. The diagnosis of acute retinal necrosis was confirmed by clinical examination and a positive laboratory test for varicella-zoster virus DNA in the aqueous humor. Occlusive retinal arteritis is visible

6.1.4.4 Diagnosis

The diagnostic criteria for acute retinal necrosis (ARN) have evolved from relying solely on clinical manifestations to incorporating a combination of clinical findings and laboratory examinations. In 1994, the Executive Committee of the American Uveitis Society defined ARN based on clinical characteristics [185]. In 2015, the Japanese ARN Study Group introduced new diagnostic criteria that combined clinical features indicative of ARN with laboratory results. These criteria included six early-stage ocular findings: [1a] anterior chamber cells or mutton-fat keratic precipitates, [1b] yellow-white lesions in the peripheral retina which appear granular or patchy in the early stage (Fig. 6.16) and then gradually merge (Fig. 6.17), [1c] retinal arteritis (Fig. 6.18), [1d] hyperemia of the optic disc (Fig. 6.19), [1e] inflammatory vitreous opacities, and [1f] elevated intraocular pressure. The clinical course aspects included [2a] rapid circumferential expansion of the retinal lesions

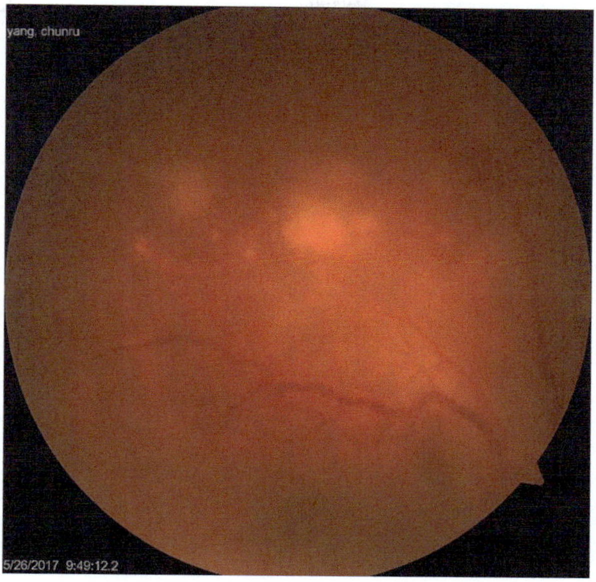

Fig. 6.16 The photograph shows the fundus of the right eye of a 54-year-old male with blurred vision for 2 weeks. The diagnosis of acute retinal necrosis was confirmed by clinical examination and positive varicella-zoster virus DNA and Goldmann-Witmer coefficient tests in the aqueous humor. Yellowish-white, granular, and patchy retinal necrosis is visible

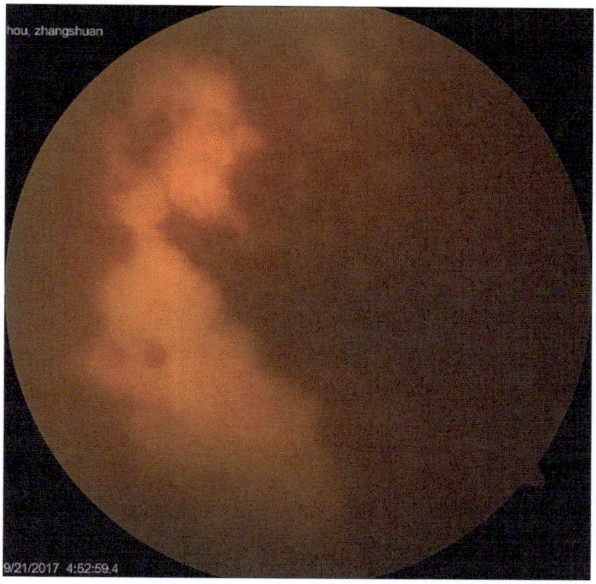

Fig. 6.17 This image depicts the fundus of the right eye of a 63-year-old male with blurred vision for 3 weeks. The diagnosis of acute retinal necrosis was confirmed by clinical examination and a positive aqueous humor varicella-zoster virus DNA test. Peripheral retinal necrosis that has merged can be seen

(Fig. 6.20), [2b] development of retinal breaks or detachment (Fig. 6.21), [2c] retinal vascular occlusion, [2d] optic atrophy, and [2e] response to antiviral agents. Laboratory analysis of intraocular fluids via polymerase chain reaction (PCR) or the Goldmann-Witmer coefficient for herpes simplex virus or varicella-zoster virus was also incorporated, enhancing the criteria,s sensitivity to 89% and specificity to 100% [186].

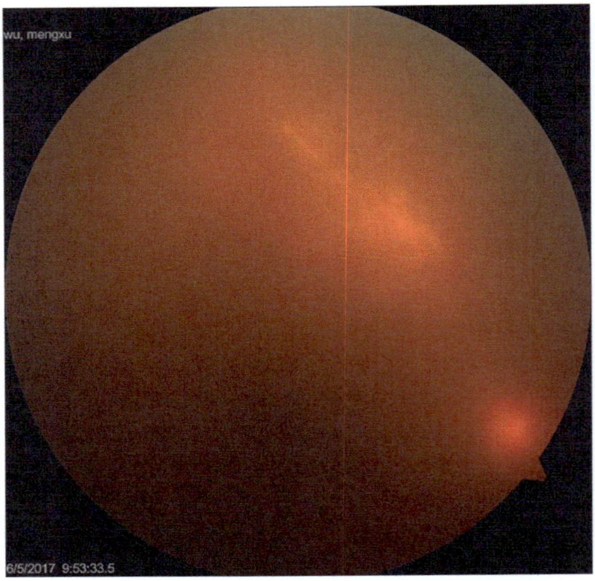

Fig. 6.18 The photograph captures the fundus of the right eye of a 54-year-old female with bilateral blurred vision for 2 months. Acute retinal necrosis was confirmed through clinical examination and a positive aqueous humor varicella-zoster virus DNA test. Retinal vasculitis and phlebitis of the superior temporal branch are observable

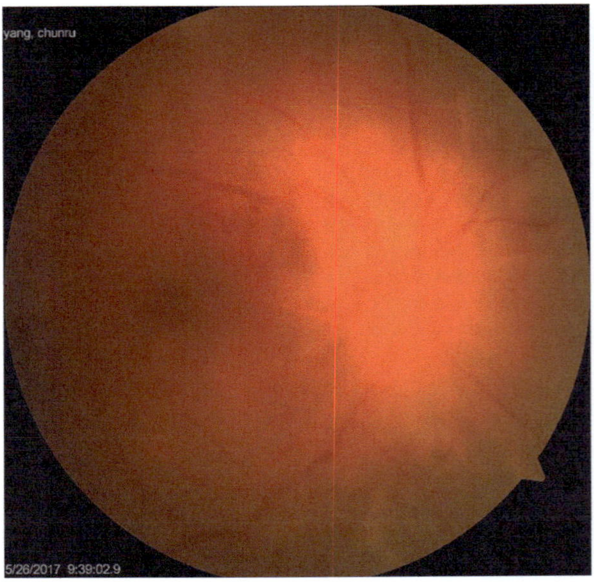

Fig. 6.19 This image shows the fundus of the right eye of the same patient from Fig. 6.16. Optic disc edema with an unclear boundary and congestion is evident

In 2017, the American Academy of Ophthalmology conducted a comprehensive review of the literature, emphasizing the importance of PCR testing of ocular fluids. The Academy recognized this test as a valuable tool to support the clinical diagnosis of ARN [187].

By 2021, the PCR assay of intraocular fluid specimens, positive for either HSV or VZV, was adopted by the Standardization of Uveitis Nomenclature (SUN) Working Group as one of the essential classification criteria for ARN [188].

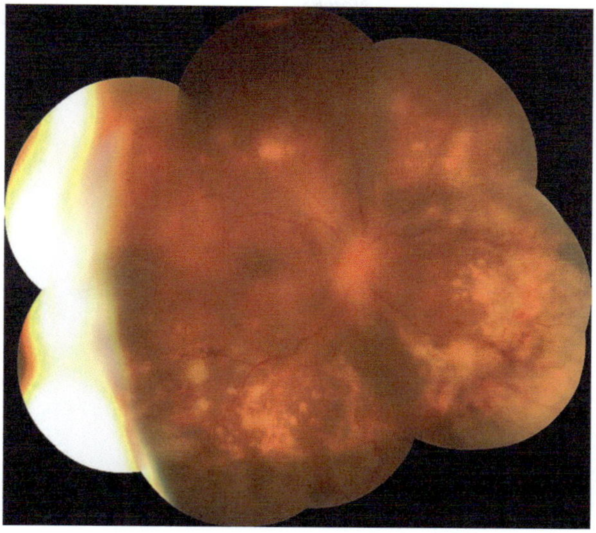

Fig. 6.20 The photograph of the fundus of the right eye of the same patient from Fig. 6.16 shows rapid circumferential expansion of retinal necrosis progressing rapidly toward the posterior pole

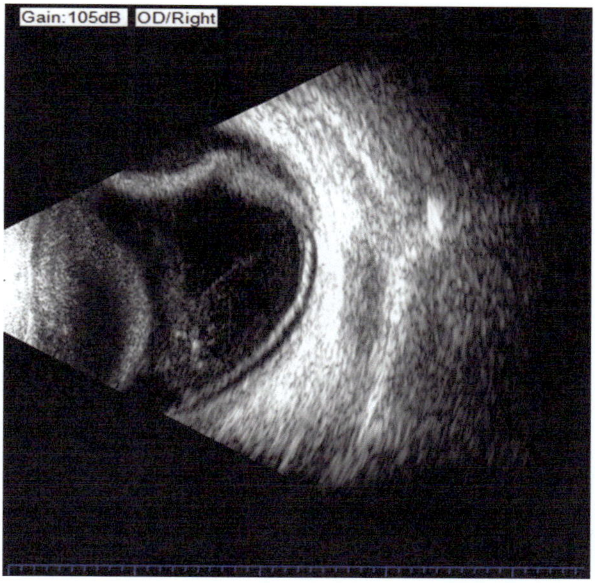

Fig. 6.21 This image depicts the fundus of the right eye of a 60-year-old male with blurred vision for 20 days. The diagnosis of acute retinal necrosis was confirmed by clinical examination and a positive varicella-zoster virus DNA test in the aqueous humor. The patient's visual acuity deteriorated rapidly from 0.3 to merely hand movements within 2 months post-antiviral treatment. B-ultrasound examination confirmed the presumed diagnosis of retinal detachment

6.1.4.5 Examination of Intraocular Fluids

Extensive research has demonstrated the efficacy of viral DNA testing on aqueous and vitreous samples in diagnosing ARN. Selected studies and their outcomes are summarized in Table 6.1.

ARN secondary to HSV-2 tended to have persistent active retinitis with a higher rate of retinal detachment despite the implementation of similar treatment protocols: retinal detachment was found to transpire in 25% of cases involving varicella-zoster virus, whereas HSV-2 cases exhibited a significantly higher rate of 75%

Table 6.1 Studies reporting viral DNA testing in acute retinal necrosis

Authors	Publication time	Total patient number	Samples	Eyes with positive examination of viral DNA		Positive rate	
Nishi et al. [164]	1992	4 eyes	Vitreous, aqueous humor and subretinal fluids	VZV	3 eyes	75.0%	3 eyes, 75.0%
Itoh et al. [189]	2000	16 eyes	Vitreous and aqueous humor	HSV-2	7 eyes	43.8%	16 eyes, 100%
				VZV	9 eyes	56.2%	
Lau et al. [190]	2007	18 eyes	Vitreous	VZV	9 eyes	50.0%	16 eyes, 88.9%
				VZV and EB	3 eyes	16.7%	
				HSV	4 eyes	22.2%	
Sugita et al. [191]	2008	16 eyes	Vitreous and aqueous humor	HSV-1	2 eyes	12.5%	16 eyes, 100%
				HSV-2	3 eyes	18.8%	
				VZV	11 eyes	68.8%	
Hillenkamp et al. [192]	2009	30 eyes	Vitreous	VZV	23 eyes	76.7%	30 eyes, 100%
				VZV and EB	2 eyes	6.7%	
				VZV and HSV	1 eye	3.3%	
				HSV	4 eyes	16.7%	
Wong et al. [193]	2010	81 eyes	Vitreous	VZV	48 eyes	59.3%	81 eyes, 100%
				HSV	33 eyes	40.8%	
Zhao et al. [194]	2017	18 eyes	Vitreous and aqueous humor	VZV	15 eyes	83.3%	16 eyes, 88.9%
				HSV-1 and EB	1 eyes	5.6%	
Alireza Hedayatfar et al. [195]	2021	19 eyes	Aqueous humor	VZV	14 eyes	73.7%	18 eyes 94.7%
				HSV	3 eyes	15.8%	
				CMV	1eye	5.3%	

[196]. For ARN patients treated with intravenous acyclovir and intravitreal injections of antiviral drugs, the intraocular VZV-DNA load decreased according to a logarithmic model, with a 50% reduction in the load achieved within an average timeframe of 3 ± 0.7 days. There was a significant viral load (>100 copies/mL) at 50 days after the onset of treatment. VZV DNA showed reproducible kinetics with a two-phase evolution: a plateau followed by a logarithmic decrease [197]. Furthermore, eyes with a quantitative PCR DNA copy number of $\geq 5.0 \times 10^6$/mL had worse final visual acuity ($P = 0.007$) compared with patients with a DNA copy number $<5.0 \times 10^6$/mL [198].

Detection of Goldmann-Witmer coefficient of HSV/VZV antibody has laboratory diagnostic value for both active stage [165] and regression stage of ARN. In cases of ARN, both VZV antibody Goldmann-Witmer coefficient and VZV nucleic acid exhibit high specificity [135, 136], and the positive VZV or HSV antibody Goldmann-Witmer coefficient could be established in 57% of the patients displaying the typical clinical manifestations of ARN, whereas none of the control subjects exhibited a positive coefficient [165].

CD8+ T lymphocytes population in AH from ARN patients were higher than in AAU patients ($p = 0.006$). CD4/CD8 ratios of T lymphocytes and the percentage of CD8 + CD25+ T lymphocytes in AH were significantly lower in ARN than in AAU ($p = 0.006$; $p = 0.012$) [199]. In ARN, proinflammatory and vascular mediators including IFN-γ, IL-6, IL-8, IL-18, MIF, MCP-1, eotaxin, IP-10, IL-15, sICAM-1, sVCAM-1, and anti-inflammatory mediator (IL-10) were significantly elevated in ARN compared to the controls [200, 201].

6.1.4.6 Management

The initial treatment most frequently mentioned in literature consists of intravenous administration of acyclovir or oral administration of valaciclovir [187]. The classic treatment regimen is intravenous acyclovir (1500 mg/m^2/day) for 5–10 days followed by oral acyclovir (800 mg, 5 times a day) for 4–6 weeks [202–205]. There exists levels II and III data supporting the use of intravenous or oral acyclovir as a preventive measure against the development of ARN in the contralateral eye [187].

The bioavailability of valaciclovir ranges from 54% to 60%, which is approximately three to five times greater than that of acyclovir. After oral administration, the substance undergoes metabolism to form acyclovir, which is responsible for its pharmacological actions. However, the bioavailability of acyclovir is limited to a range of 15%–30% [206]. The peak concentration and area of the concentration time curve of acyclovir produced by oral valaciclovir 250 mg four times a day are close to those observed with oral acyclovir 800 mg five times a day [207].

The administration of ganciclovir via intravitreal injection has demonstrated efficacy in numerous cases across diverse geographical regions [208]. It is suggested that intraocular injection of antiviral drugs should be carried out together with systemic treatment. The results of the comparison analysis demonstrated that the combination treatment approach, involving intravitreal antiviral injection and systemic antiviral medicines, yielded superior outcomes compared to the single systemic antiviral therapy. Specifically, this combined treatment approach was associated with reduced severity of vision loss and a greater likelihood of achieving a significant improvement in vision by at least two lines [209]. Intravitreal injection of foscarnet has also been reported to be used for treatment of ARN, particularly in cases resistant to acyclovir [187, 210]. A 10-year retrospective study showed that 66.12% of eyes with ARN had secondary retinal detachment when systemic antiviral drugs and glucocorticoids were used as the main treatment regimen [211]; comparatively, if the intravitreal injection of antiviral drugs be the main treatment, the proportion of secondary retinal detachment is 16% [212]. There is a lack of unanimity about the role of prophylactic laser retinopexy or early vitrectomy [187].

Antithrombotic treatment employing a modest dosage of aspirin is commonly administered due to the prevalence of occlusive retinal vasculitis and phlebitis in the majority of severe instances of the condition [205]. Oral aspirin can improve the hypercoagulable state of platelets and hereby mitigate retinal ischemia [213]. The recommended dose of aspirin for oral use is 100 mg/day for HSV-ARN and 200–300 mg/day for VZV-ARN [205].

The pathogenic mechanism of ARN includes not only the direct destruction of tissue and cells by virus but also the intense inflammatory response. Therefore, it is essential to give appropriate anti-inflammatory treatment in the process of antivirus. Oral glucocorticoids are usually given 24–48 h after the start of antiviral treatment (prednisone 1 mg/kg/day, tapered) [203]. Topical treatment includes eye drops of 0.1% betamethasone or dexamethasone six to eight times daily combined with midriatics such as atropine sulfate and tropicamide [205].

6.1.5 Progressive Outer Retinal Necrosis

6.1.5.1 Brief Introduction

Progressive outer retinal necrosis (PORN) is characterized as necrotizing retinitis predominantly caused by herpesvirus, primarily the varicella-zoster virus (VZV). This condition initially targets the outer retinal layer and is marked by rapid clinical progression. Although PORN is rare, it poses a significant risk of visual impairment [214, 215]. In 1990, Forster first described this condition in two AIDS patients, coining the term "progressive outer retinal necrosis" [215]. The disease mainly affects severely immunocompromised patients, especially those with acquired immunodeficiency syndrome (AIDS) [216, 217], with CD4+ lymphocyte counts often nearing or below 20/mm^3 [218–221]. Histological studies have revealed intranuclear inclusions consistent with viral particles in choroidal cells [222].

6.1.5.2 Epidemiology

Most PORN cases occur in AIDS patients. Reports also describe PORN in patients with lupus erythematosus undergoing immunosuppressive treatment [223, 224], individuals with microscopic polyangiitis (MPA) treated with cyclophosphamide and rituximab [225], patients post-bone marrow transplantation [226, 227], and multiple sclerosis patients on natalizumab [228]. A history of cutaneous zoster is documented in 67% of patients [218].

6.1.5.3 Clinical Manifestation

Patients typically present with painless blurred vision [216], peripheral vision loss [229], or sudden vision loss [230]. Clinically, the disease manifests as single or multifocal, irregularly sized, deep, necrotic yellowish-white retinal lesions, often without vitreous inflammation [230–232]. These lesions typically appear as outer retinal whitening observable in clinical settings (Fig. 6.22) [233] and may exhibit fusion and patchy necrosis in the periphery, showing rapid progression (Fig. 6.23) [216]. A "cherry red spot" may appear in cases affecting both maculae, accompanied by peripheral atrophy and pigmentary changes [234]. In the late stage, a diffused thin remnant of the retina and retinal holes formed post-necrosis can lead to a high rate of rhegmatogenous retinal detachment.

Fluorescein angiography may show zonal microvascular alterations, retinal pigment epithelium (RPE) destruction, and choroidal leakage. Retinal damage is closely correlated with areas of choroidal leakage. A prominent brush-fire border of intense leakage involving the retina, RPE, and choroid may indicate disease reactivation [233].

Optical coherence tomography (OCT) is a valuable tool for early diagnosis. OCT can detect edema in the outer retina, outer retinal disorganization, or areas of extremely low reflectivity with well-defined but irregular borders during active retinitis (Fig. 6.24). In later stages, OCT may reveal extremely thin remnants of the retina in areas of prior necrosis (Fig. 6.25) [231, 235, 236].

Secondary complications such as optic neuritis, cilioretinal artery occlusion, retinal artery occlusion, or combined central retinal vein and artery occlusions require careful monitoring [216, 230, 237].

6.1.5.4 Diagnosis

The diagnosis of this disease is primarily based on clinical manifestations. A presumed case of PORN should be considered if the following criteria are met: (1) immunocompromised condition, especially a history of AIDS; (2) blood CD4+ T

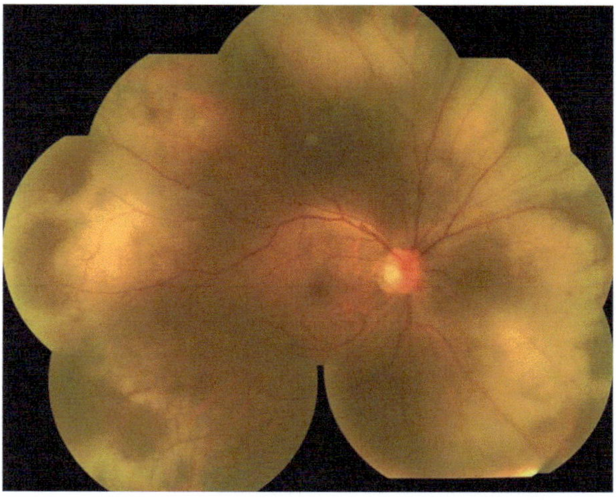

Fig. 6.22 Fundus photography of a patient with progressive outer retinal necrosis, showing deep and blurred necrotic lesions in the peripheral and mid-peripheral areas of the retina. (Courtesy of Prof. Ian Y Wong, Department of Ophthalmology, Hong Kong Sanatorium and Hospital)

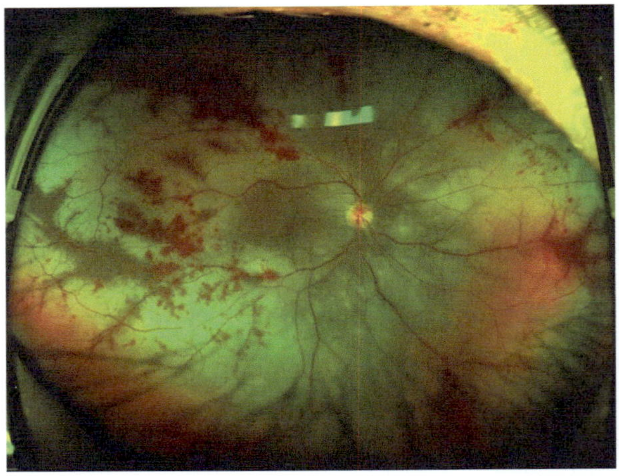

Fig. 6.23 Fundus photography of a patient with progressive outer retinal necrosis, depicting rapidly progressive necrotic retinitis with retinal hemorrhage and clear vitreous. The viral load as determined by PCR was 1.23×10^7 copies/mL for VZV. (Courtesy of Prof. Wenjun Kong, Department of Ophthalmology, Beijing Youan Hospital, Capital Medical University, Beijing, China)

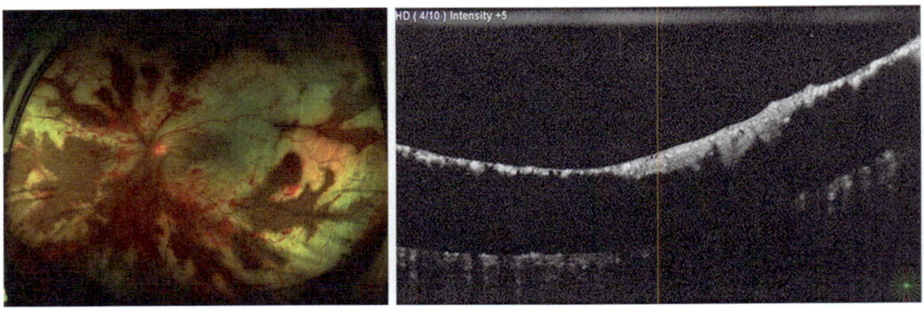

Fig. 6.24 Optical coherence tomography of a patient with progressive outer retinal necrosis, illustrating outer retinal disorganization. (Courtesy of Prof. Ian Y Wong, Department of Ophthalmology, Hong Kong Sanatorium and Hospital, Hongkong, China)

cells <50/mm^3; (3) multifocal and patchy white retinal lesions that can appear anywhere on the retina; (4) necrosis of the outer layer of the retina at the early stage of the disease, with involvement of the entire retinal and choroidal layers at the later stages; (5) little or no bleeding; (6) lack of vitritis and inflammation; and (7) rapidly progressive development of the disease. Detection of VZV in intraocular fluid is of significant diagnostic value.

This disease primarily needs to be differentiated from acute retinal necrosis. One of the main differences is the speed of progression; PORN progresses more rapidly and initially affects the outer layer of the retina without vascular inflammation or scleritis. Vitreous opacity and anterior chamber inflammatory reaction are typically unremarkable [215].

6.1.5.5 Examination of Intraocular Fluids

Polymerase chain reaction (PCR) is very useful in identifying the causative agent [222], and PCR of the viral DNA in the aqueous and vitreous humors is diagnostic for PORN [238]. Although herpes simplex virus type 1 [239], herpes simplex virus

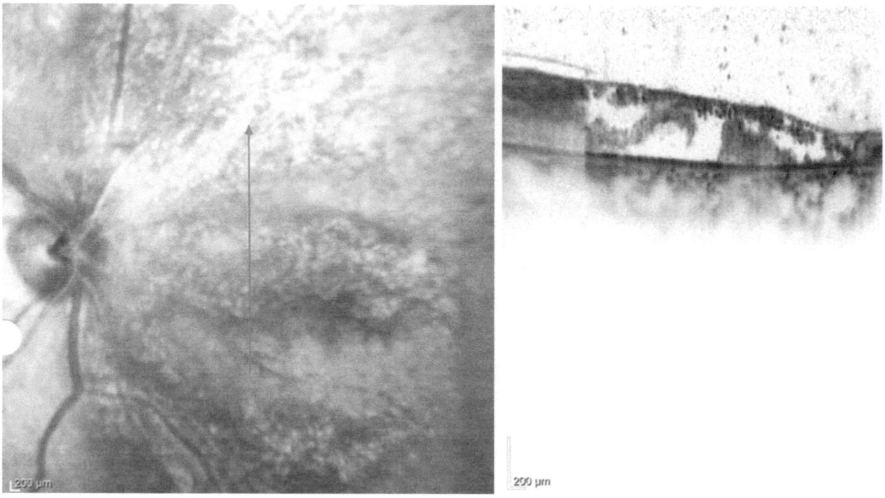

Fig. 6.25 Fundus photography (left) and optical coherence tomography (right) of a patient with late-stage progressive outer retinal necrosis, showing a diffused thin remnant of retina. The viral load as determined by PCR was 5.81 × 10^4 copies/mL for VZV. (Courtesy of Prof. Wenjun Kong, Department of Ophthalmology, Beijing Youan Hospital, Capital Medical University, Beijing, China)

type 2 [240], CMV, and *Mycobacterium avium* intracellulare duodenitis [219], as well as HIV [230, 241] and dual virus infections [242], may rarely cause PORN, the vast majority of cases are due to varicella-zoster virus (VZV) [230, 243–250]. For patients undergoing multiple intravitreal injections of antiviral drugs, serial PCR for VZV may be performed on aqueous humor to monitor the clinical course [251].

6.1.5.6 Management

The disease progresses rapidly, and once diagnosed, treatment should commence immediately [217, 224]. The typical treatment strategy combines intravenous foscarnet and acyclovir with intravitreal injections of ganciclovir. This regimen lasts for 3 weeks, followed by the administration of oral acyclovir [230]. Alternatively, sorivudine, administered orally at 40 mg daily alongside ganciclovir injections, has shown effectiveness, with retinitis improving and becoming inactive within 2 weeks [252].

Case studies have indicated that administering a single intravenous dose of foscarnet at 60 mg per kg of body weight, three times per week, did not yield satisfactory results. However, initiating treatment with intravitreal ganciclovir at a dosage of 400 mg twice per week led to the remission of retinal necrosis [253]. Intravitreal ganciclovir offers a more targeted approach and, compared with earlier reports using systemic therapy alone, may result in better visual outcomes [245]. The initiation of twice-weekly intravitreal injections using dual antiviral drugs, including ganciclovir (2 mg/0.05 mL) and foscarnet (1.2 mg/0.05 mL), has been reported to lead to remission of PORN [251].

The prognosis for this disease is generally poor [217]. Despite intensive intravenous antiviral therapy, rapidly progressive widespread retinal involvement may lead to the development of rhegmatogenous retinal detachment [232], which occurs in 51–70% of cases and significantly worsens visual outcomes [218, 245]. Visual acuity was NLP (no light perception) in 67% of eyes within 4 weeks after diagnosis [218]. Pars plana vitrectomy (PPV) and silicone oil injection may be employed to treat rhegmatogenous retinal detachment secondary to PORN [254]. Aggressive vitrectomy techniques aimed at repairing any associated detachments may help preserve useful visual acuity [255]. Currently, there is no consensus on the efficacy of early photocoagulation in preventing the development of retinal detachment, provided that retinal necrosis is effectively controlled [253].

6.1.6 HTLV-1-Associated Uveitis

6.1.6.1 Brief Introduction

Human T-lymphotropic virus type 1 (HTLV-1), the first human oncogenic retrovirus, belongs to the type C retroviruses in the *Deltaretrovirus* genus [256] and is known to cause persistent infections [257]. Ocular manifestations of HTLV-1 can be primarily classified into three groups: uveitis, opportunistic infection or malignant infiltration of the eye in adult T-cell leukemia/lymphoma (ATL) patients, and keratoconjunctivitis sicca [258].

HTLV-1 is mainly transmitted through sexual contact, blood transfusion, and from mother to child [259]. There is a trend of family aggregation in HTLV-1-associated diseases [257]. HTLV-1-associated uveitis is an infectious uveitis triggered by HTLV-1, with a documented correlation between HTLV-1 uveitis and Graves' disease [260, 261]. The transmission rate of HTLV-1 from males to females is four times higher than from females to males [262, 263]. The gender ratio (female/male) of patients with HTLV-1-associated uveitis is 2.0 [261]. The peak age of uveitis onset is in the 50s for women, followed by the 60s, and in the 60s for men, followed by the 70s [264, 265]. Recurrence of uveitis is seen in 30–52% of patients with HTLV-1-associated uveitis [261, 264–266].

6.1.6.2 Epidemiology

An estimated 5–10 million people are infected with HTLV-1 worldwide, predominantly residing in endemic areas such as Japan, Africa, Latin America, Australia, the Caribbean islands, and the Middle East, particularly in Iranian cities like Mashhad, Sabzevar, and Neyshabur [256, 267, 268]. The Kyushu region of Japan has one of the highest prevalences of HTLV-1 globally, with the highest carrier rate in the region reported at 8%, compared to 0.3–1.2% in other regions of Japan [269, 270].

The frequency of HTLV-1-associated uveitis across Japan is approximately 0.8% [270, 271]. A nationwide survey in Japan revealed that 85.5% of healthcare facilities reported no noticeable decline in the number of individuals seeking treatment for HTLV-1-associated uveitis [272]. The prevalence of HTLV-1 is significantly higher in specific groups such as sex workers, people infected with the human immunodeficiency virus, and intravenous drug users, with rates up to 20% [273]. Sociodemographic analysis shows that HTLV-1-infected individuals often have lower educational levels, and the prevalence of HTLV-1 infection increases with age [262, 263].

6.1.6.3 Clinical Manifestation

The primary symptoms of HTLV-1-associated uveitis at the initial presentation include ocular floaters (33.3%), foggy vision (34.5%), and blurred vision (15.5%) [261, 264]. Patients also report pain, burning, itching, and a sensation of a foreign body in the eye [258, 274, 275]. The inflammation can be either unilateral or bilateral [270, 274, 276, 277].

HTLV-1-associated uveitis primarily manifests as intermediate uveitis, characterized by moderate to severe vitreous opacity, including fine cells and reticular membranous opacity. Vitreous opacity (Fig. 6.26) is the most significant clinical feature, which may coexist with mild iritis and mild retinal vasculitis but without chorioretinal lesions [274]. Slit lamp examination may reveal corneal deposits, fibrin exudation, hypopyon, anterior chamber flare, floating cells, iris nodules, and posterior synechiae in the anterior chamber [278, 279]. Although anterior uveitis and retinal vasculitis may occur, they typically present in a mild form [264].

Nearly half of the patients (43.8%) experience ocular complications such as cystic macular edema, macular epiretinal membrane, and optic nerve damage [261]. Some cases may also be complicated by cataract and glaucoma [261, 274, 277, 280–282].

6.1.6.4 Diagnosis

HTLV-1-associated uveitis is typically diagnosed based on blood tests and distinct ophthalmic findings, specifically the presence of uveitis and confirmation of HTLV-1 infection [264]. Blood tests for diagnosing this condition include the detection of

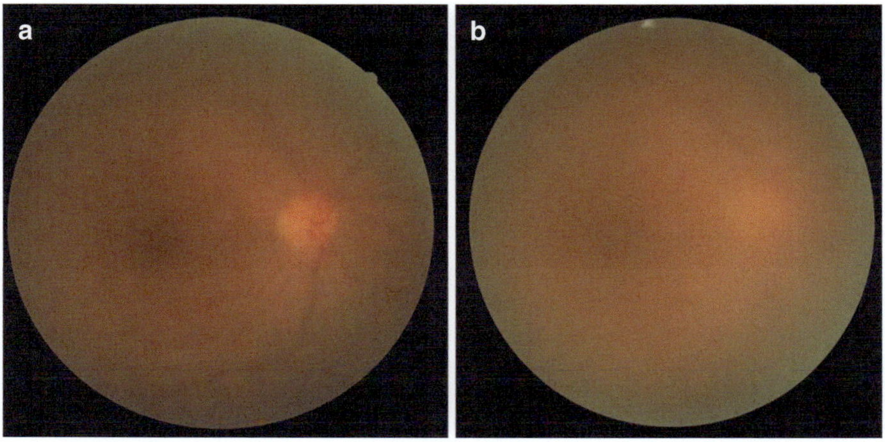

Fig. 6.26 Fundus photography of a patient with HTLV-1-associated uveitis showing the progression of vitreous opacity from a mild state (**a**) to a severe state (**b**). (Courtesy of Prof. Koh-Hei Sonoda, Department of Ophthalmology, Graduate School of Medical Sciences, Kyushu University, Fukuoka, Japan)

serum HTLV-1 antibodies by enzyme-linked immunoassay or particle agglutination, detection of HTLV-1 proteins by Western blot, or detection of the proviral pX region by polymerase chain reaction (PCR) [264, 283]. The seroprevalence of HTLV-1 infection is significantly higher in patients with uveitis of unknown cause (35%) compared to those with etiology-defined uveitis (10%) or non-uveitic ocular diseases (16%) [284]. The HTLV-1 proviral load (pVL) in peripheral blood mononuclear cells (PBMCs) is suggested as a marker of disease progression [285].

Additionally, the absence of systemic evidence of HTLV-1-related diseases such as ATL (adult T-cell leukemia/lymphoma) or HAM/TSP (HTLV-1-associated myelopathy/tropical spastic paraparesis) is required [275], and other etiologies of defined uveitis must be ruled out through comprehensive ophthalmic and systemic examinations, including Behçet's disease, Vogt-Koyanagi-Harada syndrome, and sarcoidosis [258, 264, 275].

6.1.6.5 Examination of Intraocular Fluids

In patients with HTLV-1-associated uveitis, the floating cells in the anterior chamber are predominantly lymphocytes with a small proportion of macrophages [275]. The majority of infiltrating cells in the aqueous humor are CD3+ T cells [286], indicating a specific immune response characteristic of this viral infection.

HTLV-1 proviral DNA, HTLV-1 protein, and viral particles have been detected in ocular infiltrating cells within the eyes of patients with HTLV-1 uveitis [258, 287, 288]. PCR analysis revealed the presence of HTLV-1 proviral DNA exclusively in the inflammatory cells located in the anterior chamber of all seropositive uveitis patients. In contrast, none of the patients with other forms of uveitis showed the presence of this proviral DNA, indicating that HTLV-1 is a specific causative agent for this distinct type of intraocular inflammation [284]. Advanced molecular techniques such as multiplex PCR/broad-range PCR using ocular samples have facilitated rapid and accurate diagnoses [264].

Cytokines produced by HTLV-1-infected T cell clones (TCC) established from ocular fluids of patients with HTLV-1 uveitis include high amounts of Interleukin (IL)-1 alpha, IL-3, IL-6, IL-8, TNF-alpha, IFN-gamma, and GM-CSF, with significant but lower levels of IL-2 and IL-10 [289]. These findings support the use of immunosuppressive therapy in managing HTLV-1-associated uveitis.

6.1.6.6 Management

Despite potential complications such as cystic macular edema, macular epiretinal membrane, and optic nerve damage, which can lead to visual loss, the overall visual prognosis for HTLV-1-associated uveitis is generally good. Corticosteroids, which inhibit cytokine production by T lymphocytes, are effective for mild intraocular inflammation and can be administered locally. For complications like cystic macular edema, systemic corticosteroid treatment is recommended and can restore normal vision effectively. Mild vitreous cavity inflammation may be treated with an intraocular injection of triamcinolone acetonide. More severe vitreous cavity inflammation and retinal vasculitis may require oral prednisone; however, long-term steroid use should be avoided. Typically, HTLV-1-associated uveitis is alleviated after 4 weeks of treatment, with ongoing clinical management adjusted based on the level of intraocular inflammation [258, 270]. Although most patients improve or fully resolve intraocular inflammation post-corticosteroid treatment, about 60% may experience a relapse of uveitis and develop secondary glaucoma, necessitating glaucoma filtering surgery or trabeculotomy [258, 270].

Additionally, a combination of zidovudine (AZT) and IFN-α is considered an effective treatment for HTLV-1 infections [256]. Recent studies suggest that blocking PD-1 signaling enhances the immune response during the chronic phase of HTLV-1 infection, particularly given the expression of PD-1 in ATL and HAM/TSP cases. This could provide a new direction for future treatments of HTLV-1-associated uveitis [268].

6.1.7 Fuchs' Uveitis Syndrome

6.1.7.1 Brief Introduction

Fuchs' uveitis syndrome (FUS) is a chronic, low-grade inflammatory disorder that primarily affects the anterior uvea and vitreous [290]. Originally described by Ernest Fuchs in 1906, the condition has historically been known by various names, including Fuchs' heterochromic cyclitis, Fuchs' heterochromatic iridocyclitis, and Fuchs' heterochromatic uveitis. In more recent discussions, it is commonly referred to as Fuchs' uveitis syndrome [291–293].

FUS is characterized by mild inflammatory symptoms that can lead to stellate keratic precipitates, iris atrophy (which may occur with or without heterochromia), mild flare, and minimal cellular presence in the anterior chamber, along with vitreous opacity, cataract formation, and secondary glaucoma [294]. The disease typically manifests between the ages of 20 and 45 [294–299], and most cases are unilateral [300]. Epidemiological data on gender distribution vary, with some reports indicating a balanced prevalence between men and women. For instance, Massimo Accorinti noted that men constituted 49.4% of FUS patients at a tertiary referral center in Italy, while Babu K et al. reported that men accounted for 56.9% of FUS cases in southern India. In contrast, Nasrollahi K found that 55% of FUS patients were female in Iran [301–303].

6.1.7.2 Epidemiology

Fuchs' uveitis syndrome (FUS) is reported globally and is typically ranked in the middle to upper echelon of prevalence among uveitis cases. In the Iranian population, FUS ranks as the fourth most common type of uveitis [304]. A review of 26 studies (involving 24,126 patients with uveitis) from 12 European countries found that FUS accounted for 6.1% of uveitis cases [305]. In Poland, FUS constituted 12.2% of uveitis cases [305], while a German interdisciplinary uveitis center reported that FUS made up 34.3% of the ocular syndrome subtype of uveitis [306]. In Northeast China, FUS represented 9.41% of total anterior uveitis cases [307], and in Turkey, it accounted for 14.6% of anterior uveitis cases [308].

Among anterior uveitis cases caused by cytomegalovirus (CMV), most (93.3%) displayed clinical characteristics of Posner-Schlossman syndrome, with 6.7% exhibiting keratic precipitates similar to those seen in FUS [6].

6.1.7.3 Clinical Manifestation

The most common symptoms of FUS at initial presentation are decreased visual acuity or blurred vision and floaters [299, 309, 310]. Typical findings include diffuse small, white, stellate keratic precipitates (Fig. 6.27), mild anterior chamber reaction featuring flare and floater cells, heterochromia (Fig. 6.28), and iris nodules, absence of posterior synechiae, elevated intraocular pressure, posterior subcapsular cataract (Fig. 6.29), and vitreous cells and debris (Fig. 6.30) [298, 299, 309]. Often, the classical FUS presentation is not observed at first [299], and characteristic findings may be absent at the disease onset. Secondary complications such as cataract, ocular hypertension, or glaucomatous disc damage generally emerge after an average disease duration of 10–20 years [311].

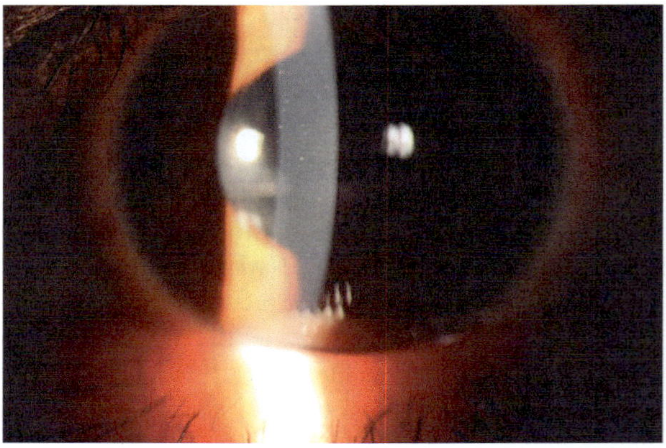

Fig. 6.27 Anterior segment photography of an eye affected by Fuchs' uveitis syndrome (FUS), displaying diffuse stellate keratic precipitates

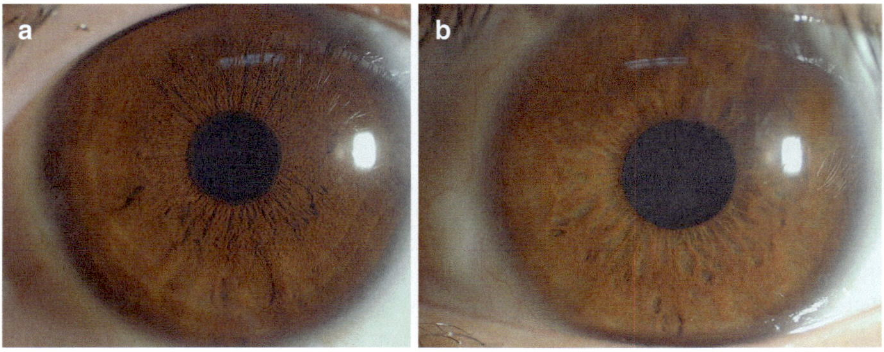

Fig. 6.28 Anterior segment photography comparing both eyes of a patient with FUS; (**a**) shows the normal iris color of the unaffected eye, while (**b**) illustrates heterochromia in the FUS-affected eye

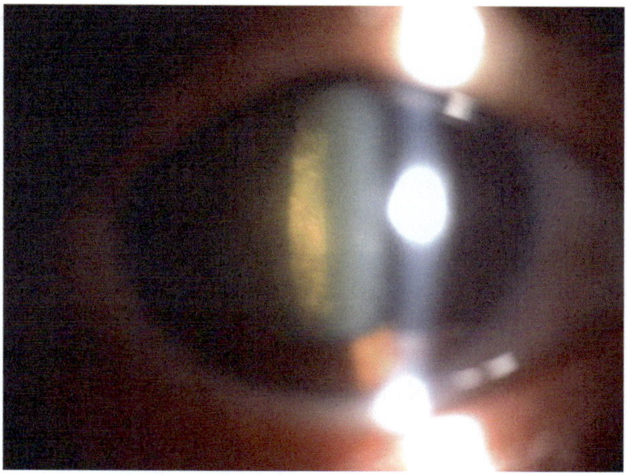

Fig. 6.29 Anterior segment photography of an eye with FUS, highlighting a posterior subcapsular cataract

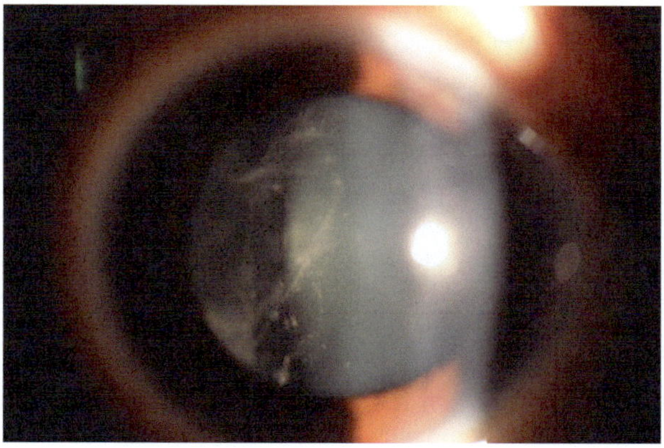

Fig. 6.30 Image showing vitreous opacity and debris characteristic of an eye with FUS

Atypical KPs in a minority of patients may appear in varied sizes from small to large with a triangular distribution over the inferior corneal endothelium [312]. KPs in FUS cause focal damage to endothelial cells, reflected in a decreased percentage of healthy hexagonal cells [313], and corneal endothelial cell density and the percentage of hexagonal cells are lower than in healthy eyes [314–316].

Auxiliary examinations contribute to the further and quantitative evaluation of lesions in FUS. Predominant morphologies of KPs shown by confocal scan were dendritiform (80.0%) and infiltrating (78.0%) [317]. Fluorophotometry can help reveal an abnormally permeable blood-aqueous barrier in FUS eyes [318]. Exudates adjacent to the ciliary body were common in patients studied by UBM [300]. In eyes with FUS, moderate but discontinuous autofluorescence in the pigment ruff, a petaloid pattern of autofluorescence in the pupillary zone, moderate autofluorescence in the collarette, and a reticular pattern of autofluorescence in the ciliary zone and optic nerve head hyperfluorescence may be observed [319, 320].

Fundus fluorescein angiography may show optic disc hyperfluorescence, mild vascular leakage, and an epiretinal membrane [303, 310, 321]. Furthermore, foveal vascular density in the superior deep capillary plexuses, radial peripapillary capillary vessel density, and the choroidal vascularity index were significantly lower in the FUS group than in normal eyes [322–325]. OCT revealed decreased mean subfoveal choroidal thickness; ganglion cell complex thickness; and RNFL thickness, with diffuse and full-thickness choroidal thinning in FUS eyes; and a more remarkable intereye subfoveal choroidal thickness difference between FUS and contralateral eyes [298, 326–329]. Electrophysiological examination contributes to the diagnosis and monitoring of FUS progression and treatment efficacy [329]. Furthermore, blood tests, including mean lymphocyte count, mean monocyte count, LMR (lymphocyte-to-monocyte ratio), PLR (platelet to lymphocyte ratio), and NLR (neutrophil to lymphocyte ratio), varied significantly between the FUS group and healthy controls [330, 331].

6.1.7.4 Diagnosis

In the current era, where there are no definitive diagnostic laboratory tests for Fuchs' uveitis syndrome (FUS), predominant clinical findings have been distinguished and combined to form clinical diagnostic criteria [293]. Essential findings, which must all be present, include the absence of acute symptoms (severe redness, pain, and photophobia), characteristic keratic precipitates and/or minimal cells and flare in the aqueous (1+ or 2+), diffuse iris stromal atrophy, and the absence of synechiae. Associated findings, of which at least two must be present, include the unilaterality of the uveitis, heterochromia, iris posterior pigment epithelium atrophy, subcapsular cataract, elevated intraocular pressure, vitreous opacities, and chorioretinal lesions [293]. The mean delay in diagnosis ranges from 4.6 to 13 years [300, 332]. Misdiagnosis of FUS, particularly among young patients, is common [321].

Recently, a set of revised diagnostic criteria, recommended for their high sensitivity (96.55%) and specificity (97.42%), has been proposed [333]. These include three essential findings required for diagnosing FUS: diffuse iris depigmentation, absence of posterior synechiae, and mild inflammation in the anterior chamber at presentation. Additionally, five associated findings that may further strengthen the diagnosis of FUS include predominantly unilateral involvement, cataract, vitreous opacities, absence of acute symptoms, and characteristic iris nodules.

The Classification Criteria for Fuchs Uveitis Syndrome, as outlined by the Standardization of Uveitis Nomenclature (SUN) Working Group, are as follows: key criteria include unilateral anterior uveitis with or without vitritis and either (1) heterochromia or (2) unilateral diffuse iris atrophy and stellate keratic precipitates. The misclassification rates for FUS were 4.7% in the training set and 5.5% in the validation set, respectively [334].

6.1.7.5 Examination of Intraocular Fluids

Several viruses, including rubella virus (RV) [335–337], herpes simplex virus [335, 338], CMV [339, 340], and chikungunya virus [341, 342], as well as parasites such as *Toxoplasma gondii* [343], have been reported to be related to FUS, with RV and CMV regarded as the main causes [25, 344].

The relationship between RV and FUS has been reported in different centers across various regions. The vitreous fluid from a 73-year-old male patient showing notable FUS alterations, including iris darkening in the left eye, was subjected to real-time RT-PCR analysis. The findings indicated the presence of RV RNA. The patient's medical history revealed an occurrence of a localized outbreak of RV infection during his adolescence at the age of 14 [345].

Among FUS eyes, the positive rate of RV by PCR was 20% [299]. However, more reports were about the detection of RV antibodies in the intraocular fluids. RV antibodies were positive in the intraocular fluids, including aqueous humor and vitreous, in 73–100% of FUS cases. However, no such antibodies were observed in the control group, and no other types of antibodies were identified [335–337]. Consistently, 91.67% (11/12) of FUS patients had a positive Goldmann-Witmer coefficient for RV [346]. Recently published literature has used "RV-associated uveitis" instead of FUS to distinctively define the enrolled patients in the study [299, 332, 347, 348]. Being positive for intraocular antibody production against RV or the Goldmann-Witmer coefficient determination and/or polymerase chain reaction of RV helps confirm the diagnosis of RV-associated uveitis [347]. Among the eyes positive for RV in aqueous fluid, 20% were by PCR, 97% by GWC, and 13% by both [299].

In the European population, occurrences of FUS are primarily linked to RV rather than CMV [6, 10, 47], whereas CMV infection is responsible for 16% to 42% of FUS cases in Asian populations [4, 294, 339]. Among the patients with confirmed intraocular infection of CMV, 10–20.8% had featured ocular lesions of FUS [16, 25]. FUS patients with CMV infection were significantly more prone to develop glaucoma eventually than those with RV infection ($P = 0.039$). Conversely, vitreous opacity was found in 25.0% of CMV patients and 66.7% of RV patients ($P = 0.038$) [344].

In addition, the expression of cytokines and immune cells in the intraocular fluid of FUS patients has also been reported. The level of IL-6 in the aqueous humor of FUS patients increased [349], as well as the levels of inflammatory cytokines; chemokines; growth factors including interleukin-1ra, −5, −8, −10, and −13; interferon-inducible 10-kDa protein; MCP-1 (monocyte chemoattractant protein 1); and macrophage inflammatory protein 1 beta, and regulated upon activation, normal T-cell expressed and secreted (RANTES) in the vitreous fluid of FUS patients who underwent vitrectomy due to vitreous opacity [350]. Moreover, a significant increase in VEGF, bFGF, IL-6, MCP-1, MMP-3, and MMP-9 levels in the aqueous humor of patients with FUS compared to controls was found [351–353]. There was a statistically significant positive correlation between the severity of cataract and IL-6 and IL-8 levels in the aqueous humor ($P = 0.001$ and $P = 0.002$, respectively) [352]. It was also reported that FUS patients with cataract showed high levels of IL-2 and IL-23 [348]. In contrast to FUS patients without glaucoma, MCP-1 and MMP-9 levels were lower in FUS with glaucoma, while the expression of MMP-2, MMP-3, and TGFβ-1 was increased [353].

Although both Posner-Schlossman syndrome (PSS) and FUS can be caused by CMV, the ocular inflammatory response of PSS patients (aqueous humor IL-1RA: 73.4 pg/mL; IL-8: 199.4 pg/mL; IL-10: 33.4 pg/mL; IP-10: 126,350 pg/mL) was stronger and more active than in FUS patients (aqueous humor IL-1RA: 4.3 pg/mL; IL-8: 72.4 pg/mL; IL-10: 1.6 pg/mL; IP-10: 57,400 pg/mL) [290].

The intraocular cell population of patients with rubella-associated uveitis primarily consisted of T-cells and monocytes/macrophages, while the presence of B-cells was found to be minimal [348]. The utilization of flow cytometry has demonstrated the existence of a concentrated clonal population of CD8(+) CD28(−) T cells in the aqueous humor of FUS [354]. This finding potentially strengthens the hypothesized viral etiology of FUS and provides a possible explanation for the lack of a significant response to steroid therapy in FUS.

6.1.7.6 Management

The anterior chamber response in FUS is usually mild, and local hormone therapy should be carefully considered as it may potentially exacerbate the patient's cataract and lead to glaucoma. In special cases, such as a dense aggregation of keratic precipitates (KPs), deposition on the anterior capsule, or an outbreak of inflammation before and after ophthalmic surgery, glucocorticoid eye drops may be considered. The author's personal approach in such situations primarily involves injecting 4 mg of triamcinolone subconjunctivally at the inferior fornix and closely monitoring intraocular pressure. Based on personal experience, intraocular inflammation may substantially subside following this treatment.

Glaucoma, cataract, and vitreous opacity are the three major vision-threatening complications of FUS. A large number of studies [355–357] have shown satisfactory prognoses for cataract extraction (phacoemulsification or small incision surgery) combined with intraocular lens implantation in FUS patients. Hydrophobic acrylic intraocular lenses [358] or heparin surface-treated intraocular lenses [359] are recommended. After cataract surgery, it is still necessary to use glucocorticoids for a few months to prevent deposits on the intraocular lens surface and increased intraocular pressure [350].

Vitrectomy is considered a safe and effective treatment for severe vitreous opacity in FUS and can be combined with cataract extraction when necessary. Most patients (67%–69%) experience at least a two-line improvement in vision, without aggravation of inflammation post-vitrectomy [360, 361].

The primary cause of untreatable visual loss in FUS is glaucoma [299]. Both trabeculectomy and the Ahmed glaucoma valve (AGV) have success rates higher than 90% over 6 months. However, at 36 months post-surgery, the success rate drops to 76% in the trabeculectomy group and to only 9% in the AGV group [362]. Encapsulated bleb formation is the most common complication, occurring in 47% of eyes [363]. Cyclophotocoagulation should be considered a safe and effective procedure if medical treatment fails to control glaucoma in FUS [364].

6.1.8 Tubercular Uveitis

6.1.8.1 Brief Introduction

Tuberculosis (TB), a chronic systemic infectious disease caused by *Mycobacterium tuberculosis*, is a public health hazard affecting about one-third of the world's population [365–367]. In human tuberculosis, the lungs are affected in 80% of cases, while the remaining 20% may involve other organs, including the organ of vision. The choroid, due to its high oxygen content, is particularly susceptible [368]. Uveal tract inflammation is the most widely recognized tuberculous manifestation in the organ of vision, attributed to its high blood supply [368–370].

There are two possible mechanisms for the occurrence of tuberculous uveitis: one is a direct inflammatory reaction to active *Mycobacterium* infection, which is induced by blood dissemination and direct invasion of *Mycobacterium tuberculosis* into ocular tissues, such as the formation of choroidal granuloma [371]; the other is an immune-mediated response driven by *Mycobacterium* and its antigens, resulting in conditions such as retinal vasculitis and creeping choroiditis [372, 373].

6.1.8.2 Epidemiology

The incidence rate of ocular tuberculosis over a 10-year period was 0.77 per 100,000 population in Australia [374]. Regarding etiology, tuberculosis accounts for 5.5–10.7% of uveitis cases in some series [375–377]. There has been a reported increase in the prevalence of tubercular uveitis across various regions [270, 378, 379], and it may represent the most common infectious cause of uveitis, accounting for 7.5–23% of cases [24, 380, 381]. Ocular tuberculosis occurs in 3.5 to 5.1% of cases, primarily among HIV-infected patients [368, 382–384]. Tubercular uveitis constituted 66% of cases of infectious uveitis [385]. In children, tuberculous uveitis accounts for 0.4–5.1% of all uveitis cases [386]. The proportion of males with tubercular uveitis is slightly higher than that of females [387].

The prevalence of tuberculous uveitis varies significantly among countries. In developed countries, the proportion is generally less than 3% [386]. In moderately developed countries, it accounts for about 5% [388]. In developing countries, tuberculosis accounts for 11% of pan-uveitis, 13.8% of anterior uveitis, 7–23.6% of intermediate uveitis, 3–35% of posterior uveitis, and 17.6% of total uveitis cases [389–391]. Moreover, even within the same geographic area, the rates of tuberculous uveitis can vary significantly between different racial groups [392].

6.1.8.3 Clinical Manifestation

The main presenting symptoms of tubercular uveitis vary and include decreased vision, ocular pain, floaters, redness, and photophobia [393]. The mean age at onset is approximately 30 years, with most patients experiencing bilateral involvement [394]. Chest X-rays/CT scans reveal findings suggestive of pulmonary TB in 25.6%–40% of patients [393, 395]. Common ocular manifestations of tubercular uveitis include mutton-fat keratic precipitates, iris nodules, iridocyclitis or anterior chamber reaction, posterior synechiae, rubeosis iridis, hypopyon, vitritis, macular edema, retinal vasculitis or periphlebitis (Fig. 6.31), retinal neovascularization, choroidal masses with or without significant intraocular inflammation (Fig. 6.32), choroiditis or chorioretinitis (Fig. 6.33), and total ophthalmia (Fig. 6.34). Other relatively rare manifestations include isolated choroidal granuloma, multifocal choroidal tuberculoma, endophthalmitis, creeping choroiditis, subretinal abscess, neuroretinitis, and tractional retinal detachment (Fig. 6.34) [393, 394, 396–398]. Multifocal choroiditis appears more frequently than focal choroiditis and

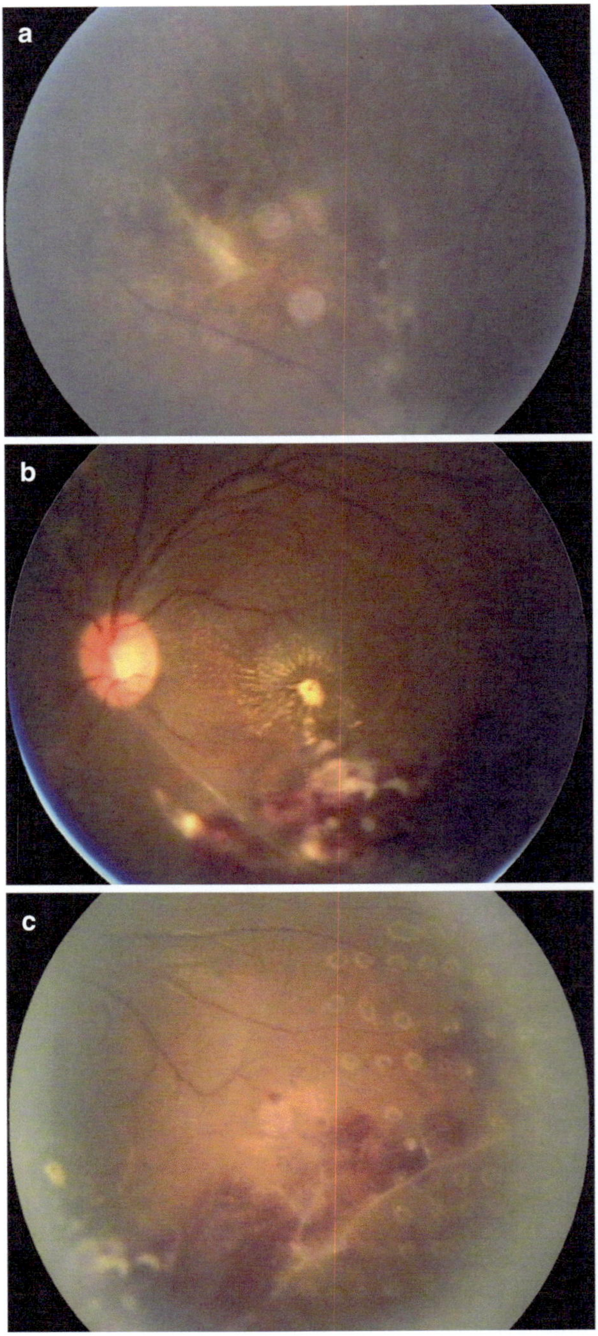

Fig. 6.31 Fundus photography of the left eye of a 32-year-old male with a positive T-SPOT.TB test. Observable features include a white sheath of retinal vessels (**a**), macular hard exudates (**b**), and retinal hemorrhage (**c**)

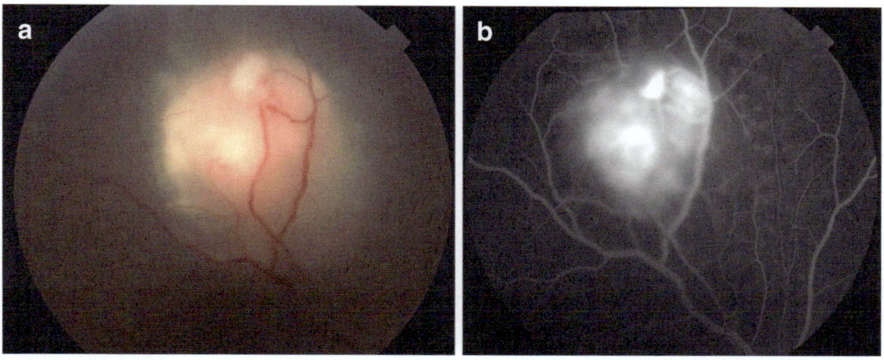

Fig. 6.32 Fundus photography (**a**) and fundus fluorescein angiography (**b**) of the right eye of a 27-year-old female with a history of pulmonary tuberculosis and a positive T-SPOT.TB test. An isolated choroidal mass under the vascular arch above the temporal optic disc and hyperfluorescence in the corresponding area could be observed

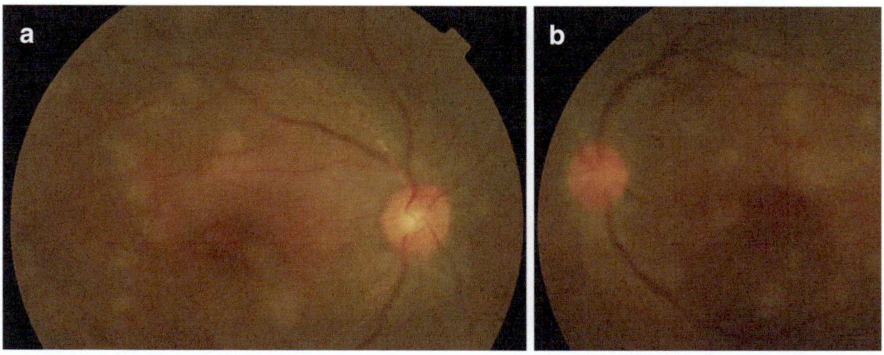

Fig. 6.33 Fundus photography of the right eye (**a**) and the left eye (**b**) of a 26-year-old female with a positive T-SPOT.TB test and a strongly positive tuberculin skin test. Bilateral multifocal choroiditis, primarily involving the posterior pole, and retinal vasculitis are evident

serpiginous-like choroiditis [393]. Macular edema is a major cause of vision loss in cases of uveitis [393, 399].

The reproduction and pathogenesis of *Mycobacterium tuberculosis* within the human body are closely related to the nutritional and health status of the individual as well as to the living environment and nutrition levels across different countries and regions. Given the remarkable worldwide variance in living standards, the ocular manifestations of tuberculous uveitis exhibit significant differences between countries and areas. For instance, in Chile, South America, the predominant manifestations of tuberculous uveitis are non-granulomatous uveitis (84.4%) and anterior uveitis (53.1%) [400]. In India, tuberculosis is an important cause of anterior chamber empyema, accounting for 23.8% of cases [401]. Conversely, in other regions, the proportion of tuberculosis in intraocular empyema is very low.

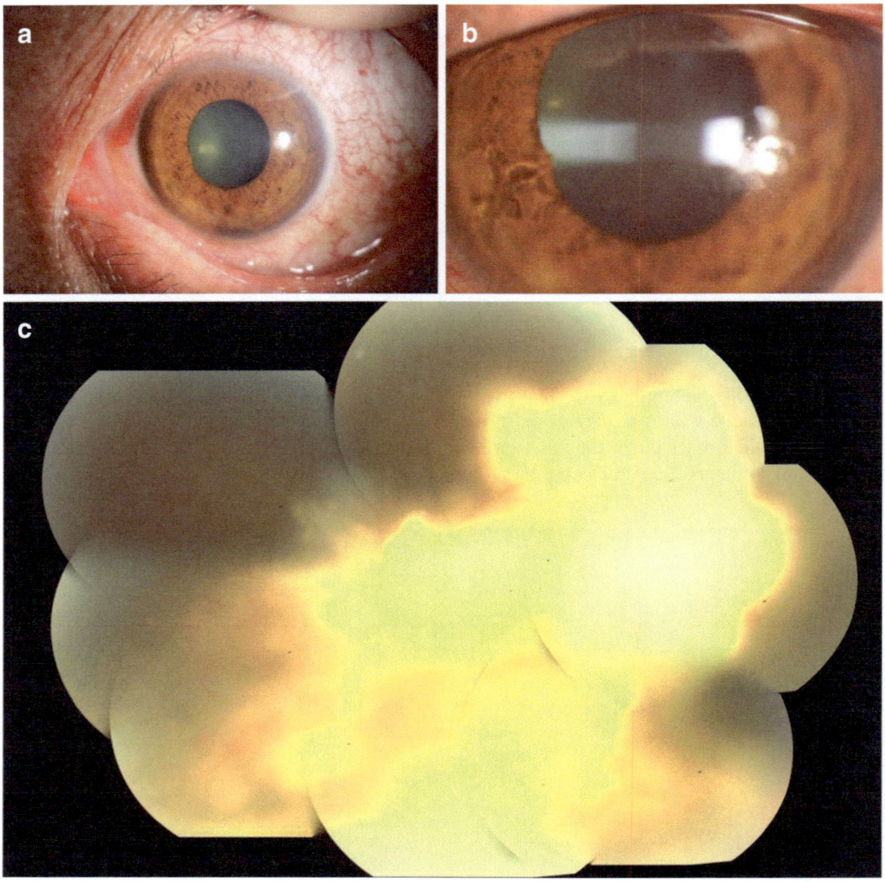

Fig. 6.34 Photography of the anterior segment (**a** and **b**) and fundus (**c**) of the left eye of a 49-year-old male with a positive T-SPOT.TB test and serum TB antibody. Ciliary hyperemia (**a**), floater cells in the anterior segment, and positive Tyndall's phenomenon (**b**), as well as severe vitreous opacity and a subretinal abscess (**c**), can be observed. PCR analysis indicated that Mycobacterium tuberculosis DNA in the vitreous fluid was 9.42×10^5 copies/mL. The presence of *Mycobacterium tuberculosis* was also confirmed by acid-fast staining

6.1.8.4 Diagnosis

Due to the complexity of clinical signs of tubercular uveitis, which may mimic other intraocular diseases, and the absence of diagnostic examinations with both high specificity and sensitivity, diagnosing tubercular uveitis remains a conundrum. The only way to determine a tubercular etiology is by using a conglomerate of clinical signs, radiologic findings, and immunologic tests [366]. A broad consensus on the diagnosis and treatment of tubercular uveitis is still lacking [402].

Goyal JL et al. developed a diagnostic criterion for ocular tuberculosis, which includes four parts (A–D): (A) clinical signs (A-1, cellular reaction in the anterior chamber/vitreous with or without posterior synechiae; A-2, snowball opacities in the inferior vitreous; A-3, perivascular cuffing of inflammatory exudates; A-4, solitary or multiple granulomas with or without exudative retinal detachment; A-5, subretinal abscess; A-6, optic disc granuloma with or without neuroretinitis; (B) ocular investigations (B-1, demonstration of AFB/culture of *M. tuberculosis* from ocular fluids; B-2, positive PCR for conserved sequences of *Mycobacterium tuberculosis*); (C) systemic investigations (C-1, positive Mantoux reaction; C-2, chest radiography suggestive of active/healed TB; C-3, evidence of extrapulmonary TB); and (D) therapeutic test (D-1, positive response to antitubercular therapy over a period of 4–6 weeks). One or more of the clinical signs (A) along with one of the positive tests (B) could be confirmatory for intraocular TB. Any one or more of the clinical signs (A), with any of the positive tests (C), or a positive therapeutic trial (D) should be presumed to have ocular TB [403].

The Standardization of Uveitis Nomenclature (SUN) Working Group established key classification criteria, including (1) anterior uveitis with iris nodules, (2) serpiginous-like tubercular choroiditis, (3) choroidal nodule (tuberculoma), (4) occlusive retinal vasculitis, and (5) in hosts with evidence of active systemic tuberculosis, multifocal choroiditis, and evidence of tuberculosis, including histologically or microbiologically confirmed infection, positive interferon-γ release assay test, or positive tuberculin skin test. The overall accuracy of diagnosing tubercular uveitis vs. other types of uveitis was 98.2% [404]. QuantiFERON-TB Gold In-Tube (QFT), an interferon-γ release assay test, is not superior to the tuberculin skin test (TST) in sensitivity as a screening test for TB-related uveitis; however, QFT is more specific than TST in identifying infections by *Mycobacterium tuberculosis* [405].

6.1.8.5 Examination of Intraocular Fluids

Identification of *Mycobacterium tuberculosis* in intraocular fluid by acid-fast staining and culture is a classic and important method for diagnosing tubercular uveitis [403]. However, typically only one or two *Mycobacterium tuberculosis* bacteria can be observed near necrotic tissue or multinucleated giant cells, requiring a high level of technical expertise from inspectors [406]. The positive rate of microscopic observation after staining vitreous humor can reach 100% (5/5) for patients with diffuse posterior endogenous tuberculous endophthalmitis [407]. Generally, obtaining aqueous or vitreous humor for acid-fast staining of *Mycobacterium tuberculosis* is less likely to be successful [371, 408]. For example, sometimes, only after enucleation of the eyeball can enough tissue samples be obtained for staining in cases of multifocal choroiditis [409]. Culturing *Mycobacterium tuberculosis* takes at least 8 weeks [403].

The advantage of using PCR to detect *Mycobacterium tuberculosis* nucleic acid in intraocular fluid lies in its high sensitivity. DNA amplification compensates for the shortcomings of traditional methods to an extent. For instance, in the study reported by Wroblewski KJ et al., in two of the three cases with positive qPCR results, acid-fast bacilli were not found in the tissue sections [406]. Detection of *Mycobacterium tuberculosis* DNA in intraocular fluid by PCR can guide clinical anti-tuberculosis treatment. The correlation between PCR detection results of Mycobacterium tuberculosis nucleic acid in intraocular fluid and clinical treatment response was 80%, with sensitivities ranging from 73.3 to 90.2%, specificities from 92.3 to 93.9%, and positive and negative predictive values from 91.7 to 93.9% and 75 to 90.2%, respectively [410, 411]. Specificity, sensitivity, and diagnostic accuracy of normalized quantitative PCR (nqPCR, where the ratio of the mpb64 gene to the RPH1 gene of the host is normalized) in ocular fluids (aqueous/vitreous) can be as high as 94.4%, 85.0%, and 89.4%, respectively [412]. The sensitivity, specificity, positive predictive value, and negative predictive value of multi-targeted PCR using three specific targets for *Mycobacterium tuberculosis* on intraocular fluid samples—IS6110, MPB64, and protein b—were 77.77%, 100%, 100%, and 88.88%, respectively [413].

The GeneXpert molecular diagnostic system is a new type of fully automated, integrated nucleic acid detection system based on the PCR method. One advantage of this method is that it can indicate drug sensitivity. Sharma K et al. applied it to the detection of *Mycobacterium tuberculosis* nucleic acid in vitreous humor, and the results showed that 84.2% were rifampicin-sensitive and 15.8% were rifampicin-resistant among patients clinically diagnosed with ocular tuberculosis [414]. Comparatively, GeneXpert and multiplex PCR were positive in 17.2% and 71.8% of patients with tubercular uveitis, respectively [415].

Instead of traditional culture of *Mycobacterium tuberculosis*, PCR is increasingly used routinely to quickly detect Mtb-specific DNA sequences such as IS6110 and MPB64, providing a specificity range of 80–100% [416–420]. It should also be noted that PCR detection of *Mycobacterium tuberculosis* nucleic acid by collecting intraocular fluid is mainly reported in developing countries, where the basic nutritional conditions and living standards are poor and the infection of tubercular uveitis is severe. Hence, *Mycobacterium tuberculosis* in the intraocular fluid is abundant. In developed areas, the manifestations of ocular tuberculosis are usually retinal vasculitis and choroiditis due to hypersensitivity with mild ocular inflammation and very few *Mycobacterium tuberculosis* in the intraocular fluid. Therefore, it is difficult to detect *Mycobacterium tuberculosis* by PCR in these cases. Examination of *Mycobacterium tuberculosis* DNA in intraocular fluid by PCR should be selectively carried out in patients with intraocular floater cells. The results of a recently published international cooperative study on ocular tuberculosis showed that only 6.13% (59/962) of patients with ocular tuberculosis worldwide underwent PCR detection of intraocular fluid, of which 33 cases were positive (56%, all Asian Indians) [418].

Flow cytometry has been used to analyze cell components in the vitreous fluid of patients with tuberculous uveitis after vitrectomy. In the vitreous humor, the proportion of CD4+ was close to that of CD8+ T cells, with higher expression of the recent activation marker CD69 and proinflammatory cytokines IFN-γ and IL-17A in CD4+ T cells compared to peripheral blood [421]. Further studies have shown that the immunophenotyping of vitreous humor samples demonstrated polyfunctional effector and central memory CD4+ T helper cells coexpressing IFN-γ, TNF-α, and IL-17, with both ESAT-6 (*Mycobacterium tuberculosis*-specific antigen early secreted antigenic target-6) and RCE (retinal crude extract, autoreactive) specificity found in T cells extracted from TB uveitis samples [422].

Studies on cytokine concentrations in the aqueous of TB uveitis patients have shown that the TAU group exhibited significantly higher levels of interleukin-6 (IL-6), interleukin-8 (CXCL8), monokine induced by interferon-gamma (CXCL9), and interferon-gamma-induced protein 10 (IP-10 or CXCL10), compared to cataract controls [423]. Additionally, intraocular levels of IFN-γ, IL-17/IL-17A, GRO-α, IL-8, MIG, IP-1, and IL-10, IL-15, TNF-α were also found to be elevated in the tubercular uveitis group [424, 425].

Validated by real-time quantitative PCR, miR-423-5p, miR-328-3p, miR-21-5p, and miR-16-5p are significantly dysregulated miRNAs in the aqueous humor from tubercular uveitis patients compared with cataract controls, and these four miRNAs might play an important role in IOTB pathogenesis via tuberculosis-associated pathways: PI3K-Akt signaling, autophagy, and MAPK pathway [426]. MicroRNAs (miRNAs) shed light on future candidates to diagnose tubercular uveitis [416].

6.1.8.6 Management

Given the limited available evidence, including the lack of randomized controlled trials, the Collaborative Ocular Tuberculosis Study (COTS) consensus has concluded that treating patients with features suggestive of tubercular choroiditis with antitubercular therapy (ATT) is potentially of significant benefit [427]. A recently published international literature meta-analysis, which included results from 28 studies and involved treatment outcomes of 1917 patients, showed that 84% of patients with tubercular uveitis did not relapse after receiving anti-tuberculosis treatment [365]. The treatment strategies and durations varied across different reports. In the 18 studies reviewed, the standard treatment regimen included isoniazid, rifampicin, ethambutol, and/or pyrazinamide for at least 2–4 months, followed by two drugs (isoniazid and rifampicin) for at least 4–15 months (Table 6.2) [365, 428]. Patients with uveitis and latent TB who were treated with anti-tuberculosis therapy for more than 9 months experienced an 11-fold reduction in the likelihood of recurrence [429].

Liver and kidney function should be monitored during anti-tuberculosis treatment [403, 430]. Corticosteroids are used to reduce intraocular inflammation and

Table 6.2 Dosage scheme of commonly used anti-tuberculosis drugs [403]

	Daily dose			
Drugs	Child	Adult	Route of administration	Maximum daily dose
Isoniazid	10–20 mg/kg	5 mg/kg	Oral/intramuscular injection	300 mg
Rifampicin	10–30 mg/kg	10 mg/kg	Oral	600 mg
Pyrazinamide	15–30 mg/kg	15–30 mg/kg	Oral	2 g
Streptomycin	20–40 mg/kg	15 mg/kg	Intramuscular injection	1 g
Ethambutol	15–25 mg/kg	15–25 mg/kg	Oral	2.5 g

tissue damage since tubercular uveitis is hypothesized to occur due to a type IV hypersensitivity reaction to tubercular proteins [366, 403, 431]. These are typically administered in the initial weeks or months of anti-tuberculosis therapy [393, 403]. The effectiveness rates of anti-tuberculosis treatment alone and anti-tuberculosis combined with systemic glucocorticoid treatment are similar, at 85% for the former and 82% for the latter [365]. Systemic glucocorticoids alone should be avoided to prevent the risk of triggering systemic tuberculosis and activating latent lesions. Prednisolone acetate eye drops can be used to alleviate ocular inflammation, and peribulbar injections of glucocorticoids can be administered if intraocular inflammation is severe [403]. After anti-tuberculosis treatment and systemic corticosteroid therapy, macular edema may show clinical improvement [393].

Regarding creeping choroiditis caused by intractable tuberculosis, it has been reported that intravitreal injections of methotrexate (400 μg/0.1 mL), administered once a month for 2 months, achieved good therapeutic effects [432]. Retinal vasculitis with retinal ischemia can be treated with scatter laser photocoagulation [393]. Reported recurrence rates vary from 10% to 29.5% [433, 434]. The recurrence rate for patients with anterior and intermediate uveitis (14.29%) is relatively higher compared to those with posterior and pan-uveitis (8.59%) [435].

6.1.9 Ocular Toxoplasmosis

6.1.9.1 Brief Introduction

Toxoplasma gondii is an obligate intracellular parasite that can invade almost all nucleated cells and proliferate within them. Toxoplasmosis is a type of zoonosis. Ocular infection with *T. gondii* often results from ingesting bradyzoites in undercooked infected meat or drinking raw water contaminated with oocysts. These oocysts can survive for extended periods in the environment, and water contaminated with oocysts is a significant source in toxoplasmosis epidemics [436]. The excrement of cats and other feline animals contains egg sacs of *Toxoplasma gondii*, which can pollute water sources. These oocysts can survive for a long time and are resistant to standard industrial disinfection methods [437–439].

Toxoplasma gondii invades the eye, disrupting the blood-eye barrier, which then allows immune cells to enter the eye tissue and cause inflammation [436, 440]. *T. gondii* may cross the vascular endothelium to reach the human retina through at least three routes: via leukocyte taxis, as a transmigrating tachyzoite, or after infecting endothelial cells [441]. Ocular toxoplasmosis is a type of retinitis that is almost always accompanied by vitritis and choroiditis [441], and it is the leading cause of infectious posterior uveitis worldwide, often resulting in visual impairment [439, 442]. Congenital toxoplasmosis is transmitted through the maternal placenta. The transplantation of organs containing *Toxoplasma* cysts can also transmit toxoplasmosis [439].

6.1.9.2 Epidemiology

Approximately 25–30% of the human population is infected with *T. gondii* [443], and the prevalence of *T. gondii* cysts and oocysts in the environment contributes to this prevalence [444, 445]. However, the group infection rate of *Toxoplasma gondii* varies greatly in different countries and regions. For example, in Brazil and Latin America, serum *Toxoplasma* antibody was positive in nearly 50% of school-age children and 80% of women [446]. In Africa, the seropositive rate ranged from 23.9% to 46% [447, 448], while in the Netherlands of Europe, the positive rate of *Toxoplasma gondii* antibody in serum among women of childbearing age was 18.5% [449]. The overall positive rate of *Toxoplasma* antibody in mainland China was 12.3% [450]. In recent years, with the increase in iatrogenic immunosuppression, organ transplantation, and AIDS patients, the incidence rate of toxoplasmosis has been increasing [451–453].

It is estimated that about 2% of people infected with toxoplasmosis will have eye manifestations, meaning that about 1 in every 400 people is infected with ocular toxoplasmosis [439, 454, 455]. A retrospective chart review in India identified ocular toxoplasmosis as the most common cause of posterior uveitis, accounting for 12% of cases [456]. Ocular toxoplasmosis accounts for 7.7% of uveitis cases in children [457]. Among adults, the annual incidence of symptomatic ocular toxoplasmosis is 0.3–0.8 per 100,000 population [458].

6.1.9.3 Clinical Manifestation

Congenital toxoplasmosis is usually caused by *Toxoplasma gondii* infection of the placenta during pregnancy in the mother, which is then transferred to the fetus through blood flow. It can manifest as spontaneous abortion in pregnant women, intrauterine fetal death, intrauterine growth retardation, infant hydrocephalus, encephalitis, neuropsychiatric diseases, eye diseases, abnormal hearing, cardiovascular abnormalities, or asymptomatic normal infants [459]. Congenital toxoplasmosis is mainly characterized by invasion of the central nervous system. The primary ocular manifestation is retinochoroiditis, which can present as monocular or binocular lesions, mostly in the macular region. Fetal infection can cause congenital malformations, including microphthalmos, anophthalmia, congenital aniridia, choroidal defect, persistent primitive vitreous hyperplasia, and optic atrophy. Congenital cataract is a complication of retinochoroiditis, which can also be secondary to severe iridocyclitis, leading to strabismus and low vision [460–463]. Congenital toxoplasmosis may also complicate with tractional retinal detachment [464].

Acquired toxoplasmosis is mainly characterized by chronic recurrence in clinical practice. Most patients present with uveitis secondary to ocular toxoplasmosis in their second to fourth decade of life [445]. Severe initial toxoplasmosis often begins between the ages of 10 and 20 years. Long-term follow-up has found that the 5-year recurrence rate is 79% [465, 466].

The most common symptoms include simple blurred vision (36.8%) and blurred vision with floating objects in front of the eyes (21.1%) [455]. The primary manifestation is focal necrotizing retinitis, often accompanied by vitritis and anterior uveitis [467]. Inflammation can be granulomatous (Fig. 6.35) or non-granulomatous [466]. Vitritis is usually most prominent near the site of active chorioretinitis. Severe vitritis may induce secondary vitreoretinal traction of the preretinal membrane and adjacent parts [466], occasionally accompanied by optic papillitis. The

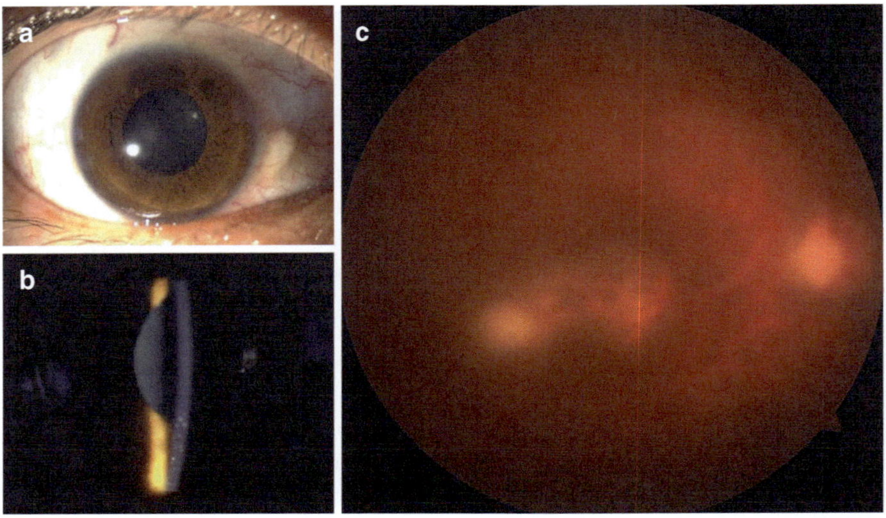

Fig. 6.35 Photography of the anterior segment (**a** and **b**) and retina (**c**) of a 33-year-old male with recurrent pan-uveitis in his right eye for 1 year. Ocular toxoplasmosis was confirmed by positive *Toxoplasma gondii* DNA in vitreous fluid, and the intravitreal concentration of *Toxoplasma* IgG was 935.21 U/L, with a *Toxoplasma* antibody Goldmann-Witmer coefficient of 3.26. Granulomatous anterior uveitis (fatty keratic precipitates) with old chorioretinal lesions in the macula and fresh lesions on the temporal side can be observed

inflammation of anterior uveitis can range from mild to severe, with manifestations ranging from mild anterior chamber reaction to severe anterior uveitis masking the posterior segment. Chorioretinal lesions located outside the macular region may be asymptomatic (Fig. 6.36).

Complications of ocular toxoplasmosis include chronic iridocyclitis, cataract, secondary glaucoma, corneal banded degeneration, macular cystoid edema, retinal detachment, optic nerve atrophy, and late secondary choroidal neovascularization. Manifestations of retinal vascular involvement include segmental retinal artery occlusion and retinal phlebitis [466]. Less typical manifestations comprise large, eventually multiple and/or bilateral lesions, endophthalmitis-like presentations, punctate outer retinitis, neuroretinitis, and scleritis [442, 468–472].

6.1.9.4 Diagnosis

The diagnosis of ocular toxoplasmosis is typically based on typical clinical manifestations. Atypical presentations, especially in immunocompromised patients, may pose diagnostic challenges and lead to misdiagnosis and inappropriate treatment [445]. If the ocular changes do not lead to a definitive diagnosis, serological examination is required, including serum anti-*Toxoplasma* IgM and IgG titers to support the diagnosis. Molecular biology techniques for diagnosing ocular toxoplasmosis have been available for many years and are now accessible as standard laboratory tests in many countries. Aqueous humor or vitreous evaluation to detect parasite DNA by polymerase chain reaction (PCR) or intraocular Toxoplasma antibody titer

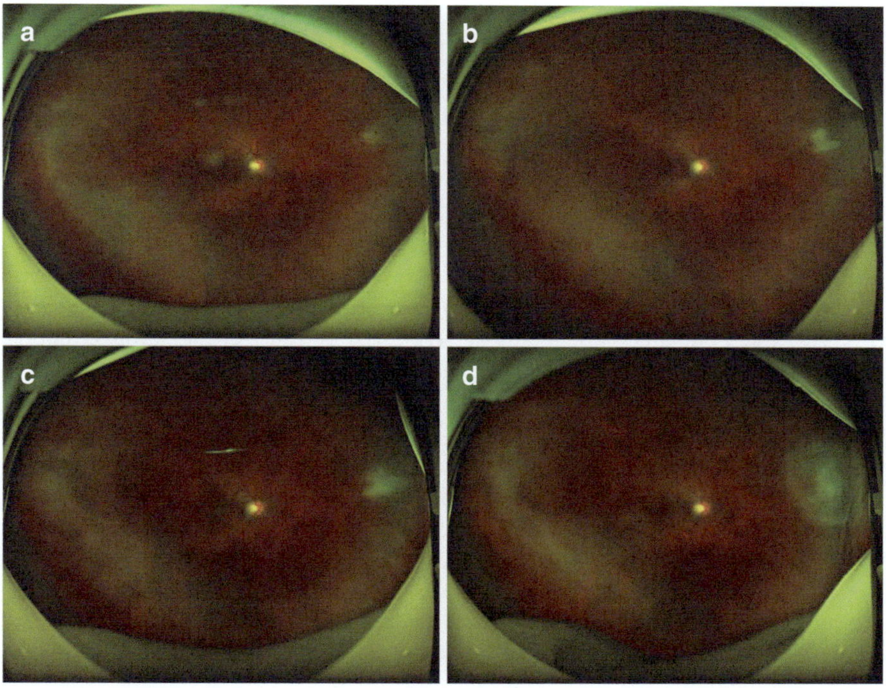

Fig. 6.36 Fundus photography of the right eye of a 55-year-old female. Ocular toxoplasmosis was confirmed by positive *Toxoplasma gondii* DNA in vitreous fluid (790 copies/mL), and the intravitreal concentration of *Toxoplasma* IgG was 38.87 IU/mL, with a Goldmann-Witmer coefficient of *Toxoplasma* antibody at 31.21. The white necrotized lesion at the peripheral nasal part of the retina kept expanding within 2 months (**a**–**d**)

may provide definitive evidence for rapid diagnosis with high sensitivity and specificity [473, 474].

6.1.9.5 Examination of Intraocular Fluids

Seropositivity for *T. gondii* infection indicates previous systemic exposure to the parasite, but this finding is not sufficient to confirm the diagnosis of ocular toxoplasmosis [445]. *T. gondii* antibody titers in ocular fluids or PCR of aqueous and vitreous samples are tools with high sensitivity and specificity to confirm the diagnosis [473, 474].

So far, the Goldmann-Witmer coefficient (GWC) of *Toxoplasma gondii* IgG is considered the gold standard for the laboratory diagnosis of ocular toxoplasmosis [475]. However, due to the limitations of a single method (the sensitivity is not high enough, with many studies reporting sensitivities of 39%–81% [476–482]), more scholars currently tend to conduct combined detection to improve sensitivity. For example, Mathist et al. found that the positive rate of single GWC for suspected ocular toxoplasmosis was only 47.6% (while the specificity is 100%), whereas the sensitivity of combined detection of *Toxoplasma gondii* antibody IgA and IgG in aqueous humor by Western blot is 71.4%, and the sensitivity of the combination of the two methods is increased to 76.2% [475]. Additionally, in the early stage of toxoplasmosis (within 3 weeks of symptoms), the sensitivity of GWC detection in aqueous humor was only 23.5%, while after 3 weeks, the proportion increased to 64% [475].

When PCR was used to detect *Toxoplasma gondii* DNA, vitreous humor (95.7%) was found to be more sensitive than aqueous humor (81.5%) [483]. Moreover, the detection of the 96 BP B1 gene by nested PCR could increase the positive rate from 58% to 71% [483]. Furthermore, the level of IFN-γ in the aqueous humor of patients with ocular toxoplasmosis was negatively correlated with the level of serum IFN-γ ($p < 0.05$), and patients with an aqueous IFN-γ/IL-10 ratio <1 had a longer course of the disease and more severe complications [484].

6.1.9.6 Management

Ocular toxoplasmosis treatments aim to prevent further retinal damage by controlling parasite reproduction, reducing inflammation, and preventing recurrence [485]. Recurrent ocular disease occurs at a high rate (79% of cases), and the time between recurrences shortens with ongoing disease [486]. However, so far, no unified plan has been reached for drug treatment [487]. In general, oral glucocorticoids and anti-*Toxoplasma* drugs are mainstream for immunocompetent patients [488]. Pyrimidine combined with sulfadiazine has a synergistic effect on interfering with Toxoplasma gondii reproduction [489, 490]. Therefore, the combination of pyrimidine, sulfadiazine, and glucocorticoid has become the "traditional triple therapy." The therapeutic dose includes a 100 mg loading dose of pyrimidine on the first day, followed by 50 mg/day; sulfadiazine 1 g/every 6 h (total 4 g/day); prednisone 40 mg/day (starting from the third day for 1 week and then gradually reduced). Additionally, folic acid 15 mg/day is used to counteract pyrimidine's folic acid antagonist side effect [491, 492]. The compound sulfamethoxazole (trimethoprim and sulfamethoxazole) may be the best choice among many alternative drugs, because the recurrence rate of ocular toxoplasmosis is the lowest in this group: compared with the traditional pyrimidine sulfadiazine group, the odd ratio of ocular toxoplasmosis recurrence rate was 0.61 in azithromycin group, 0.72 in clindamycin group, and 0.98 in the compound sulfadiazine group, which means that the compound sulfadiazine group and the traditional pyrimidine sulfadiazine group have the closest efficacy in reducing the recurrence of ocular toxoplasmosis [493]. Medication was stopped after monitoring the eye lesions until the activity of the lesions subsided, but it should last at least 1 month [491].

However, traditional treatment presents certain limitations, notably drug toxicity and side effects. The classic drug regimen for ocular toxoplasmosis treatment, including sulfadiazine, pyrimidine, folic acid, and glucocorticoid, could induce drug side effects in 85% of patients. The incidence of side effects was higher in women (95%) compared to men (77%), with 82% of the side effects being mild. Common side effects included gastrointestinal reactions, skin issues, and neurological/psychiatric abnormalities, with rare cases of serious complications such as Stevens-Johnson syndrome. The majority of side effects (90.3%) occurred during the second week after treatment [492]. In the presence of the following side effects, prompt cessation of the medication is advised: leukopenia, blood platelet count lower than 120,000/μL, blood creatinine higher than 25%, blood liver enzyme levels twice the normal limit, rash, or other life-threatening complications [491, 494].

The azithromycin group exhibited significantly fewer side effects than the traditional treatment group (both groups received a 100 mg loading dose of pyrimidine on the first day, followed by 50 mg/day; folic acid 15 mg/day; prednisone 40 mg/day, starting from the third day, and gradually decreasing after a week; the difference being that the azithromycin group was administered azithromycin 250 mg/day, or 500 mg orally every other day, while the traditional treatment group was given sulfadiazine 4 g/day) ($P < 0.04$). There was no significant difference between the two groups in terms of the regression of inflammatory activity, the reduction of the range of chorioretinal lesions, and the best-corrected visual acuity [491].

There is no definitive evidence supporting the notion that glucocorticoids combined with anti-*Toxoplasma gondii* therapy are more effective than anti-*Toxoplasma gondii* therapy alone [495]. Vitrectomy combined with silicone oil tamponade for treating secondary rhegmatogenous retinal detachment caused by toxoplasmosis has shown positive outcomes. The success rate after one operation is 68.2%, and the overall success rate is 90.9%. It's important to note that postoperative high intraocular pressure is the main complication, accounting for 22.7% of cases [496].

6.1.10 Ocular Toxocariasis

6.1.10.1 Brief Introduction

Human toxocariasis is a worldwide zoonotic helminthiasis caused by infection with *Toxocara canis* or *Toxocara cati* larvae [497]. Ocular toxocariasis is an inflammatory disease caused by the invasion of toxocarina larvae into various ocular tissues. The disease can invade patients of all age groups, but most of them are children. It is one of the main causes of leukocoria [498].

The reason why humans are infected with toxocariasis is that they eat food contaminated by embryonated eggs due to fecal oral transmission [499]. Close contact with cats and dogs, pica, inattention to personal hygiene, and eating contaminated food can cause infection. It should be noted that many patients with ocular toxocariasis do not have a history of close contact with cats and dogs, but the vast majority of patients with ocular toxocariasis resided in rural areas with poor sanitary conditions (83.3%) [500], because there are embryonated eggs in the nearby soil where they live, which is easy to pollute their food.

The second-stage larvae enter the blood flow from the intestine and transfer to the lungs, heart, liver, and peripheral circulation. When the larvae reach the arterioles whose diameter is smaller than their body, they pass through the tube wall and enter organs, most commonly the lungs, muscles, and eyes. Larvae can remain silent in the surrounding tissues without symptoms, while acute visceral worm larva migration can occur during its migration. Large organs (such as the liver) can tolerate many larvae without symptoms, but a single larva can cause visual loss. The larvae can enter the eyes directly through the choroid, ciliary body, or central retinal artery, causing ocular toxocariasis. Patients with ocular toxocariasis are not contagious. Ocular toxocariasis accounts for 1% of uveitis [501].

6.1.10.2 Epidemiology

Totally 800 soil samples were collected from parks across the UK and found that 24.4% of them had *Toxocara* embryonated eggs [498]. Even in developed countries, such as the United States, the proportion of serum *Toxocara* antibody-positive is as high as 2.8%; therefore, the dominant/recessive infection of *Toxocara* is not uncommon [502]. In developing area such as South Iran, toxocariasis was the most common infectious etiology among the pediatric population with uveitis (7.4%) or posterior uveitis (40%) [503]. The lower middle-income level countries had the highest prevalence (2–12%) as well as the African region (7–13%), and the highest infection rate (2–7%) was detected in the 1–25 mean age group [504].

6.1.10.3 Clinical Manifestation

Ocular toxocariasis is unilaterally involved in almost all cases [501, 505–507] and occurs predominantly in children (the median patient age was 8.5 years [508]). Right eye is more likely to be affected (65.79%) [509]. The most common causes of consultation included decreased vision (29.9%), strabismus (26.7%), and leukocoria (19.7%). The most common findings included peripheral or central chorioretinal granuloma, peripheral granuloma with traction bands or retinal fold [510], vitritis, and chronic endophthalmitis [501, 505, 511, 512]. Yellow-and-white dot-shaped lesions and perivascular white sheath can be commonly observed [513]. Delayed diagnosis (>8 months) seemed to be associated with higher rate of macular edema [514].

According to the manifestation, ocular toxocariasis can be classified into three categories: peripheral chorioretinal granuloma (50%, Fig. 6.37a), macular granuloma (25%, Fig. 6.37b), and pseudoendophthalmitis (moderate to severe vitreous opacity, 25%, Fig. 6.37c) [501]. The causes of visual impairment included vitritis (52.6%, Fig. 6.38), cystoid macular edema (47.4%), and traction retinal detachment (36.8–43.9%, Fig. 6.39) [501, 515]. Most of intraocular inflammation was intermediate uveitis (68.42%) [509]. Most juvenile patients with ocular toxocariasis have mild anterior segment inflammation and may have posterior pupillary adhesion, while the rate of adult patients with ocular toxocariasis is less than half (45.8%) [500]. Floaters in the anterior chamber may appear in the early stage of the disease, but it is often not obvious in patients with a long course of disease.

Vitreous opacity indicated by B-scan ultrasound (Fig. 6.40) may assist the diagnosis of this disease. The most consistent ultrasound finding in the eye with toxocariasis was a high-reflectivity retinal mass [516], located in posterior pole or periphery, which may be calcified, and the fibrous band extending from the periphery to the posterior pole or optic disc may also be demonstrated [517, 518]. For children with long course of disease and younger age, B-scan ultrasound may reveal multiple hyper-reflective onionskin-like membrane-shape foci within the vitreous chamber. In fundus fluorescein angiography, leakage of fluorescein in the

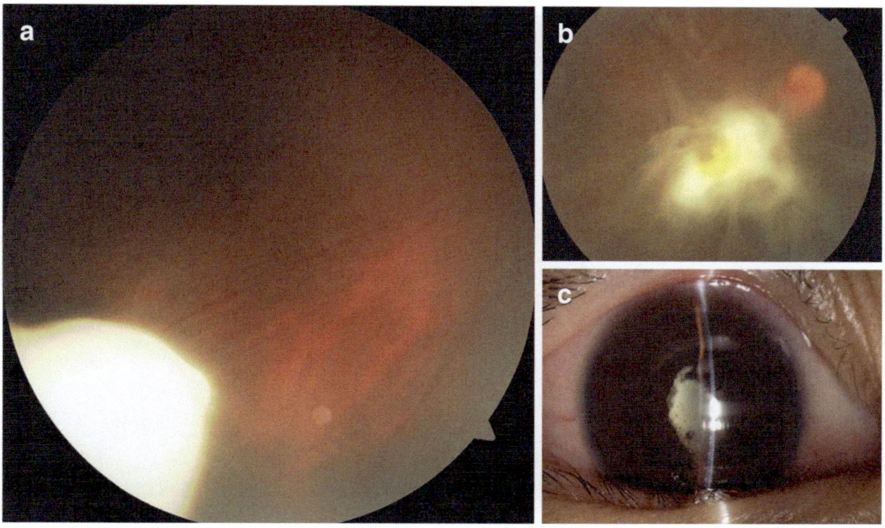

Fig. 6.37 Photography of the retina (**a** and **b**) or anterior segment (**c**) of patients with ocular toxocariasis. Peripheral chorioretinal granuloma (**a**), macular granuloma (**b**), or pseudoendophthalmitis-like changes (**c**) can be observed

Fig. 6.38 Photography of the anterior vitreous (C) of one patient with ocular toxocariasis. Dense white granular opacity in the vitreous can be observed

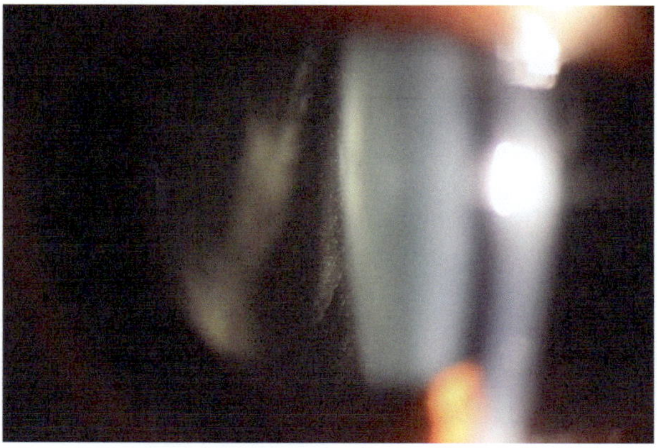

small- and medium-branch veins of the retina and a "bristle-like" change indicating increased permeability of the vessels and staining of the granuloma can be observed (Fig. 6.41) [500, 513].

6.1.10.4 Diagnosis

A clinical diagnosis of OT was made based on the criteria as follows: unilaterally involved–clinical features including the presence of a peripheral granuloma (focal, white peripheral nodule with pigmentary scarring or traction retinal detachment), posterior pole granuloma (focal, white nodule with or without posterior pole variable pigmentation), or vitritis with unknown cause, generally without inflammatory

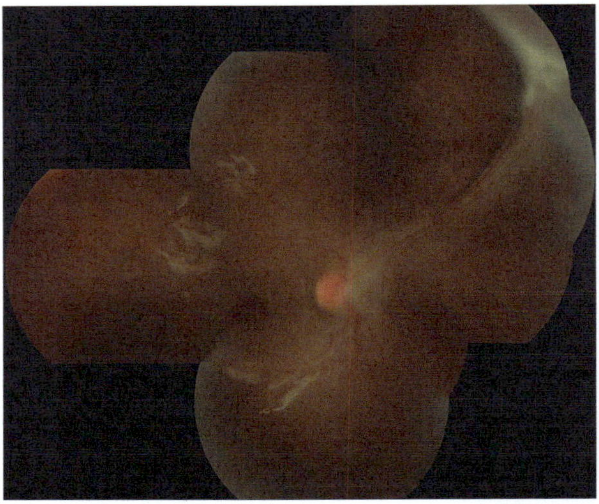

Fig. 6.39 Fundus photography of one patient with ocular toxocariasis. Traction retinal detachment in the nasal peripheral area and retinal fold can be observed

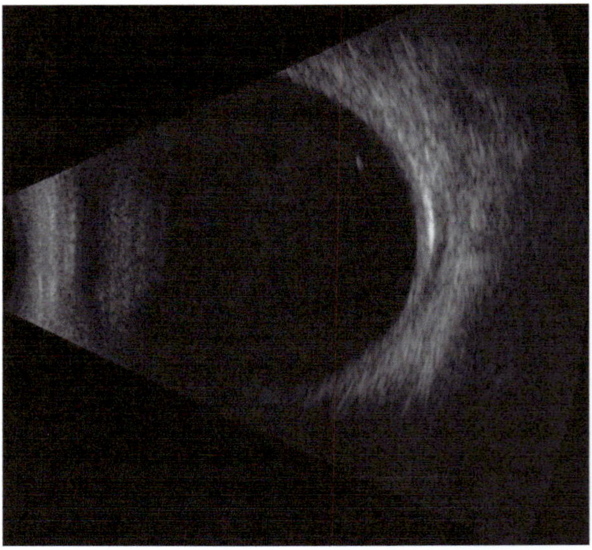

Fig. 6.40 B-scan ultrasound image of one patient with ocular toxocariasis. Medium to high reflective spots in the vitreous cavity can be observed

signs in the anterior chamber, positive *Toxocara* antibody in the intraocular fluids, and exclusion of other intraocular granulomatous diseases such as ocular toxoplasmosis, sarcoidosis, ocular tuberculosis, and other fungal infections [500, 507].

The mean levels of serum *Toxocara* antibody in patients with suspected ocular toxocariasis is significantly higher than that in other patients ($p = 0.0001$) [519]. However, serological examination of *Toxocara* antibody is only helpful for the diagnosis of ocular toxocariasis in the regions with low population *Toxocara* infection rate. It should be noted that in countries and regions with underdeveloped economic level and large soil exposure area, the proportion of group serum *Toxocara*

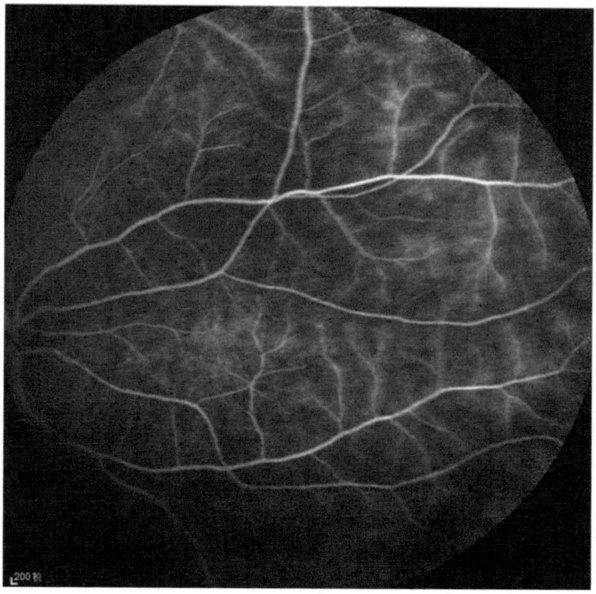

Fig. 6.41 Fundus fluorescein angiography of the right eye with ocular toxocariasis. Leakage of fluorescein in capillary and staining of capillary and small- and medium-size retinal vein at the nasal peripheral area of retina can be observed

antibody-positive can be as high as 37.3%; hereby simple positive serum *Toxocara* antibody cannot lead to the diagnosis of ocular toxocariasis [520].

6.1.10.5 Examination of Intraocular Fluids

Negative serological examination of *Toxocara* antibody cannot exclude the diagnosis of ocular toxocariasis, and intraocular fluid samples may be necessary to confirm a clinical diagnosis [521]: in Sri Lanka, serum *Toxocara* antibody was positive in only 62% of the patients with presumed ocular toxocariasis [522]. Examination of intraocular fluids provides more value than serum examination: in Inchauspe S et al.'s study, positive *Toxocara* antibody in the vitreous fluid was found in the 6 patients (15%) with negative serum *Toxocara* antibody among the 40 patients with presumed ocular toxocariasis [521]. In a domestic study of 72 cases with ocular toxocariasis, the positive rate of *Toxocara* antibody in the intraocular fluid was 84.72% which was much higher than the positive rate of *Toxocara* antibody in the serum (54.17%). Furthermore, there were 34.72% of the patients with positive *Toxocara* antibody in the intraocular fluids and negative *Toxocara* antibody in the serum [523]. A recently published study suggested that diagnostic cutoff values of anti-*Toxocara* IgG for ocular toxocariasis in the serum and intraocular fluids to be 8.2 U (sensitivity 80.2%, and specificity 94.0%) and 1.8 U (sensitivity 88.4%, and specificity 96.4%), respectively [524].

Temptation to detect *Toxocara* DNA in intraocular fluid of patients with ocular toxocariasis by PCR ended in negative results [525, 526]. It is regarded that *Toxocara* body is beneath retina and does not release nucleic acid into vitreous body [499]. With regard to the patients with ocular toxocariasis who come to ocular clinic, the intraocular *Toxocara* worms are dead, the intraocular inflammation is caused by the release of allogeneic proteins, and the nucleic acids of Toxocara have disappeared.

Usually, the duration of children with presumed ocular toxocariasis is long, and intraocular inflammation extend from vitreous cavity to anterior segment; hereby the examination of *Toxocara* antibody in aqueous humor of children is valuable. However, adult patients usually come to clinic because of visual symptoms in early stage, and the anterior segment is quiet. Therefore, for presumed ocular toxocariasis in the adults, biopsy of vitreous fluid but not aqueous humor is recommended [500].

There were 66.7 and 77.3% cases with ocular toxocariasis that showed increases in eosinophil cationic protein (ECP) and total Ig E in serum, respectively [527]. Comparatively, the sensitivity of intraocular fluid to detect IgE is higher. Comparing the titer of IgE in intraocular fluid and serum can further confirm the intraocular parasitic infection, and the positive rate is as high as 92.75% [523]. Eosinophils can be detected in the vitreous humor of 76.92% of patients with ocular toxocariasis [523].

Compared with the controls without intraocular inflammation, the intraocular levels of VEGF, IL-6, IL-8, and IL-10 in the eyes with ocular toxocariasis were significantly higher [509]. In addition, there were five cytokines exhibited significantly increased expression in the ocular toxocariasis group than in non-ocular toxocariasis uveitis group, including IL-5, IL-9, IL-10, IL-13, and PDGF-AA [528].

6.1.10.6 Management

No consensus is reached on whether patients with ocular toxocariasis should use antiparasitic drugs systematically [499]. The drugs recommended for administration include thiabendazole and albendazole. Despreaux et al. arranged oral albendazole for all patients diagnosed with toxocariasis [514] Ahn et al. decide whether to give antiparasitic drugs according to whether the serum IgE level is increased and whether the blood eosinophils are increased (for adult patients with toxocariasis: albendazole 400 mg/ time, twice a day, a total of 2 weeks) [507].

Steroids are often reported to be used to control the progress of ocular inflammation and prevent the proliferation of intraocular fibrous membranes in ocular toxocariasis [507]. Despite that systemic use of steroids such as methylprednisolone was reported to treat ocular toxocariasis in children [529], remarkable side effects led to broad concern. Peribulbar or subconjunctival injection of triamcinolone during/after vitreous surgery can reduce the probability of recurrence of intraocular inflammation of ocular toxocariasis ($P = 0.031$) [509]. Repeated doses of intravitreal dexamethasone implants showed effects including reattached retina and improved vision in a case with exudative retinal detachment secondary to ocular toxocariasis [530]. It was reported that the recurrence rates in the combination treatment group with albendazole and corticosteroids were significantly lower than those in the steroid-alone group during the mean follow-up of 27.6 months ($P = 0.001$) [527].

Indications of vitrectomy for ocular toxocariasis include (1) severe and persistent intraocular inflammation despite the use of glucocorticoids and (2) pre-macular membrane or traction that endangers vision [514]. Despreaux R et al. found that the mean visual acuity of adult patients with toxocariasis treated by vitrectomy significantly improved ($P = 0.01$) with significantly lower mean macular foveal thickness ($P = 0.017$) [514]. Relapsed intraocular inflammation in the child with ocular toxocariasis can be successfully controlled after vitrectomy [531]. It has been reported to use intravitreal injection of anti-VEGF drugs to treat choroidal neovascularization close to granuloma of toxocariasis. After injection, choroidal neovascularization subsided and vision improved [532].

For patients with toxocariasis, attention should be paid to prevention, to eat the imported food after cooking. Personal hygiene is recommended, and those who raise cats and dogs should pay more attention not to be too close. Domestic animals shall be quarantined in time.

6.1.11 Lyme-Associated Uveitis

6.1.11.1 Brief Introduction

Lyme disease is the most common tick-borne disease [533] and zoonotic infectious disease [534]. It is a natural focal disease caused by genospecies of the *Borrelia burgdorferi* sensu lato complex infection with ticks as the main vector [534]. In recent years, novel pathogenic *Borrelia* species such as candidatus *Borrelia mayonii* was identified to be the pathogen [535]. In 1991, Smith JL et al. first reported two cases of retinal vasculitis with *Borrelia burgdorferi* seropositivity, which were relieved by systemic administration of antibiotics and glucocorticoids [536].

6.1.11.2 Epidemiology

The number of cases of the disease in more than 70 countries in Asia, Europe, the United States, Africa, Oceania, and other countries has increased year by year to an estimated annual number of about 300,000 people [537]. With 85,000 cases estimated annually in Europe, it is the most common tick-borne disease in the northern hemisphere [535]. In China mainland, more than 10,000 cases every year have been reported [538, 539]. In the 1990s, Finnish scholars reported that the annual incidence rate of Lyme-associated ocular disease was about 0.3 cases/100,000 population [540].

6.1.11.3 Clinical Manifestation

The clinical manifestations of Lyme disease are diverse. In addition to the clinical types of cutaneous chronic migratory erythema, meningitis, meningo-radiculitis, cranial neuritis, arthritis, acrodermatitis chronica atrophicans, carditis, and so on, etiology and therapeutics have confirmed that Lyme disease spirochete can cause human mental abnormalities and serious harm to the population [539, 541–543]. But death is rare [533].

Ocular involvement of Lyme disease includes conjunctivitis, superficial scleritis, keratitis, uveitis, neuroretinitis, retinal vasculitis, and cranial nerve paralysis [544]. The early manifestations of Lyme disease are cold-like symptoms, lymphadenopathy, and migratory erythema. At this stage, ocular involvement is usually asymptomatic, or red eye, tears, etc. Less than 11% of patients can have follicular conjunctivitis, periorbital edema, and mild photophobia [545].

The dissemination period occurs about 3–10 weeks after infection. Patients may have general discomfort and neurological and cardiac manifestations. Advanced

Lyme disease occurs months to years later and may include recurrent arthritis, which usually affects the knee, chronic acrodermatitis, atrophic rash, and neurological diseases such as encephalopathy and dementia. Conjunctivitis may also occur, although neuro-ophthalmic findings are more common, such as cranial nerve paralysis, Horner syndrome [546], and Argyll-Robertson pupil [544, 547]. Optic neuritis has also been reported, and papilledema associated with meningitis is more common than optic neuritis. Optic papillitis with or without neuroretinitis may occur under normal intracranial pressure [548, 549]. Direct spirochete infiltration was found in cases of extraocular myositis, dacryocystitis, eyelid edema, etc. [550]. Keratitis is also relatively common in advanced Lyme disease. Although spirochetes have been detected in the cornea of keratitis patients, immune-mediated interstitial keratitis may be a more common pathogenic mechanism [550]. Superficial scleritis, anterior [551] and posterior scleritis [552], uveitis, retinal vasculitis (Fig. 6.42), branch retinal vein occlusion, and abducens nerve paralysis [544] have also been reported to be manifestations of ocular Lyme disease.

6.1.11.4 Diagnosis

Diagnosis of Lyme disease uveitis is based on the medical history, systemic symptoms and manifestations compatible with systemic Lyme borreliosis, ocular signs, laboratory findings, and the exclusion of other causes such as tuberculosis and syphilis that may cause the patient's disease [553].

The medical history that needs to be collected includes the history of erythema migrans, the history of tick exposure, the history of neurological or joint symptoms, and the history of acrodermatitis chronica atrophicans. Detailed ophthalmic examinations include indirect ophthalmoscopy and three-mirror examination. The patients with choroiditis, retinitis, and optic neuritis should be examined with fluorescein angiography, electroretinogram, visual-evoked response, and color vision. Invite neurologists to consult patients with neuroretinitis or optic neuritis and conduct cerebrospinal fluid puncture. Magnetic resonance imaging of the brain was performed in patients with uveitis who had cerebrospinal fluid abnormalities and/or central nervous system symptoms [540].

Treponema pallidum hemagglutination test should be performed to exclude syphilis. In addition, more serological tests should be carried out to exclude infections caused by *Toxoplasma gondii*, toxocarina larvae, human immunodeficiency virus, cytomegalovirus, Epstein-Barr virus, herpes simplex virus, and measles virus. Sarcoidosis can be ruled out by chest X-ray, tuberculin test, and measurement of angiotensin-converting enzyme level [540].

Laboratory tests include Western blot or ELISA for IgG and IgM of *Borrelia burgdorferi* in serum and the IgG titer ratio of *Borrelia burgdorferi* in cerebrospinal fluid and serum (>4 is positive) [540, 554].

6.1.11.5 Examination of Intraocular Fluids

In ophthalmic clinic, laboratory diagnosis of Lyme disease generally depends on the positive detection of *Borrelia burgdorferi* antibody in serology. However, in epidemic areas, due to the high proportion of natural people infected with *Borrelia*

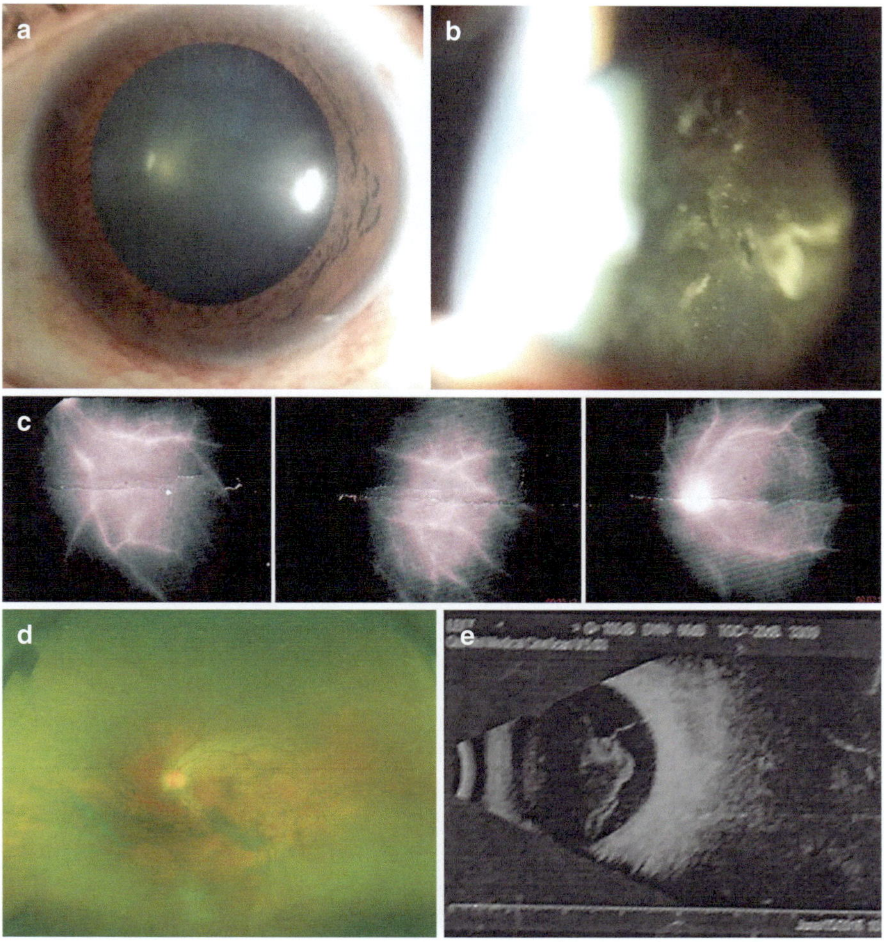

Fig. 6.42 Photograph of anterior segment (**a**) and vitreous (**b**), fundus fluorescein angiography (**c**), wide-filed fundus photograph (**d**), and B-scan ultrasound (**e**) of the eye with Lyme-associated uveitis. The patient was female, 57 years old with blurred vision in the left eye for 3 months. Past history included skin erythema for 3 years and arthritis history for 2 years. The anterior segment photography indicated that the inflammatory reaction in the anterior segment is mild (**a**), but the vitreous opacity was remarkable (**b**). Fundus fluorescein angiography indicated that the widely fluorescein leakage of retinal vascular wall and the optic disc, indicating retinal vasculitis (**c**). Fundus photography shows that the white cloudy inferior vitreous (**d**) and the B-ultrasound revealed the high reflective band in the vitreous cavity (**e**). (Courtesy of Dr. Ma Weimei, ophthalmologist of Xi'an Fourth People's Hospital)

burgdorferi and the number of persons with positive *Borrelia burgdorferi* antibody in serum is large, this method is unspecific. Bernard A et al. of France carried out a serological study on 430 patients with uveitis of unknown cause, and found that 34 patients (7.9%) were positive for *Borrelia burgdorferi* antibody, and the group survey of the French population found that 6–8.5% of the natural population were positive for *Borrelia burgdorferi* antibody. It means that in areas with high infection rate of *Borrelia burgdorferi*, it is of little significance to check serum *Borrelia burgdorferi* antibody for diagnosis [555].

Additionally, serological *Borrelia burgdorferi* antibody test may also have a false-positive reaction, because after infection with *Treponema pallidum* and oral spirochete, or mononucleosis and some autoimmune diseases, the test may also be positive [556, 557]. Moreover, serum *Borrelia burgdorferi* antibody detection may also show false-negative reaction, i.e., there are some Lyme disease patients with negative serum *Borrelia burgdorferi* antibody. In Karma A's report, there are three typical Lyme disease patients with ocular involvement whose serum *Borrelia burgdorferi* antibody are negative, and the examination results of the other two patients are close to the critical value [540].

Steere [558] and Schubert [559] successively used cytological analysis to find evidence of existence of *Borrelia burgdorferi* from vitreous fluid of patients with presumed diagnosis of Lyme-associated uveitis. Preac Mursic et al. separated *Borrelia burgdorferi* from the iris of patients suspected of Lyme-associated uveitis [560]. However, the number of *Borrelia burgdorferi* in most clinical samples is very small, which hinders direct detection [561].

Detection of *Borrelia burgdorferi* DNA by PCR directly depends on the methodology, sequencing fragment, and primer design [561–565]. O'Rourke et al. showed that the positive rate of direct detection of skin biopsy samples by PCR (77.7%) was higher than that of culture (55.1%) [565]. Mikkila et al. detected *Borrelia burgdorferi* by PCR, ELISA, and western blot in the vitreous fluid of a 40-year-old male patient with suspected Lyme-associated uveitis, who was mainly characterized by vitreous inflammation. The examination results were all positive [553] Karma A et al. performed laboratory examination of intraocular fluids for a 15-year-old girl with retinitis pigmentosa-like fundus changes in the left eye, optic neuropathy in the right eye, and demyelinating brain disease caused by advanced Lyme disease. The examination of *Leptospira* antibodies in serum and cerebrospinal fluid was negative, so the diagnosis was delayed. A specific gene fragment of *Borrelia burgdorferi* encoding 41 kD endoflagellin in vitreous fluid and cerebrospinal fluid was detected by PCR, which confirmed the diagnosis. However, another lab subsequently reported that the antibody of *Borrelia burgdorferi* of the patient's pre-treatment serum was positive. Hereby, it may imply that PCR may still be effective for cases with negative antibody detection [566].

6.1.11.6 Management

Borrelia burgdorferi belongs to gram-negative bacteria [567], and antibiotics are required for treatment. Intravenous ceftriaxone or cefotaxime is usually used to treat Lyme disease eyes, but excessive use of ceftriaxone may cause biliary complications [568]. Other commonly used drugs include tetracycline, amoxicillin, etc. The dosage and duration of antibiotic drugs should be based on the course of disease, clinical symptoms, and age of patients. The specific medication method is determined by the doctor according to the patient's situation. Randomized treatment trials have invariably failed to show any benefit of prolonged antibiotic treatment [569].

6.1.12 Ocular Brucellosis

6.1.12.1 Brief Introduction

Brucellosis is a zoonotic disease caused by the *Brucella*, one kind of gram-negative coccobacillus, and the hosts are usually cows, camels, sheep, and goats [570, 571]. It is transmitted from animals to human beings through the ingestion of unpasteurized milk and milk products (most common, 47%) [572], or uncooked meat, uncooked raw meat or by contact through infected carcasses or abortus, skin, blood, conjunctiva, gastrointestinal, or airborne spread by respiratory tracts [571, 573, 574].

Human brucellosis may be caused by four of totally six genetically and phenotypically closely related *Brucella* species, i.e., *Brucella* melitensis, *Brucella* abortus, *Brucella* suis, and *Brucella* canis [575], most cases in the world are caused by *B. melitensis* [576, 577]. The rate of patients with ocular brucellosis among patients with brucellosis was about 4–26% [578–580], and cases involving dacryoadenitis, episcleritis, keratitis, uveitis, optic neuritis, papilloedema, and diverse ocular presentations associated with brucellosis have been reported since the 1940s [581–583]. Direct presence of brucellae and immune complexes that depended on pathogenesis are regarded as two possible pathogenesis of ocular brucellosis [578, 584–586].

6.1.12.2 Epidemiology

Human brucellosis remains an important health problem in endemic areas such as the Middle East such as Turkey, the Mediterranean, Mexico, Asia, and Central and South America such as Peru [570, 578, 587, 588]. Most of the patients were rural [572]. The 5-year mean incidence of brucellosis in Iran was 46.5/100,000 [572]. Male to female ratio was 0.53–1.37/1 [572, 578]. Half of the infected population was 16–35 years of age with 21.2% being 36–55 years of age and 26.9% being >55 years of age [578]. The monthly incidence of human brucellosis in China showed a significant seasonal pattern peaking in the spring and summer seasons, especially in the month of May each year [588].

6.1.12.3 Clinical Manifestation

The main clinical manifestations of brucellosis were mainly fever, fatigue, arthralgia, and muscle pain [589]. The most common symptom of ophthalmic brucellosis was blurred vision that in most cases occurs bilaterally [578, 584]. Besides, other ocular symptoms reported included red eyes, ocular pain, foreign body sensation, scotoma, loss of vision, double vision, and lacrimation [578]. The onset can be acute or insidious, generally beginning within 2 to 4 weeks after inoculation.

Ocular involvement in brucellosis occurs in different forms including dacryoadenitis, conjunctivitis, episcleritis, nummular keratitis, iritis, iridocyclitis, cataract, glaucoma, neuroretinitis, retinitis, exudative retinal detachment, maculopathy, multifocal chorioiditis, panuveitis (Fig. 6.43), pars planitis, hyalitis, and optic neuritis [574, 578, 580, 584, 585, 590–593]. The most frequent manifestations were either conjunctivitis [580] or uveitis [578, 579]. The rate of anterior uveitis (15.8–41%) is higher than posterior uveitis or choroiditis (2.7–32%) and panuveitis (9%) [579, 580]. Usually, the patients with anterior uveitis were in the acute stage, and the

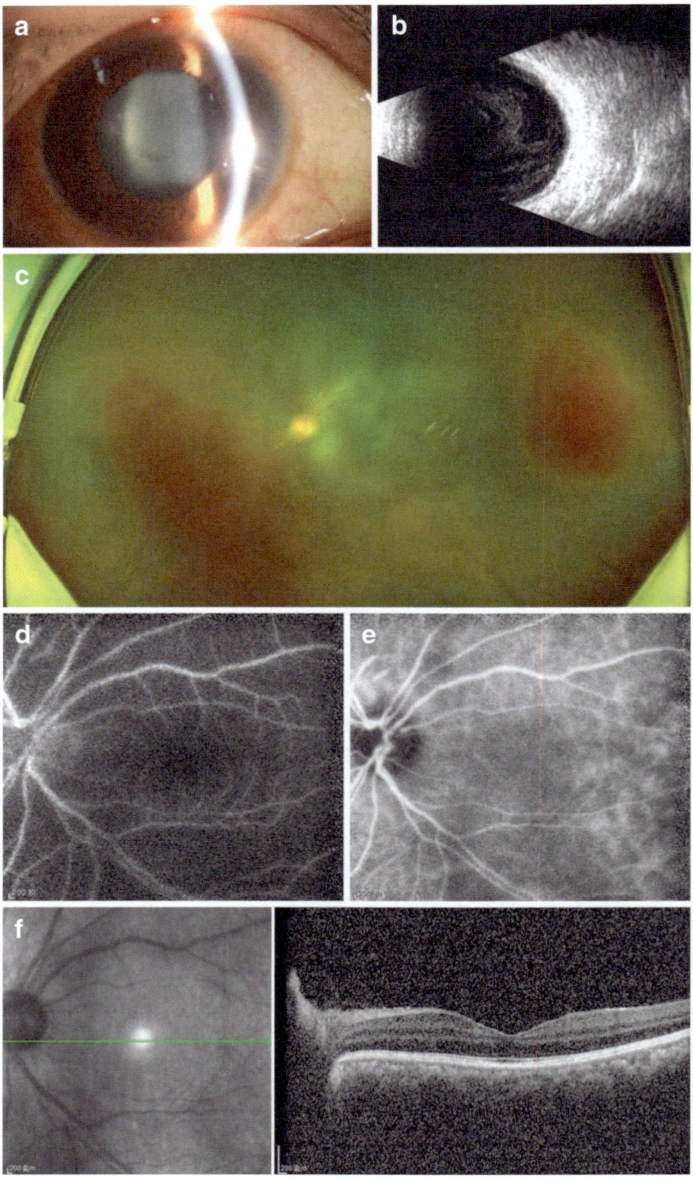

Fig. 6.43 Photograph of anterior segment (**a**), B-ultrasound scan (**b**), fundus photograph (**c**), fundus fluorescein angiography (FFA; **d**), indocyanine green angiography (ICGA; **e**) and optical coherence tomography (OCT; **f**) of the eye with ocular brucellosis. The patient was a 38-year-old male with blurred vision, photophobia, and red eye in the left eye for 9 days. Past history included type 2 diabetes mellitus. He raised sheep. The anterior segment photography indicated that the inflammatory reaction in the anterior segment is mild with ciliary conjunctiva congestion and pigment ring on the surface of lens (**a**). Fundus photograph (**c**) showed medium vitreous opacity, which was confirmed by B-ultrasound scan (**b**). Mild staining of retinal veins can be observed on the FFA (**d**) but not ICGA (**e**). Blurred retinal reflective image due to unclear refraction media without macular edema can be observed on OCT (**f**). (Courtesy of Dr. Ding Enliang, ophthalmologist of Handan Eye Hospital)

patients with posterior segment involved were in the chronic stage [579]. During vitrectomy for vitritis induced by brucellosis, the vitreous can be gel-like instead of liquefaction which is commonly secondary to other type of uveitis or vitritis (unpublished data).

6.1.12.4 Diagnosis

The diagnosis of systemic brucellosis is clinically suggested in patients with fever, arthralgia, myalgias, anorexia, sweating, headache, and malaise [585], and the diagnosis of ocular brucellosis is usually made by clinical examination and laboratory tests such as standard agglutination tests (SAT), Coombs Wright/SAT, 2-mercaptoethanol (2ME), blood culture, and bone marrow culture [584, 586], or through confirmation of etiology in other organ systems [578, 580]. The most common diagnostic method was the SAT within 1/160 and 1/320 titers [572]. Usually, the serum agglutination test is used for first screening and complement fixation or Coombs' test is used to confirm the results. It has been recommended that at least two serological tests should be combined to avoid false-negative results [575].

6.1.12.5 Examination of Intraocular Fluids

Positive isolation or finding of *Brucella melitensis* from intraocular fluids may provide direct evidence to prove in situ infection of *Brucella melitensis* and confirm the diagnosis of ocular brucellosis, particularly for the cases from pastoral area in which the other types of uveitis needs to be excluded. However, *Brucella* species are slow-growing microorganisms, whose isolation can take up to 4 weeks [577]. Hereby, rapid lab tests are demanded.

The sensitivity and specificity of the agglutination test in the aqueous humor or vitreous fluids were 66.7% and 100% for the patients with ocular brucellosis [586]. Despite that no control cases had positive agglutinations of intraocular fluids for brucellosis, there were 33.3% patients who had negative ocular agglutinations, although they were serum-positive [586]. Goldmann-Witmer coefficient of intraocular agglutinations can be further calculated to help confirmation of intraocular in situ infection of *Brucella melitensis* if the intraocular agglutinations were positive [586]. For the patient with negative culture in aqueous and humor, culture for *Brucella melitensis* in the subretinal fluid may still be positive [586].

Unbiased high-throughput sequencing approach shed light on the laboratory diagnosis of clinical diseases with unknown cause [594]. Metagenomic sequencing which could detect the total DNA or RNA has been reported to identify the *Brucella melitensis* in the intraocular fluids from a case without presumed diagnosis of ocular brucellosis and with mild increased blood titer of *Brucella* standard tube agglutination (1:25). Furthermore, the result of cytokine detection of the same sample of intraocular fluid showed a severe inflammatory reaction [595].

6.1.12.6 Management

For the patient who was diagnosed with brucellosis or ocular brucellosis, systemic antibiotic treatment along with topical or systemic corticosteroid treatment should be given to control inflammation. Oral rifampin 600 mg/day and doxycycline

100 mg/twice daily were reported most frequently [570, 584, 585, 596]. Intramuscular streptomycin sulfate, 1 g/d in an injection for 2 weeks [585]; co-trimoxazole adult two tablets, three times a day (tid) for 2 months [570]; and intravenous ceftriaxone [596] as part of combination therapy were also reported to be used sometimes. Dexamethasone phosphate drops four times a day serves as topical corticosteroid treatment [585], and oral prednisolone 1 mg/kg being tapered and stopped during a 2-month period serves as systemic corticosteroid treatment [585]. Treatment duration of antibiotics and corticosteroid were usually 2 months [570, 579, 585]. Patients with panuveitis had the worst visual prognosis, and the rate of patients with legally blind or with no light perception can be as high as 89% (8/9) and 56% (5/9) [578]. A vaccination and culling in animals should be taken in to consideration for control of regional rate of human brucellosis [597].

6.1.13 Endophthalmitis

6.1.13.1 Brief Introduction

Endophthalmitis refers to intraocular infection caused by bacteria or fungi. The intraocular inflammation induced by viruses, parasites, or other microorganisms should be regarded as other types of uveitis rather than endophthalmitis. The progress of endophthalmitis is often rapid, which may occur within a few hours or days after the symptom onset. Delay of management of endophthalmitis usually leads to irreversible blindness [598].

There are many mechanisms for endophthalmitis to cause damage to intraocular tissues. Take *Staphylococcus aureus* as an example; intraocular inflammation comes from the direct damage of bacteria to tissues and cells, dead bacteria and bacterial walls, and toxins secreted. Dead bacteria and bacterial walls only cause inflammation, but do not directly damage the retina, while toxins can damage the retina [599, 600].

6.1.13.2 Epidemiology

Endophthalmitis can be exogenous, with microorganisms on or outside the eye surface entering the eye, or endogenous, disseminated by blood. Exogenous factors include cataract surgery, trauma, intraocular implants [601], or filtering bleb-related factors. The risk factors of endogenous endophthalmitis are mainly diabetes (60.0%–88.2%) [601–603], followed by urinary tract infection (17.5%–29.4%) [601, 602], AIDS [604], cholecystitis [605], colonoscopy [606], genitourinary surgery [607], rheumatic cases such as granulomatosis with polyangiitis [608], infectious endocarditis [609], liver abscess [610], etc. In developed countries, the main causes of endophthalmitis are secondary after cataract surgery and intravitreal drug injection [598].

6.1.13.3 Clinical Manifestation

The most common symptom of endophthalmitis is blurred vision, and almost all patients have this symptom [598]. The initial symptom of all patients with endophthalmitis caused by candida is decreased vision, which can be sudden loss of vision, or partial blurred vision with or without dark spots [611]. In terms of endophthalmitis, eye pain, eye discomfort, and redness are also common. Patients with endogenous endophthalmitis may also have fever [612], but those with exogenous endophthalmitis are basically absent.

The ocular signs include ciliary congestion, anterior chamber floating cells, aqueous flare, hypopyon (about 80% of patients after cataract surgery) [613], vitreous opacity (Fig. 6.44), etc. The retinal vessels cannot be seen because of the opacity of refractive stroma [614]. When endogenous endophthalmitis spreads into the eye through choroid, subretinal abscess [615] or chorioretinal lesion may be observed (Fig. 6.45). Bacterial endophthalmitis is usually acute and occurs within a few days of an induced event, such as cataract surgery. Fungal endophthalmitis is subacute. Fungal infection of aqueous humor or vitreous tends to form clusters of inflammatory turbidity (Fig. 6.46), while bacterial endophthalmitis shows diffuse changes (Fig. 6.47). Among the patients with endophthalmitis caused by candida, 52% showed panuveitis, and 30% had retinal or papillary edema [611].

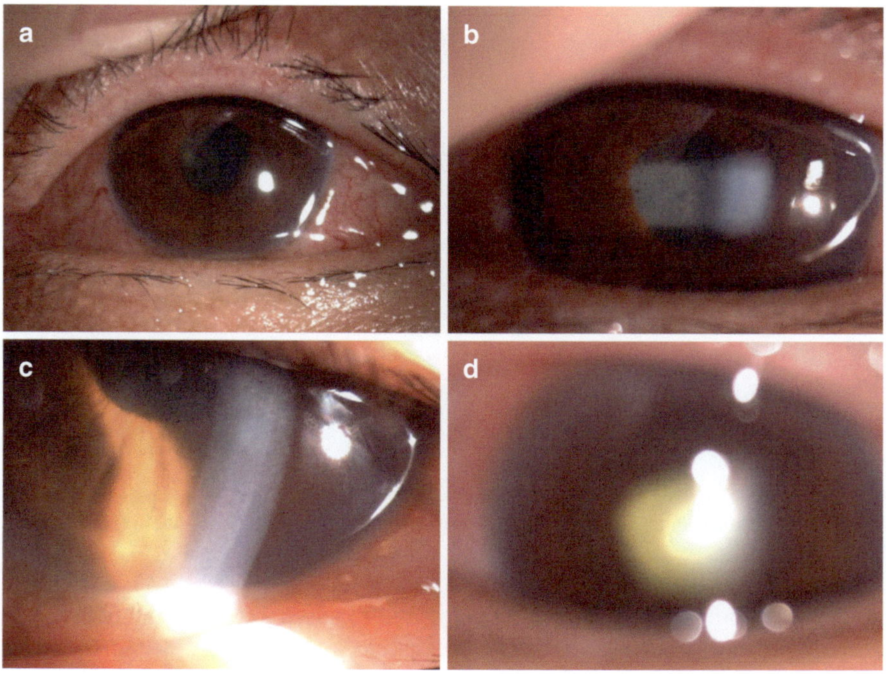

Fig. 6.44 A 48-year-old female with unexplained thrombocytopenia suffered from redness and pain in her left eye and decreased vision after continuous infusion of dexamethasone in the local hospital for 1 month. *Aspergillus fumigatus* was cultured positive in the vitreous fluid, which proved to be endogenous fungal endophthalmitis. Ocular signs included ciliary congestion (**a**), aqueous humor flare (**b**), hypopyon (**c**), and vitreous opacity (**d**)

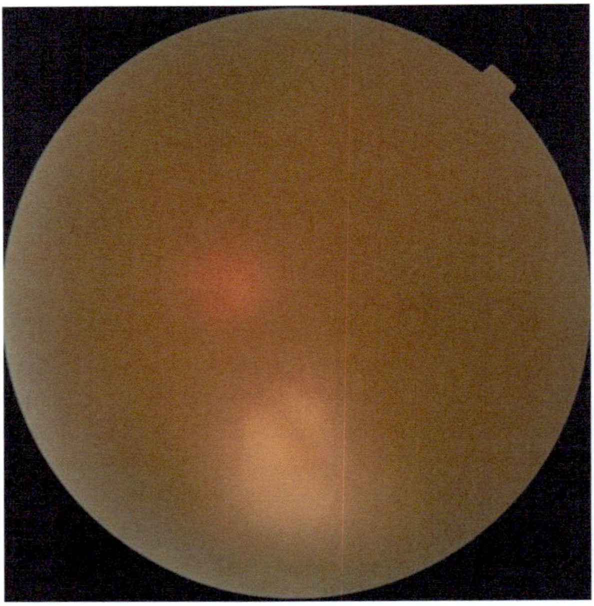

Fig. 6.45 A 62-year-old male with unsatisfactory control of diabetes came to clinic due to blurred vision in the left eye for 5 days. *Candida albicans* was detected positive by LAMP (loop-mediated isothermal amplification) in the vitreous fluid of the left eye, and hereby the diagnosis of endogenous fungal endophthalmitis was confirmed. Vitreous opacity in the left eye and white chorioretinopathy with unclear boundary beneath the optic disc can be observed

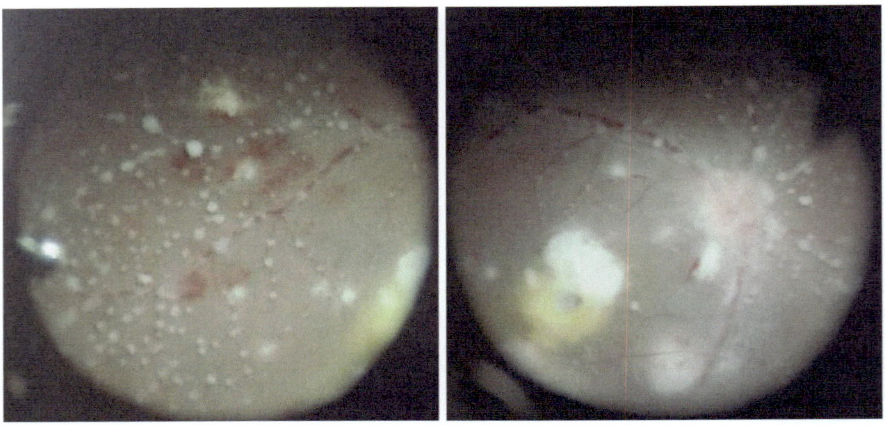

Fig. 6.46 Fundus photo of the right eye of a 54-year-old male. White vitreous opacity in clusters in the vitreous attached to surface of retina can be observed. Candida albicans was identified from the vitreous fluid

The development speed of endophthalmitis caused by different pathogenic microorganisms varied. Generally, bacteria progress fast (usually within 15 days), and fungi progress slowly (about 21–62 days) [616]. There are also differences between different species of bacteria, such as endophthalmitis caused by *Pseudomonas aeruginosa* for 1 day [617], *Staphylococcus epidermidis* for 3 days [618], *Stenotrophomonas maltophilia* for 1–3 days [619], and *Nocardia* for 24.23 ± 17.15 days [620].

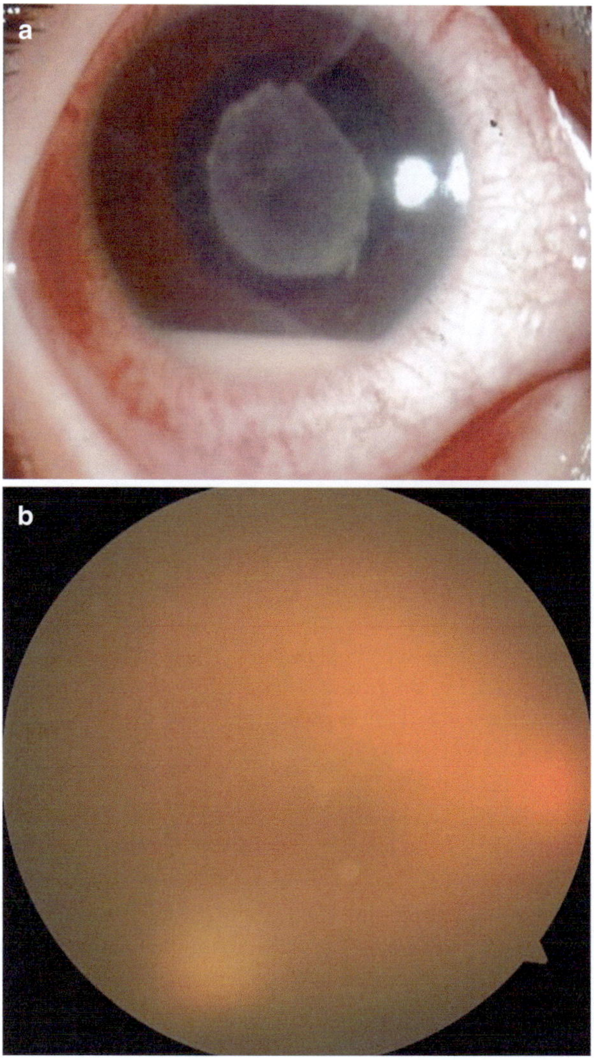

Fig. 6.47 Fundus photography of the right eye of a 7-year-old male. He complained of red and painful eye and blurred vision after 1 day of fever. Ciliary congestion, hypopyon (**a**), and diffuse vitreous opacity (**b**) can be observed. *Streptococcus pyogenes* was identified from the aqueous humor by loop-mediated isothermal amplification (LAMP), and hereby the diagnosis of bacterial endophthalmitis was confirmed

6.1.13.4 Diagnosis

Endophthalmitis is a clinical diagnosis based on clinical manifestations, which can be determined through microbial culture and blood culture of vitreous and/or aqueous humor (when endogenous endophthalmitis occurs) [598]. The possibility of endophthalmitis should be considered if the patient has obvious symptoms and signs of intraocular inflammation, with a recent history of open ocular trauma or intraocular surgery, or with low immunity and systemic risk factors that may cause endogenous endophthalmitis. Relevant laboratory tests should be carried out in time, but at least 20–30% of endophthalmitis were negative by various traditional microbial identification methods [598]. For example, for endogenous endophthalmitis, a positive culture from ocular fluid or other body fluids was obtained in 68.9% of patients with the blood being the highest source among all culture-positive results (42.0%) [602].

Considering the rapid progress and poor prognosis of endophthalmitis, even if the microbiological identification results are negative or it takes time to wait for the examination results, if the clinical manifestations are typical, it should still be actively treated. Molecular tests or relevant auxiliary antigen/antibody tests, if available in the laboratory, can provide evidence for clinicians to make diagnosis in the early stage.

6.1.13.5 Examination of Intraocular Fluids

For patients with presumed endophthalmitis, it is a traditional laboratory method to take out aqueous humor or vitreous fluid for smear staining, microscopic observation, and subsequent microbial culture for identification. PCR method was used to identify the nucleic acid sequence of pathogenic microorganisms in intraocular fluid, which was reported in different countries and showed more advantages than traditional methods (Table 6.3).

Because there are a large number of bacteria which can be the pathogens for endophthalmitis, PCR method is used to detect the common sequence nucleic acid of different kinds of bacteria—broad-spectrum bacterial nucleic acid, which has been studied by different scholars. This method was first reported for endophthalmitis in 1994, but the results at that time were not very satisfactory: PCR detection of the conservative region of bacterial 16S rRNA gene showed that 74% of patients with delayed endophthalmitis were positive, but 14% of the normal control group's intraocular fluid was also positive [627]. With the progress of technology, the results reported in the later stage are getting better and better: Mishra D et al. used broad-spectrum PCR to detect bacterial 16S rRNA in the vitreous fluid of patients with endophthalmitis; the positive rate was 65.13% (127/195), compared with 8.7% (17/195) and 30.76% (60/195) in traditional microbial culture and automatic microbial culture, with a statistically significant difference ($P < 0.0001$) [628]. In addition, for the broad-spectrum bacterial nucleic acid detection of 16S rRNA gene, the bacterial species can also be determined by analyzing the sequence. Research shows that the consistency rate of genus level is 96%, and the consistency rate of species

Table 6.3 Comparison of PCR detection of pathogenic microorganisms in intraocular fluid and microbial culture reported in different countries

Authors	Year	Country	Case number	Positive rate of PCR	Positive rate of culture
Pongsachareonnont et al. [621]	2017	Thailand	41	26.8%	11.2%
Bispo et al. [622]	2011	Brazil	21	95.3%	47.6%
Sowmya et al. [623]	2009	India	72	62.5%	37.5%
Seal et al. [624]	2008	England	20	95.0%	70.0%
Chiquet et al. [625]	2007	France	30	61%	32%
Anand et al. [626]	2000	India	57	91.2%	56.1%

level is 87.5% [629]. Ogawa et al. reported to conduct broad-spectrum detection of 28S rRNA gene of fungi. Their results showed that among 11 patients with positive 28S rRNA gene detection of fungi, 10 patients were fungal endophthalmitis which was confirmed by further examination, and the correct rate was as high as 90.9% [630].

Budding AE et al. developed an automated method for the detection of 16S–23S rRNA gene broad-spectrum bacteria—IS pro. In 66 samples, IS pro and microbial culture were positive in 20 (30%) samples. In addition, in 31 (47%) samples, IS pro identified more bacterial species than microbial culture. In addition, in five samples with negative microbial culture, IS pro was positive. Hereby, this automated broad-spectrum bacterial detection method shows advantages and brings hope for rapid identification of endophthalmitis bacteria in the future [631].

To carry out high-throughput sequencing to analyze all nucleic acid sequences of intraocular fluid samples and then compare the data in the gene library to obtain microbial information, meta-genomic sequencing which is unbiased and hypothesis-free shed light on laboratory diagnosis of complicated endophthalmitis. Deshmukh D et al. collected the vitreous bodies of 34 patients with suspected endophthalmitis and carried out high-throughput sequencing (metagenomic next-generation sequencing, mNGS). Only 44% (15/34) of patients were positive for traditional culture, while 88% (30/34, 26/30 for bacteria, 2/30 for fungi, and 2/30 for mixed infection) of patients were positive for NGS. Moreover, NGS in intraocular fluid samples of 30 patients with negative control was negative [632]. In one our preliminary study including 15 eyes of 15 patients, 8 samples were identified as positive for different kinds of pathogens by mNGS and were also confirmed by other laboratory examinations or effective diagnostic treatment; however, despite that the final diagnosis was still intraocular infection in 4 (included 1 fungi, 1 *Brucella melitensis,* and 2 tuberculosis-induced intraocular infection) of the 7 cases with negative mNGS results. Hereby, mNGS could be helpful in determining pathogens in cases of suspected intraocular infection, and the mNGS protocols should be optimized for the detection of intracellular bacterial and fungal pathogens [633].

Although blood or tissue culture and histological examination are the gold standard for diagnosis of systemic invasive fungal infection, many auxiliary tests are used to assist diagnosis [634, 635]. It is a routine practice to smear intraocular fluid specimens, identify *Candida* spp. with Gram stain method and methyl blue for the presence of filamentous fungi and India ink staining for *Cryptococcus* spp. under light microscope. For microbial culture, the samples are inoculated on Sabouraud medium and incubated at 37 °C and 27 °C for 7–10 days. Check the culture dish every day, and then conduct macroscopic and microscopic evaluation on the colonies. Other diagnostic methods include detection of specific antigens, such as *Candida* mannan antigen, *Aspergillus* galactomannan antigen, and *Cryptococcus* antigen [636].

β-D-glucan (BDG, G test) is a polysaccharide cell wall component found in many fungi, which is released during invasive fungal infection [637]. Under the situation of infection by *Candida, Aspergillus, Fusarium,* and other fungi, the BDG content in serum can be measured quantitatively [634]. However, not all pathogenic fungi produce BDG (or only at a very low level). Therefore, the G test is not applicable when the intraocular tissues are infected by *Cryptococcus*, Zygomycetes, and *Blastomycetes* that usually cause dermatitis. The overall sensitivity, positive predictive value, specificity, and negative predictive value of Fungitell kit (a G test kit) for the diagnosis of invasive fungal infection were 64.3%, 91.1%, 86.6%, and 74.1%, respectively [634]. Although BDG levels were reported to be measured in pleural effusion [638], cerebrospinal fluid [639], bronchoalveolar lavage samples [640], and joint fluid [641], the normal range of intraocular fluid BDG concentrations has not been determined [634]. We previously reported the G test results in a series of fungal endophthalmitis cases and non-fungal intraocular inflammation cases including bacterial endophthalmitis and acute retinal necrosis, the mean data were 1875 ± 612.7 pg/mL (range: 859 pg/mL–4109 pg/mL) and 45.1 ± 13.34 pg/mL (range: <10 pg/mL–97.1 pg/mL), respectively. Remarkably, there was a gap between the positive and negative measurement results [642]. Shimbo et al. quantitatively measured the vitreous fluid BDG level of 26 patients and found that the vitreous fluid BDG level of two patients with fungal endophthalmitis was significantly increased, while the vitreous fluid BDG level of other patients was lower than 10.0 pg/mL [643]. In addition, because BDG is easy to be contaminated when it is submitted for examination, in the diagnostic guidelines for some invasive fungal infections in internal medicine, it is required that the G test and GM test of blood samples are positive for two consecutive times [644]. The situations as follows may lead to false negative of G test: (1) having received antifungal treatment and (2) Zygomyces (cephalosporium, mucor, and calcaneus) infection. The situations as follows may lead to false positive of G test: (1) hemodialysis; (2) intravenous infusion of immunoglobulin, albumin, and blood transfusion; (3) using β-lactamase inhibitor; (4) streptococcemia; and (5) contamination exists when the operator handles the specimen. Therefore, in the process of G test detection, attention must be paid to aseptic operation, and the operation standards must be strictly followed. When making diagnosis, the above influencing factors should also be taken into account, so as to reduce the unreasonable use of antifungal drugs [645].

Galactomannan (GM) is a polysaccharide component of cell wall of most *Aspergillus* species, which is released when invading tissues or blood vessels. GM test is of great value in the diagnosis of pulmonary aspergillosis. The meta-analysis results showed that serum GM in patients with impaired immunity suspected of having suspected invasive aspergillosis had sensitivity of 0.71 and specificity of 0.89 [646].

Lipopolysaccharide (LPS) is an endotoxin released by gram-negative bacteria. If LPS was added to human retinal pigment epithelial cell line in culture, the expression levels of MCP-1 and IL-6 increased significantly [647]. An animal model of endophthalmitis can be created by injecting LPS into the eyes of rabbits [648]. In our experience, spectroscopic examination of LPS in intraocular fluid can be assisted to provide an objective evidence for clinical diagnosis of gram-negative bacterial endophthalmitis in a short time which usually may be less than 2 h. We have ever reported the examination of LPS in the aqueous humor for a case with hypopyon and inflammation signs in the anterior segment at 10 days after cataract surgery. Spectroscopic examination of aqueous humor revealed LPS level of >2.5 (normal value <0.053, suspected or early infection 0.053–0.109, and positive value >0.109) and interleukin (IL)-6 level of 70186.8 pg/mL, which was highly positive and strongly implied a severe intraocular infection by gram-negative bacteria. Antibiotics sensitive to gram-negative bacteria were given rapidly. Five days later, the Gram-negative bacillus *Stenotrophomonas maltophilia* was cultured, which confirmed the diagnosis despite the prolonged report. Comparatively, the level of LPS in the aqueous humor samples collected from cataract surgery for five patients were all negative [649].

Cells in the vitreous cavity, especially those related to retinal components, may be activated when bacterial infection occurs and secrete immune-related cytokines, including IL-1 β, IL-6, CXCL1, CXCL2, SLPI, INF γ, MIP2, IL-17A, cathelicidin-related peptide (CRAMP), hBD-1, and hBD-2 [600, 650–657]. Deshmukh et al. tested the titers of 16 kinds of cytokines in vitreous humor of endophthalmitis with positive microbial culture, including GCSF, GRO and IFN-γ, IL-1 α, IL-1 β, IL-1 RA, IL-6, IL-8, IP-10, MCP-1, MCP-3, MIP-1 α, IL-1 β, TGF-α, and TNF-α. The study found that IL-1RA, IL-6, IL-8, GRO, and G-CSF are independent predictors of endophthalmitis and non-endophthalmitis diseases. Initial vision was significantly associated with intraocular levels of TGF- α, IL-1 β, and IL-8 [658].

For laboratory examination of endophthalmitis, vitreous specimen is more accurate and reliable than aqueous humor specimen. It was reported that 48% of endophthalmitis patients with negative aqueous humor microbial culture had positive microbial growth [659]. Similar results were repeated in the Chinese study: three cases of endophthalmitis with no microorganism in aqueous humor were found positive in vitreous fluid; however, none of the intraocular fluid patients with negative vitreous fluid test had positive aqueous humor results [660]. In order to identify the pathogen, vitrectomy and diagnostic vitrectomy are often used for sampling, but the culture-positive rate of vitreous samples collected from vitrectomy is higher than that of vitreous paracentesis (92% vs. 44%) [661]. One of the possible reasons is that the specimen of vitrectomy is closer to the retinal surface [662].

6.1.13.6 Management

The prognosis of endophthalmitis is related to many factors, majorly the types of infectious pathogens. For instance, in patients with endogenous endophthalmitis, the prognosis caused by gram-negative bacteria is worse than that caused by gram-positive bacteria [602]. The prognosis of endophthalmitis caused by candida is better than that caused by mold. The regression of retinal exudation is the earliest manifestation of treatment, which can occur within 1–2 weeks after treatment [611].

Intravitreal injection of antibiotics is an effective means to treat bacterial endophthalmitis. For endophthalmitis caused by gram-positive bacteria, vancomycin injection is highly sensitive (97.14%, 34/35). If the bacterial flora of endophthalmitis is from oral and upper respiratory tract, the prognosis is worse [663]. In the consensus of experts on the treatment of acute bacterial endophthalmitis after cataract surgery in China in 2010, the drug regimen for vitreous injection of suspected cases and early cases was given: (1) 10 g/L vancomycin 0.1 mL + 20 g/L ceftazidime 0.1 mL, (2) 10 g/L vancomycin 0.1 mL + 4 g/L amikacin 0.1 mL, and (3) 10 g/L vancomycin 0.1 mL + 22.5 g/L ceftazidime 0.1 mL. Inhale the dissolved diluent of the above preparation method into a 1 mL syringe, and inject 0.1 mL intravitreally. It is recommended to inject once every 3 days [664].

The recommended scheme for anterior chamber lavage of bacterial endophthalmitis is as follows: vancomycin (0.02 g/L) + ceftazidime (0.04 g/L), inhale 1 mL syringes respectively, add 1 mL of each into 500 mL infusion balanced salt solution or other perfusion solutions, and perform anterior chamber lavage [664].

It is proposed that phased treatment plans be taken for control of infectious endophthalmitis after cataract extraction in different stages. In the first stage with only anterior chamber floater cells 2+ and without hypopyon and vitreous opacity, intensive observation is required, and if necessary, anterior chamber antibiotic irrigation and/or adjuvant therapy can be given. In the second stage with hypopyon and without vitreous opacity shown by B-ultrasound, antibiotic lavage in the anterior chamber and intravitreal injection combined with adjuvant therapy should be given. In the third stage with hypopyon and vitreous opacity, vitrectomy and intravitreal injection combined with adjuvant therapy should be given. In clinical practice, the patient should be monitored every 4–6 h. For patients with rapid progression disease, the patient should be monitored every 2 h, and the treatment plan should be constantly adjusted according to the stage of the disease [665].

For bacterial endophthalmitis, it is regarded that early vitrectomy results in better prognosis such as improvement of visual acuity [666] or preservation of the anatomical integrity of eyeballs [667]. A randomized study including 108 cases of endogenous endophthalmitis showed that vitrectomy combined with silicone oil tamponade led to better prognosis, i.e., lower risk of retinal detachment and better final visual acuity. In vitrectomy-combined silicone-oil group and single vitrectomy group, the successful rates were 63.7% and 43.4%, respectively [668].

For fungal endophthalmitis, vitrectomy is also considered necessary. Celiker H et al. showed that vitrectomy can improve the vision of 85.7% (6/7) of the affected eyes, and 28.6% (2/7) of the affected eyes need to be operated again, but all the affected eyes kept the retina attached at the last follow-up visit without occurrence of atrophia bulbi [669]. Similar research results can also be observed in the report of Ghoraba et al. 70% (7 eyes) of ten eyes with endogenous fungal endophthalmitis after urinary surgery had improved vision after vitrectomy. All patients kept the retina attached without occurrence of atrophy eyeball [670]. Lee et al.'s research results suggest that early vitrectomy led to better visual prognosis [671].

Mithal et al.'s treatment plan for fungal endophthalmitis was as follows: all eyes underwent pars plana vitrectomy with injection of antifungals, comprising daily intravitreal voriconazole (100 μg/0.1 mL) and alternate day intravitreal amphotericin B (5 μg/0.1 mL), until resolution of vitreous exudates [616]. In the treatment of cases of exogenous fungal endophthalmitis reported by Wykoff CC, most of them used at least three different antifungal drugs, in consideration of the high drug resistance of fungi [672]. The combination of different antifungal drugs may enhance the overall effect of treatment.

In general, although the prognosis of endophthalmitis is generally poor, if early diagnosis and correct intervention can be made, a considerable number of cases can still achieve good results [671].

6.2 Noninfectious Intraocular Inflammation

6.2.1 Diabetic Retinopathy

6.2.1.1 Brief Introduction

Diabetic retinopathy (DR) is a significant contributor to global visual impairment, defined as a crucial microvascular consequence of diabetes that impacts around 30 to 40% of individuals with diabetes [673–675]. Diabetes-induced hyperglycemia can trigger metabolic pathways, leading to impaired functioning of mitochondria in retinal cells, loss of pericytes, and thickening of basement membranes in retinal blood vessels. The subsequent occurrence of ischemia and inflammatory conditions in the retinal tissue might result in retinal neurodegeneration, the formation of microaneurysms, retinal edema, neovascularization, and the growth of glial cells [676].

6.2.1.2 Epidemiology

In 2021, the prevalence of diabetes mellitus reached 529 million individuals globally, reflecting the increasing global trend of this condition [677]. As a result, the prevalence of people experiencing diabetic retinopathy (DR) or diabetic macular edema (DME) has similarly risen over time. DR is expected to increase from 103 million cases in 2020 to 161 million cases in 2045 [678]. A prior meta-analysis examined the epidemiology of DR, finding that the overall occurrence of any DR in individuals with diabetes mellitus was estimated to be 34.6%, with PDR at 6.96% and DME at 6.81% [674]. Approximately 60.0% of patients will receive a diagnosis of DR after enduring 20 years of type 2 diabetes mellitus (T2DM) [679]. As the duration of the follow-up period increases, the severity of DR advances in 34–41% of patients, and 7–11% of patients experience the development of PDR [680, 681].

DME is an important complication of DR and can greatly impact the vision of diabetes mellitus patients. It can occur at any stage of DR, and the risk for DME increases over time. The occurrence of DME in patients with T2DM rises from 3% within 5 years of diagnosis to 28% after 20 years [682]. By 2045, it is projected that there would be around 29 million patients worldwide with clinically significant diabetic macular edema (CSDME) [678].

For each year before puberty, the likelihood of clinical retinopathy increased by 28%, and for each year beyond puberty, it increased by 36% [683]. Hyperglycemia is the main systemic factor that impacts the progression of early DR. It has been proposed that there is a strong correlation between HbA1c levels and the probability of encountering complications [684]. Nevertheless, when blood pressure and total serum cholesterol are taken into account, HbA1c alone may only account for a maximum of 10% of the risk of DR [685].

6.2.1.3 Clinical Manifestation

DR is characterized by specific observations such as intraretinal hemorrhages, which can appear as dot-, blot-, or flame-shaped, as well as hard exudates, cotton-wool spots, intraretinal microvascular abnormalities (IRMAs), and beading of retinal veins [686]. The categorization of DR is determined on the observable characteristics of the disease. Non-proliferative diabetic retinopathy (NPDR) is characterized by alterations in the blood vessels within the retina, without the appearance of fibrovascular tissue outside the retina (Fig. 6.48). NPDR is classified into three categories: mild, moderate, and severe.

If intraretinal hemorrhages and microaneurysms can be observed in four quadrants of the retina, venous beading can be observed in two or more quadrants of the retina, and moderate intraretinal microvascular abnormalities (IRMA) can be observed in at least one quadrant of the retina, there is a very high chance of progression to proliferative DR (PDR) [686]. Proliferative diabetic retinopathy (PDR) is characterized by the formation of new blood vessels due to reduced blood supply caused by diabetes and its related consequences. PDR can be categorized as either early, high-risk, or advanced [687].

When retinopathy advances to PDR, one can see the presence of newly formed retinal arteries or fibrous tissue that intersect and extend beyond the retina (Fig. 6.49). Vitreous hemorrhage and tractional retinal detachment can occur due to bleeding from retinal arteries or the contraction of fibrovascular tissue. Neovascular proliferation can be classified into two categories: neovascularization of the disc (NVD) and neovascularization elsewhere (NVE), depending on its location [688].

In eyes with CSDME, hard exudates and thickening of the retina at or within 500 micrometers of the center of the macula can be observed, and patients have a higher chance of experiencing blurred vision [689].

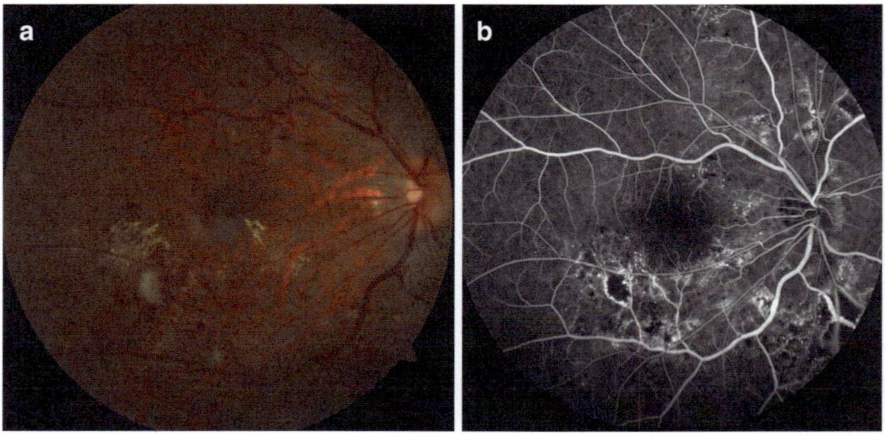

Fig. 6.48 Fundus photography of right eye (**a**) and fundus fluorescein angiography (**b**) of non-proliferative diabetic retinopathy. Microaneurysms, retinal hemorrhages, hard exudates, and small areas of retinal capillary non-perfusion without neovascularization can be observed

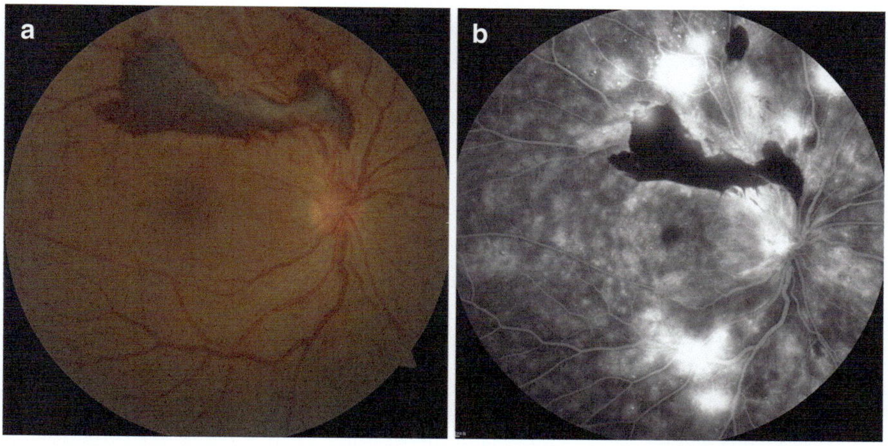

Fig. 6.49 Fundus photography of right eye (**a**) and fundus fluorescein angiography (**b**) of proliferative diabetic retinopathy. Vitreous hemorrhage, retinal neovascularization, and remarkable leakage of fluorescence can be observed

6.2.1.4 Diagnosis

Direct and indirect ophthalmoscopy, along with fundal photography, are the most popular methods for diagnosing DR [690]. Retinal hemorrhages, soft and hard exudates, and fibrovascular membranes commonly found in the eyes of diabetic patients are indicative of the existence of DR. Non-mydriatic digital cameras, while effective for DR screening, exhibit lower sensitivity when compared to ultra-wide-field fundus photography and indirect ophthalmoscopy [691]. DME is diagnosed when slit lamp biomicroscopy or optical coherence tomography (OCT) reveals retinal thickness, intraretinal cysts, subretinal fluids, hyper-reflective foci, and disorganization of retinal inner layers (DRIL) in patients with DME. Research has demonstrated a strong correlation between retinal thickness, intraretinal cysts, and DRIL with patients' visual acuity [692].

Moreover, FA is valuable for the diagnosis of DR. During FA, the presence of tiny hyperfluorescent dots, with or without mild leakage of dye in the late phase, indicates the presence of microaneurysms. Additionally, areas of hypofluorescence, known as hypofluorescent non-perfusion areas, can be noticed in the peripheral or posterior pole of the retina. Neovascularization exhibits initial intense fluorescence and subsequent release of fluid in FA. FA is a valuable technique for visualizing the disruption of the blood-retinal barrier through the detection of leakage from retinal capillaries, while it is not suitable for assessing the presence or absence of macular edema. The presence of leakage shown on the angiography does not necessarily indicate macular edema, as it can occur even without thickness of the macular retina. Therefore, it is not considered a definitive diagnostic sign of macular edema [690]. OCT-angiography (OCTA) is an innovative diagnostic method that allows for the noninvasive examination of retinal vascular networks. It is particularly effective in identifying foveal and macular ischemia in eyes affected by DR [693].

6.2.1.5 Examination of Intraocular Fluids

Angiogenic and pro-inflammatory factors play a crucial role in the formation and progression of DR and DME. Presently, the utilization of intraocular fluid analysis in DR is predominantly employed as a supplementary technique. The test can provide insights into the presence of neovascularization, proliferative fibrosis, and immune-inflammatory activity, which can serve as indicators of the disease's severity and help predict therapy outcomes. Furthermore, it serves as a guide for choosing suitable therapies.

As early as 1994, the Aiello and Adamis teams reported an increased concentration of vascular endothelial growth factor (VEGF) in the vitreous of patients with PDR [694, 695]. Angiopoietin-2 (Ang-2) in Tie-2 pathways may be associated with the breakdown of the blood-retinal barrier, increased leakage from retinal vessels, aggregation of leukocytes, and development of neovascularization in DR [696, 697]. Other angiogenic factors, such as transforming growth factor-β (TGF-β), placental growth factor (PlGF), erythropoietin (EPO), matrix metalloproteinase-9 (MMP-9), and apelin, have also been reported to be related to the severity of DR [698–704].

Following the administration of ranibizumab treatment through monthly injections into the eye, the levels of ICAM-1, VEGF, PlGF, IL-6, and MCP-1 reduced. The levels of VEGF were decreased by 97%, subsequently followed by reductions in IL-6, PlGF, ICAM-1, and MCP-1, which were lower by 63%, 51%, 15%, and 6% correspondingly [705]. Additionally, a significant decrease in IP-10, IL-1β, IL-1RA, IL-5, eotaxin, FMS-like tyrosine kinase-3 ligand (Flt-3 L), IL-12p40, IL-12p70, and growth-related oncogene (GRO) levels was observed after five monthly injections of aflibercept, while fractalkine and granulocyte macrophage colony-stimulating factor increased after therapy [706]. Intravitreal bevacizumab injection significantly reduced the concentration of VEGF in the aqueous humor of patients with PDR 1 week after treatment [707]. A study found that the concentration of IL-8 in the aqueous humor (16.81 ± 13.15 pg/mL) in DME patients with a favorable response to anti-VEGF was significantly lower than in patients with a poor response (30.82 ± 23.96 pg/mL) [708]. Additionally, an increase in baseline ICAM-1 levels was associated with a favorable anatomical response following intravitreal ranibizumab [705]. A previous study found that the concentration of VEGF in the vitreous was significantly higher in the progressive group (770.43 ± 229.04 pg/mL) compared to the stable group (506.49 ± 228.84 pg/mL) after vitrectomy for PDR ($P = 0.001$) [709].

Inflammation is another crucial aspect of DR pathogenesis. Elevated levels of various inflammatory and pro-inflammatory cytokines have been observed in patients with DR. These cytokines play a role in the breakdown of the blood-retinal barrier, damage to blood vessels, neuroinflammation, and the development of pathological angiogenesis in DR, which can be further complicated by the presence of DME and PDR [710]. Tumor necrosis factor (TNF) and various interleukins (IL) have been found to be upregulated in the aqueous and vitreous of DR patients [711–713]. The concentrations of intercellular adhesion molecule-1 (ICAM-1), vascular cell adhesion molecule-1 (VCAM-1), IL-1β, IL-6, IL-8, and TNF-α are significantly increased in the aqueous humor and vitreous fluid of DR patients and are closely correlated with disease severity [714–717]. The concentration of IL-6 in the aqueous humor continues to increase from the background stage to NPDR and further to PDR [718]. Furthermore, MCP-1 levels in the vitreous of DR patients are elevated and higher than in serum, increasing with the progression of DR [719].

Among the patients with DME, there was a positive correlation between increased levels of intercellular adhesion molecule-1 in the aqueous humor and greater macular volume ($P = 0.002$). Additionally, higher levels of IL-10 were associated with improved best-corrected Snellen visual acuity ($P = 0.03$) [720]. After receiving an intravitreal implant injection of dexamethasone for DME, the levels of IP-10 and MCP-1 reduced considerably 8 weeks later [721]. In relapsed DME cases, significantly higher levels of IL-6, IL-8, IP-10, and MCP-1 were found [721]. The effectiveness of intravitreal dexamethasone implants in reducing DME is correlated with the baseline levels of MCP-1 in the aqueous humor ($P = 0.028$). Higher baseline levels of MCP-1 are associated with better anatomical responses to treatment [722].

In conclusion, analyzing intraocular fluid in DR can provide valuable insights into the present angiogenic and inflammatory status of the patient. This information can guide the selection of optimal treatment options and help predict the outcomes following various therapeutic interventions.

6.2.1.6 Management

The management of diabetic retinopathy (DR) and diabetic macular edema (DME) may encompass diverse strategies, contingent upon the gravity and progression of the ailment. An essential element of treatment involves maintaining strict glycemic control. Research has established a correlation between HbA1c levels and the occurrence of diabetic retinopathy (DR) and diabetic macular edema (DME). Controlling blood sugar levels through dietary choices, physical activity, and medication is crucial for slowing down the advancement of diabetic retinopathy and retinal edema. Optimal glycemic management can mitigate the likelihood of ocular impairment linked to these ailments [723].

Patients with resistant diabetic macular edema (DME) can undergo laser photocoagulation to treat the specific areas of focused leakage and edema. Laser therapy is employed to precisely target and treat specific regions of the retina that are impacted by anomalous blood vessels. Laser photocoagulation reduces the risk of vision loss and preserves or enhances eyesight by closing leaking blood vessels and regulating the formation of aberrant ones. Despite the Protocol-S trial conducted by DRCR.net demonstrating comparable outcomes between continuous intravitreal administration of anti-VEGF and pan-retinal photocoagulation, the latter remains the recommended treatment in numerous guidelines for patients with severe non-proliferative diabetic retinopathy (NPDR) and proliferative diabetic retinopathy (PDR) [724].

Intravitreal injections of anti-vascular endothelial growth factor (anti-VEGF) drugs are frequently employed to treat both diabetic macular edema (DME) and diabetic retinopathy (DR). Empirical research has shown that aflibercept is effective in treating diabetic macular edema (DME) [706]. Aflibercept had superior efficacy compared to laser therapy in enhancing visual acuity and reducing central retinal thickness in individuals with diabetic macular edema, as evidenced by the VIVID and VISTA trials [725].

In recent times, the FDA has granted approval for two novel anti-VEGF medicines to be used in the treatment of DME in numerous countries. Brolucizumab is a monoclonal antibody fragment that is specifically engineered to attach to and block the activity of vascular endothelial growth factor (VEGF). By using smaller molecules and increasing the molecular dosage, it has shown a treatment response that is just as effective as aflibercept in treating DME [726]. Faricimab is a novel drug that operates by employing a dual mode of action. It has the ability to block both VEGF-A and Ang-2. Faricimab seeks to provide improved effectiveness in lowering retinal vascular leakage and enhancing visual outcomes by obstructing both causes simultaneously [727].

In the context of the development of diabetic retinopathy (DR) and diabetic macular edema (DME), corticosteroids can be employed as an alternative treatment to manage and regulate the inflammatory process. Subtenon or intravitreal corticosteroid injections have demonstrated efficacy in the management of diabetic macular edema (DME) [728]. Triamcinolone acetonide, dexamethasone implants, and fluocinolone acetonide implants are the three most common intravitreal medications for DME [729–731]. The main treatment methods for diabetic macular edema (DME) generally involve administering anti-vascular endothelial growth factor and corticosteroids through injections into the eye.

Vitreous hemorrhage or tractional retinal detachment in advanced cases of DR may require a surgical treatment known as vitrectomy. Following anti-VEGF treatment, there was a notable rise in the levels of fibrinogen and fibrinogen precursor in the vitreous fluid of PDR patients, which further intensified fibroproliferation [732]. A separate study discovered a notable reduction in VEGF levels following intravitreal anti-VEGF treatment for 2–5 days in patients with proliferative diabetic retinopathy (PDR). Conversely, the number of actively dividing cells experienced a considerable increase after 21 days of treatment [733]. These findings indicate that the most favorable timing for vitrectomy in individuals with proliferative diabetic retinopathy (PDR) is within a week following anti-vascular endothelial growth factor (anti-VEGF) medication.

6.2.2 Retinal Vein Occlusion

6.2.2.1 Brief Introduction

Retinal vein occlusion (RVO) is a prevalent retinal vascular disorder that ranks second in terms of frequency. It affects both sexes equally around the globe. RVO occurs when the retinal venous system becomes obstructed due to the formation of a blood clot, and it can manifest as central retinal vein occlusion (CRVO), hemi-central retinal vein occlusion (HRVO), or branch retinal vein occlusion (BRVO) [734, 735].

RVO can be broadly classified into ischemic or nonischemic types, mostly based on the extent of capillary non-perfusion. This differentiation holds significant clinical relevance in guiding therapeutic interventions. The extent of retinal ischemia resulting from the inadequate perfusion of retinal capillaries exhibits variability and is mostly influenced by the severity of retinal vein thrombosis [736]. These alterations result in an elevation in the synthesis of vascular endothelial growth factor (VEGF) and other cytokines, thereby promoting the formation of novel blood vessels. This phenomenon predominantly affects the iris and angle in CRVO and the retina in BRVO, but other regions may also be involved to some extent [737]. These aforementioned concerns have the potential to lead to neovascular glaucoma, vitreous hemorrhage, and tractional retinal detachment, all of which can cause substantial visual impairment [738].

6.2.2.2 Epidemiology

Prior studies have demonstrated that RVO ranks as the second most prevalent retinal vascular disorder, following diabetic retinopathy [739, 740]. BRVO exhibits a higher incidence rate but is associated with less severe visual impairment compared to CRVO [741–743].

Age and hypertension were significant risk factors for RVO [744–746]. For any RVO, the prevalence increased from 0.26% in individuals aged 30–39 years to 0.44% among those aged 40–49 years and to 3.39% in those aged 80–89 years [741]. With global aging trend, it is logical to anticipate a rise in the overall prevalence of RVO [747]. In 2008, among individuals aged 30 and above, the population of any RVO, BRVO, and CRVO were estimated to be 16.4 million, 13.9 million, and 2.5 million, respectively [748]. In 2015, the global prevalence of any RVO, BRVO, and CRVO in people aged 30–89 years was 0.77%, 0.64%, and 0.13%, equivalent to an overall of 28.06 million, 23.38 million, and 4.67 million affected people, which is remarkably more than 2008 [741].

Besides age and hypertension, diabetes is in correlation with incidence of both BRVO and CRVO [749]. Although the prevalence of diabetes in patients with RVO is not much higher than that in the general population, doing diabetes testing at the time of RVO diagnosis has proven to be an efficient method for identifying undiscovered cases of diabetes [750]. RVO has been associated with dyslipidemia, smoking, and renal illness as well. Glaucoma and elevated intraocular pressure are ocular-associated risk factors for CRVO that may impede venous outflow at the level of the lamina cribrosa [743].

Up to 34% of eyes with nonischemic CRVO converted to ischemic CRVO over a 3-year period [751]. Nevertheless, nonischemic CRVO may potentially undergo spontaneous resolution without the occurrence of any associated problems.

In the rare patient with simultaneous bilateral CRVOs, the possibility of hyperviscosity should be considered [747]. There is an annual increase of 0.9% in the likelihood of developing any vascular obstruction in the unaffected eye of individuals with unilateral CRVO [747, 752]. The occurrence of bilateral BRVO is observed in approximately 4.5% to 6.5% of patients upon initial diagnosis. Moreover, there is an elevated likelihood of developing BRVO in the unaffected eye, ranging from 7% to 10% [753].

6.2.2.3 Clinical Manifestation

The clinical examination of BRVO reveals the presence of sectoral hemorrhages, both retinal and intraretinal, as well as edema, cotton-wool patches, venous dilations, and tortuosity [754]. Nonischemic CRVO (Fig. 6.50) exhibits a lower probability of presenting with disc or macular edema, many hemorrhages, cotton-wool patches, and pronounced tortuosity compared to ischemic CRVO [755].

Macular edema (ME) is the primary etiology of visual impairment in retinal vein occlusion (RVO), often accompanied by subsequent foveal ischemia [734, 750]. ME represents a significant consequence that can arise from both ischemic and nonischemic CRVO. It is possible for ME to have spontaneous resolution, and the resolution of ME in ischemia CRVO varied between 0% and 73% within a timeframe of 2 to 15 months. In comparison, the corresponding proportion for nonischemic CRVO was 30% [751]. During a 1-year period, a range of 5% to 15% of eyes diagnosed with BRVO without ME at the beginning of the study subsequently acquired ME. Conversely, among those eyes that initially presented with ME, around 41% saw resolution of ME without any therapeutic intervention within a timeframe of 7.5 months [753].

Vitreous hemorrhage (VH) is another prevalent condition leading to visual impairment in patients with untreated ischemic RVO accompanied with posterior segment neovascularization. It ranks as the second most frequent cause of vision loss, following ME, with a reported occurrence rate ranging from 61% to 73%. The occurrence of VH in untreated ischemia CRVO was estimated to be 10% and 13% at 9 months and 10 years of follow-up, respectively [756].

In the later stages, distinctive observations may include the presence of hard exudates, microaneurysms, vein sclerosis, vascular shunts at the optic disc, arterial constriction and sheathing, VH, tractional retinal detachment, as well as neovascularization affecting the retina, optic disc, or iris [757]. The incidence of neovascular

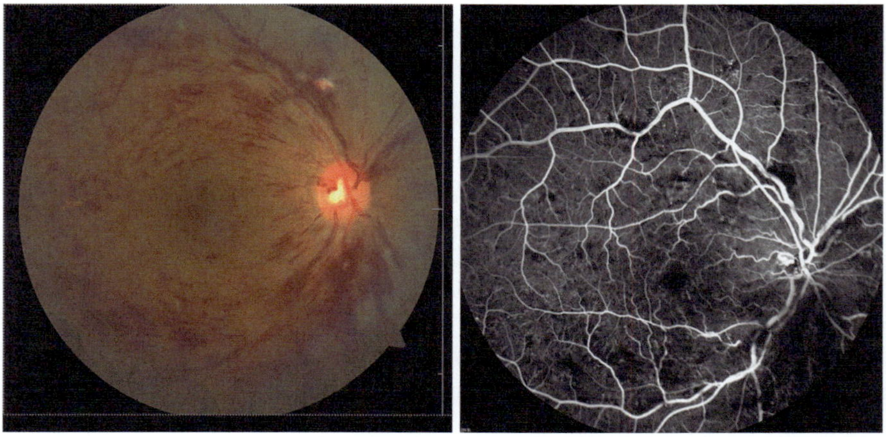

Fig. 6.50 The fundus photography (left) and fluorescein angiography (right) of the right eye with central retinal vein occlusion. Pan-retinal hemorrhages, cotton-wool patches, venous dilation and tortuosity, and hypofluorescence area due to retinal hemorrhage can be observed

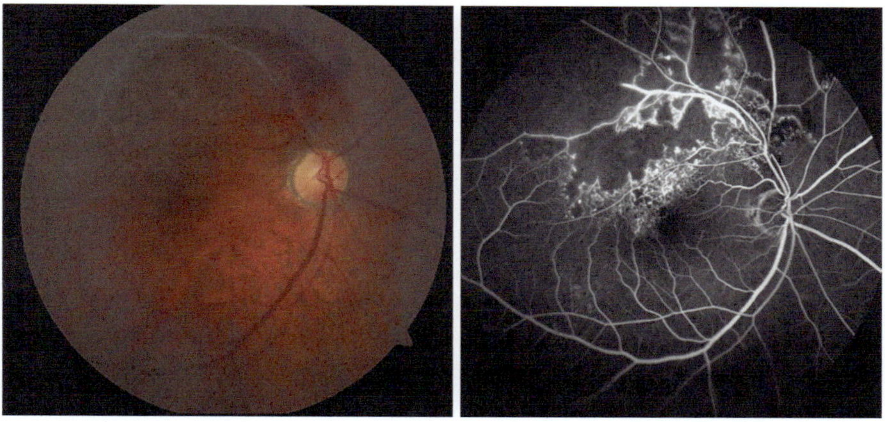

Fig. 6.51 The fundus photography (left) and fluorescein angiography (right) of the right eye with branch retinal vein occlusion in the late stage. Occlusion retinal superior temporal branch vein and corresponding non-perfusion area without remarkable retinal neovascularization can be observed

complications is significantly reduced in cases of BRVO due to the limited extent of capillary non-perfusion (Fig. 6.51). The prevalence of retinal neovascularization exceeds that of anterior segment neovascularization [735]. The risk of developing neovascular glaucoma (NVG) is elevated in individuals with an expanded area of retinal non-perfusion, and this risk is strongly associated with the likelihood of developing anterior segment neovascularization [758]. However, it should be noted that not all eyes exhibiting anterior segment neovascularization (NV) will always develop NVG [759].

Vascular leakage may be observed in the early or middle stages of fluorescein angiography (FA), but cystic space filling may be characteristic of late-stage FA. Nevertheless, optical coherence tomography (OCT) remains the most efficacious approach for the diagnosis and evaluation of ME caused by RVO [760]. FA or optical coherence tomography angiography (OCTA) is commonly advised for the assessment of retinal non-perfusion in order to facilitate the identification of eyes afflicted with ischemic RVO [750]. In the realm of RVO, the utilization of optical coherence tomography angiography (OCTA) has facilitated a comprehensive examination of the superficial capillary plexus (SCP) and deep capillary plexus (DCP) [761]. Both the SCP and DCP of RVO eyes may exhibit a larger foveal avascular zone (FAZ) [762, 763]. Given its proximity and stronger association with the retinal arterioles, the SCP has a higher prevalence of non-perfusion zones compared to the DCP [764]. Moreover, when comparing with FA or OCT, cystoid pockets, which are characterized by black circular regions lacking flow signal, exert a more pronounced influence on both plexuses and are more readily discernible [765].

6.2.2.4 Diagnosis

Clinical diagnosis of RVO mainly depends the fundus appearance including retinal hemorrhage, edema, dilated and torturous retinal vein, impaired blood flow, etc.

These manifestations may occur in an asymptomatic eye [760]. When RVO is suspected, it is recommended to do a comprehensive ophthalmologic assessment, specifically including a test of visual acuity (VA), an examination of the iris to exclude neovascularization, thorough examination of the fundus, diagnostic tests including color and red-free fundus photography, OCT/OCTA, FA, ultrasonography in the presence of severe vitreous hemorrhage, and systemic evaluation including blood pressure, serum glucose, FBC, and ESR [766, 767].

6.2.2.5 Examination of Intraocular Fluids

The physiological alterations associated with retinal vein occlusion (RVO) exhibit similarities to those observed in diabetic retinopathy (DR). There is a growing body of information in the field of intraocular fluid detection that indicates an increase in the expression of vascular endothelial growth factor (VEGF), along with other pro-angiogenic growth factors and inflammatory mediators, which play a significant role in the pathogenesis of RVO.

The levels of both vascular endothelial growth factor (VEGF) and interleukin-6 (IL-6) in the aqueous humor of patients with ME secondary to CRVO significantly elevated, particularly in those with ischemic CRVO ($P < 0.0001$ and $P = 0.0003$) [768]. Similarly, the severity of ME secondary to BRVO was correlated with the concentrations of VEGF in both the aqueous humor and vitreous body fluid ($P = 0.0001$ and $P = 0.0272$) and also correlated with the levels of interleukin-6 (IL-6) ($P = 0.0331$) in the vitreous fluid [769].

Distinct variations can be observed in the cytokine expression within the intraocular fluid across various forms of RVO. It has been observed that the aqueous humor turbidity in patients with ischemia CRVO is much greater than that observed in nonischemic CRVO patients [770]. In addition, the levels of VEGF in the aqueous humor were considerably elevated in individuals with ischemic CRVO compared to those with nonischemic CRVO ($P = 0.01$). Furthermore, there was a positive correlation between the concentration of VEGF, as determined via logarithmic quantification, and the duration of arterial and venous blood flow ($P = 0.0001$) [771]. There exists a positive correlation between the severity of obstruction resulting from BRVO and CRVO and an upregulation of VEGF together with a down-regulation of VEGF165b, which is an antiangiogenic factor. The disruption of angiogenic equilibrium occurs as a consequence of the widening of the obstruction range, leading to a shift toward the promotion of angiogenesis [772]. The levels of MCP-1 and VEGF-A in the aqueous humor or vitreous fluid of individuals newly diagnosed with and suffering from HRVO were shown to be significantly elevated compared to those with BRVO [773]. Nevertheless, within the old RVO type, only MCP-1 was significantly different for CRVO or HRVO versus BRVO [774]. There exists a positive correlation between the levels of VEGF, intercellular adhesion molecule-1 (ICAM-1), and IL-6 in the aqueous humor of patients with CRVO and the extent of aqueous humor turbidity [770].

Additional angiogenic factors, such as pigment epithelium-derived factor (PEDF), angiopoietin 4 (Ang 4), platelet-derived growth factor (PDGF), and several inflammatory factors, including intercellular adhesion molecule-1 (ICAM-1), interleukin-8 (IL-8), IL-1β, serum amyloid A (SAA), and growth factor such as bFGF and TGF-β, present in the intraocular fluid, have also been documented to exhibit associations with the severity of different forms of RVO [768, 775–780]. Specifically, a notable decrease in the concentration of PEDF in the vitreous humor of patients with CRVO compared to the control group (17.5 ng/mL vs. 28.4 ng/mL) was observed ($P = 0.0298$). Similarly, the vitreous PEDF level was significantly lower in BRVO patients than controls ($P = 0.026$) [781]. Moreover, there was a significant positive correlation between perifoveal capillary blood flow velocity and the vitreous level of PEDF in patients with BRVO and macular edema ($P = 0.013$), which implied that the vitreous level of PEDF may influence macular microcirculation in patients with BRVO [782]. Additionally, the levels of IL-6, IL-8, and MCP-1 in both the vitreous and aqueous humor were found to be greater in the CRVO patients compared to the control group. Furthermore, it was shown that the inflammatory factor ICAM-1 exhibited a substantial rise in the vitreous of patients with CRVO compared to the control group (20.5 vs. 5.0 ng/mL, $P < 0.001$) [768, 776, 777]. Similarly, the concentration of ICAM-1 in the aqueous humor of patients with BRVO was shown to be considerably greater (6.90 vs. 3.30 ng/mL) compared to the control group. Furthermore, there was a significant correlation between the concentration of ICAM-1 and the severity of ME ($P = 0.005$) [778, 779]. The concentrations of IL-8 (63.5 vs. 5.1 pg/mL) and MCP-1 (1522.4 vs. 746.5 pg/mL) in the vitreous fluid of patients with BRVO were found to be considerably elevated compared to those of the control group ($P = 0.001$, $P = 0.001$) [776].

Furthermore, the findings derived from the analysis of metabolomics and proteomics offer novel insights into the investigation of the pathophysiology of RVO. A notable elevation in the oxidative stress index and lipoprotein 2 levels in the aqueous humor of patients with RVO ($P = 0.04$ and $P = 0.021$) was found. Conversely, a significant decrease in the glucose metabolism-associated protein glutamine was observed ($P = 0.017$). In addition, an elevation in the expression levels of 49 protein sites associated with angiogenesis, oxidative stress, and collagen formation in the aqueous humor of individuals diagnosed with BRVO was also observed [768, 783–785].

Intraocular levels of some cytokines were reported to relate with anatomic retinal structure. Specifically, a significant correlation was observed between the concentration of bFGF and the inner central macular thickness (CMT) of BRVO patients ($r = 0.688$; $P = 0.02$); a significant correlation was observed between the concentration of SAA and both the full and outer CMT of the ischemic group ($r = 0.545$ and 0.683, respectively; $P = 0.04$ and 0.01, respectively); and in the nonischemic group, the level of IL-6 was significantly associated with inner CMT ($r = 0.560$; $P = 0.03$) [780].

Patients with BRVO who were subjected to vitrectomy as a treatment modality and got benefit from substantial improvement in their vision exhibited considerably higher levels of VEGF and ICAM-1 in the vitreous fluid at baseline. However, these levels reduced significantly following vitrectomy. The initial concentration of pigment epithelium-derived factor (PEDF) exhibited a notable reduction, followed by a substantial increase subsequent to vitrectomy [786]. Nevertheless, the visual prognosis of patients with CRVO following vitrectomy is associated with the concentrations of VEGF and PEDF in the vitreous fluid, rather than the levels of intercellular adhesion molecule-1 (ICAM-1) [787]. In another study, a notable association was observed between the visual prognosis after to vitrectomy for BRVO and the levels of interleukin-6 (IL-6) in the vitreous fluid [788].

Significant reductions in the amounts of vascular endothelial growth factor (VEGF), soluble vascular endothelial growth factor receptor-1 (sVEGFR-1), platelet-derived growth factor (PDGF), placental growth factor (PlGF), interleukin-6 (IL-6), and monocyte chemoattractant protein-1 (MCP-1) were observed in the aqueous humor of patients with macular edema (ME) attributable to CRVO 1 month following intravitreal injection of ranibizumab (IVR). The regression of ME was found to be associated with the levels of VEGF and IL-6, whereas an inverse correlation was observed between the concentration of VEGF and improvements in eyesight [789]. Patients diagnosed with BRVO have a significant association between aqueous flare and the levels of soluble vascular endothelial growth factor receptor-1 (sVEGFR-1), placental growth factor (PlGF), soluble intercellular adhesion molecule-1 (sICAM-1), monocyte chemoattractant protein-1 (MCP-1), interleukin-6 (IL-6), and interleukin-8 (IL-8). There exists a correlation between the alterations observed in aqueous flare and the subsequent improvement of eyesight in individuals who have undergone IVR treatment after a period of 6 months [790]. Nevertheless, there exists a notable correlation between the initial PDGF-AA levels in patients with BRVO and the likelihood of experiencing recurrent ME. This correlation can serve as an autonomous indicator for determining the required number of IVR injections [791]. Following the administration of intravitreal bevacizumab (IVB) to patients with BRVO, the unresponsive group exhibited significantly elevated levels of VEGF (491 ± 231 vs. 250 ± 112 pg/mL, $P < 0.001$) and PEDF (32 ± 4 vs. 25 ± 5 ng/mL, $P < 0.001$) compared to the responsive group. Furthermore, these elevated levels of VEGF and PEDF persisted at 6 weeks posttreatment [792].

For patients with BRVO, IVB treatment led to a significant decrease in VEGF titers ($P < 0.001$), while intravitreal injection of triamcinolone acetonide (IVTA) resulted in decreased levels of IL-6, IL-17, IP-10, PDGF-AA, and VEGF in the aqueous humor ($P = 0.012$, $P < 0.001$, $P < 0.001$, $P < 0.001$, $P = 0.015$, $P < 0.001$). These findings suggest that anti-inflammatory therapy not only reduces the levels of inflammatory factors but also influences the expression of VEGF [793]. One week following IVTA, there was a substantial drop in the levels of MCP-1 and macrophage inflammatory protein-1 (MIP-1) in the aqueous humor of patients with BRVO ($P < 0.001$, $P = 0.044$). Additionally, there was a correlation between the level of MIP-1 and the improvement of ME ($r = 0.58$, $P = 0.020$) [794]. Initial levels of VEGF and IL-6 in the aqueous humor of patients who did not exhibit a positive response to IVTA treatment for BRVO with subsequent ME were significantly elevated compared to the levels observed in the group of patients who did respond to the treatment (VEGF: 511 ± 245 vs. 230 ± 108 pg/mL, $P < 0.001$; IL-6: 38 ± 31 vs. 16 ± 13 pg/mL, $P < 0.001$). After a period of 3 months following IVTA treatment, it was observed that the nonresponders exhibited a higher concentration of VEGF (312 ± 64 pg/mL) compared to the responders (86 ± 21 pg/mL, $P < 0.001$). However, the concentration of interleukin-6 (IL-6) decreased to a level within the normal range [795].

It is evident that in cases when patients with ME related to RVO have not responded well to anti-VEGF or anti-inflammatory treatments, the measurement of intraocular fluid can provide valuable information regarding elevated cytokine levels. This information can aid in the precise selection of therapeutic agents that target the specific cytokines involved.

6.2.2.6 Management

Before treatments are performed, one should notice that RVO may regress naturally. Therefore, comparison between the further damage due to any invasive therapy and the harm by RVO blindness complications should be considered carefully. In non-ischemic CRVO eyes with an initial visual acuity of 20/70 or worse, visual acuity demonstrated improvement in 32% of cases at the 3-month follow-up period. Furthermore, throughout the 2- to 5-year follow-up, visual acuity improvement was observed in 47% of these cases. In contrast, for ischemic CRVO eyes, visual acuity improvement was observed in 10% and 23% of cases at the 3-month and 2- to 5-year follow-up periods, respectively [796]. Correspondingly, within a span of 3 months from the initial occurrence, it was observed that the visual acuity of eyes with an initial measurement of 20/60 or higher either improved or stayed stable in 75% of cases for major BRVO and in 86% of cases for macular BRVO [797].

Mainstream therapy for macular edema (ME) resulting from RVO is the administration of anti-vascular endothelial growth factor (anti-VEGF) agents, which effectively suppress vascular leakage. Aflibercept, ranibizumab, and bevacizumab have undergone extensive evaluation in numerous clinical trials, demonstrating significant promise in terms of functional improvement or a more limited scope of regeneration [798–801]. The addition of anti-vascular endothelial growth factor (anti-VEGF) therapy to pan-retinal photocoagulation (PRP) may provide potential benefits for patients diagnosed with anterior segment neovascularization resulting from ischemic CRVO [802]. One of the major drawbacks of anti-VEGF therapy for RVO is the repeated injections. Compared with anti-VEGF therapies, the burden of retreatment is reduced by sustained releasing of local injection of steroid, such as the use of a dexamethasone intravitreal implant and triamcinolone [803–805]. Despite that meta-analysis study showed that intravitreal injection of triamcinolone led to 68.1 μm greater CMT reduction than bevacizumab [806], however, BCVA and CMT at 4, 12, and 24 weeks after treatment did not vary significantly between the IVB groups and IVTA groups [807]. Furthermore, the rate of intraocular pressure rise after intravitreal injection was significantly higher in the IVTA groups ($P < 0.001$) [807].

The available evidence does not provide support for the notion that there are any benefits associated with the combination of intravitreal anti-VEGF therapy with macular grid laser or PRP for the treatment of ME related to CRVO [750]. In addition, it should be noted that despite the prompt administration of anti-VEGF medication, the advancement of retinal non-perfusion in eyes afflicted with CRVO cannot be completely halted. Following the discontinuation of anti-vascular endothelial growth factor (anti-VEGF) therapy, individuals diagnosed with ischemic CRVO continue to face the potential for neovascularization, necessitating vigilant surveillance [808].

Surgical evacuation may be necessary for eyes with non-clearing vitreous hemorrhage resulting from secondary retinal neovascularization. During the vitrectomy procedure, it is possible to simultaneously address the hemorrhage by removing epiretinal membranes, fibrovascular proliferations (if present), and applying complete PRP [809]. While this particular approach has the potential to prevent or assist in the regression of neovascularization in the anterior region, it is important to note that visual outcomes may be constrained by the degree of retinal non-perfusion that underlies the condition [810].

6.2.3 Coats' Disease

6.2.3.1 Brief Introduction

Coats' disease is a relatively rare condition affecting the retinal vessels, which is distinguished by the presence of retinal telangiectasia, subretinal exudation, and exudative retinal detachment with unclear pathogenesis [811]. Coats' disease is typically unilateral and male predominance, with median age at the diagnosis is 5 years [811–814]. Advanced cases of the condition may result in the development of a complete detachment of the retina and the occurrence of neovascular glaucoma, both of which frequently contribute to a significant decline in visual acuity.

Coats' disease is infrequently observed in the adult population and has a comparatively slower progression when compared to its manifestation in children [815, 816]. It is widely believed among experts that individuals with Coats' disease in their later years are typically those who were asymptomatic during childhood and hence diagnosed at a later stage [817]. The occurrence of bilateral Coats' disease is infrequent, and the unaffected eye may remain asymptomatic and exhibits minor peripheral telangiectatic veins [813, 814, 818].

6.2.3.2 Epidemiology

Based on a prospective study conducted in the United Kingdom, the estimated prevalence of Coats' disease is 0.09 cases per 100,000 individuals [819] Coats' disease was ever described in a preterm child born at 31 weeks gestational age and a 3-week-old boy [820, 821]. It is characterized by its sporadic and nonhereditary nature, devoid of any accompanying systemic abnormalities or racial predilection [813].

A comprehensive analysis of 351 consecutive patients diagnosed with Coats' disease at a singular medical institution revealed that 295 individuals (84%) were identified as male, whereas all 351 patients (100%) exhibited unilateral manifestations of the condition [813]. Prior studies have indicated that the manifestation of this particular ailment commonly occurs on one side, with a range of 0% to 10% of persons with Coats' disease suffering the condition bilaterally [822, 823].

6.2.3.3 Clinical Manifestation

Main clinical features of Coats' disease include unilateral dilated retinal capillaries, retinal telangiectasia, and aneurysms with retinal exudation in eyes [824, 825]. Although the exact pathophysiology of Coats' disease remains unknown, a few studies have indicated that telangiectatic blood vessels exhibit increased permeability, hence facilitating the influx of lipoproteins into the retina. The accumulation of lipoproteins has the potential to cause a disruption in the external limiting membrane of the retina, leading to the occurrence of non-rhegmatogenous retinal detachment, and further develop into a bullous retinal detachment as a result of the accumulation of lipoproteinaceous debris [826, 827].

The staging of Coats' disease is facilitated with the utilization of Shields criteria [814]. Stage 1 involves only retinal telangiectasia; stage 2 involves telangiectasia and exudation with 2A representing extrafoveal exudation, and stage 2B representing exudation involving the macular fovea (Fig. 6.52a). Additionally, Daruich et al. proposed an updated classification system introducing two subcategories within stage 2B, namely, stage 2B1 (without subfoveal nodules) and stage 2B2 (with subfoveal nodules) [828]. Stage 3 involves exudative retinal detachment, in which stage 3A1 does not involve the fovea, stage 3A2 involves the fovea, and stage 3B involves total retinal detachment; stage 4 involves total retinal detachment with glaucoma; and stage 5 involves severe end-stage disease [811]. Late complications include neovascular glaucoma, retinal detachment, anterior chamber cholesterolosis, vitreous hemorrhage, macular fibrosis, and retinal bleeding from abnormal blood vessels [827, 829].

While clinical examination alone may be sufficient for diagnosis in certain circumstances, further tests such as fluorescein angiography (FA), OCT, OCTA, ultrasonography, computed tomography (CT), and magnetic resonance imaging (MRI) are typically necessary in the majority of cases [830]. The FA examination indicates increased brightness in the venous phase of the retina due to anomalous blood vessels, areas of reduced blood flow in the capillaries, and early reduced brightness in areas with fluid leakage in the retina, followed by late staining and leaking from abnormal blood vessels (Fig. 6.52b, c). Additionally, there is swelling in the central part of the retina (macular edema) and the growth of new blood vessels in the optic disc, retina, and iris [813]. OCT is utilized for the detection and measurement of several ocular conditions, including cystoid macular edema, epiretinal membrane, vitreomacular traction, subretinal/intraretinal fluid, central macular thickness, and subfoveal choroidal thickness [828, 831]. Coats' disease is characterized by vascular abnormalities that impact both the deep and superficial retinal plexuses. OCTA scans allow for comprehensive assessment of both of these plexuses; however, FA is unable to visualize the deep vascular plexus [832–835].

Ultrasonography, CT, and MRI can aid in differentiating malignant lesions that exhibit similar clinical symptoms to Coats' disease by enabling the visualization of calcification, such as in retinoblastoma [836]. Ultrasonography reveals characteristic indications, including exudate masses that appear bright on the scan, a distinct space beneath the retina without significant thickening of the choroid or traction on the vitreoretinal interface, and a detachment of the retina around the optic nerve

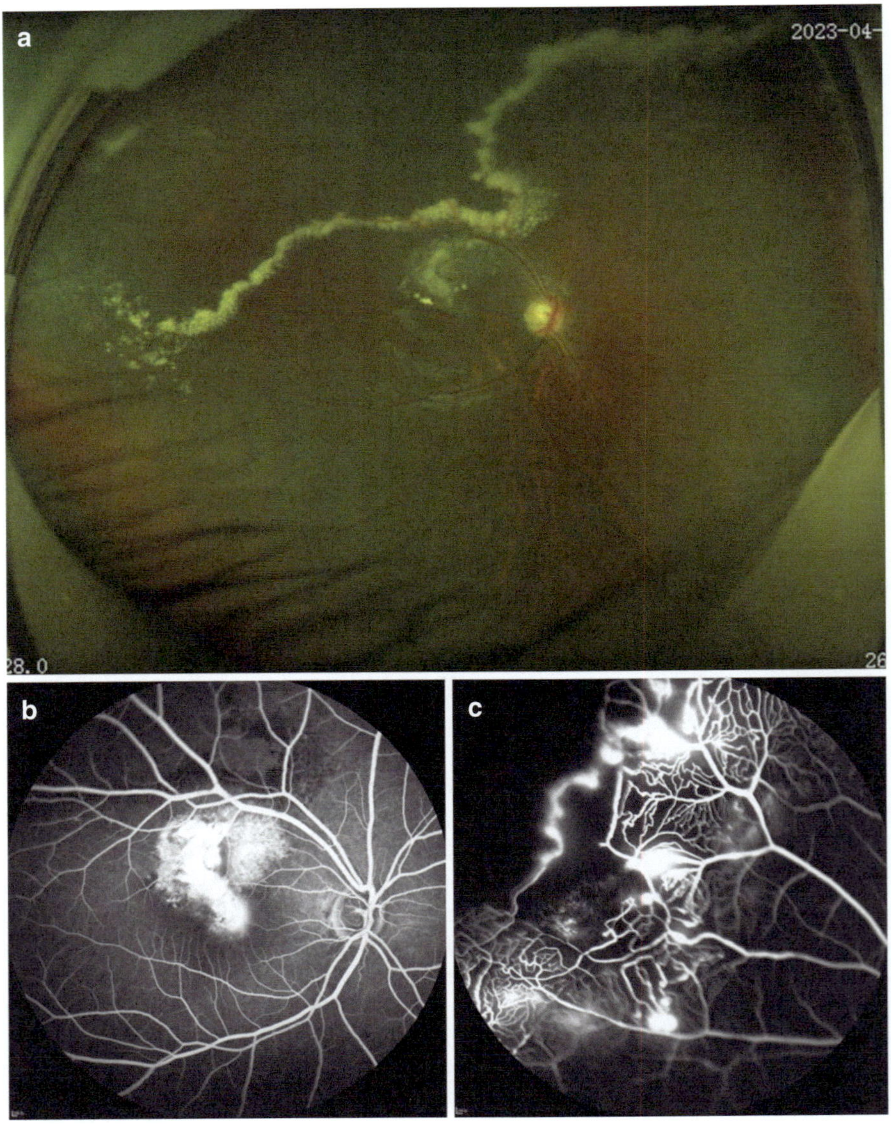

Fig. 6.52 The fundus photography (**a**) and fluorescein angiography (**b** and **c**) of the right eye with Coats' disease. Dilated peripheral retinal capillaries, retinal telangiectasia, aneurysms with macular-involved retinal exudation (**a**), leakage of fluorescence at macula (**b**) and the peripheral new vessels (**c**), and non-perfusion area (**c**) can be observed. (Courtesy of Dr. Jingjing Fan of Department of Ophthalmology, The First Affiliated Hospital of Zhengzhou University, Zhengzhou, Henan, China)

head that contains fluid. Ultrasound can detect linear echo, which is a clear sign of retinal detachment in severe situations. In Coats' disease, the fluid behind the retina is acoustically transparent, but there may be vitreous echoes of moderate reflectivity. Additionally, it can be utilized to exclude the possibility of retinoblastoma, as calcium in retinoblastoma is dispersed in a random manner, while calcium in Coats' disease exhibits a curved pattern [837]. CT is useful for excluding retinoblastoma when there is a solid tumor with calcification; however, it becomes perplexing when dealing with retinoblastoma cases lacking calcium. Calcification regions on a CT scan may be observed in around 20% of advanced Coats' cases, due to bone development along artery walls and the presence of calcified sub-macular nodules [830]. MRI is particularly advantageous in facilitating diagnosis in complex instances. In retinoblastoma, the exudate appears brighter than normal on both T1 and T2 images, whereas the tumor appears brighter than normal on T1 but darker than normal on T2. Additionally, the tumor shows increased brightness when a gadolinium contrast is used [838].

6.2.3.4 Diagnosis

Indirect ophthalmoscopy is a reliable method for diagnosing Coats' disease by examining the fundus [817]. Retinal telangiectasia is consistently observed in all instances. The term "light bulb telangiectasias" has been used to describe these growths due to their bulbous shape and the noticeable yellow exudation that accompanies them [839]. The anomalous blood arteries, characterized by their elongated and tapered shape, are commonly observed in the peripheral regions located between the equator and ora serrata [811]. In virtually all cases, intraretinal exudation is apparent, and it can be extensive and far from the telangiectasia. The exudate moves downward toward the macular region [840–842]. Retinal hemorrhage may infrequently manifest in proximity to a vascular anomaly. Possible complications of a chronic retinal detachment include the development of retinal macrocysts, vasoproliferative tumors, and vitreous bleeding [811].

In addition, patients with Coats' disease typically do not have a previous history of being born prematurely or a family history of prematurity. The presence of vitreoretinal and retinal drag is only seen in rare cases that have not been treated. This characteristic sets Coats' disease apart from other exudative retinopathies in children, such as retinopathy of prematurity, familial exudative retinopathy, and Norrie disease [817].

6.2.3.5 Examination of Intraocular Fluids

Reported in 2007, the VEGF content in the vitreous humor of a 2-year-old child with Coats' illness was found to be dramatically elevated, reaching 908 pg/mL, which is over ten times higher than the average value of 100 pg/mL in healthy individuals. After 8 weeks of anti-VEGF medication, the concentration of VEGF levels decreased to 167 pg/mL [843]. Additional case series have since provided further confirmation that the levels of VEGF within the eye are elevated in children with Coats' disease, and these elevated levels of VEGF are positively associated with the severity of the condition [844–847]. Specifically, in stage 3B, the intraocular VEGF concentration in children with stage Coats' disease was significantly higher than that in stage 3A ($P = 0.010$) [847]. Continuous case reports have also shown the effectiveness and safety of anti-VEGF therapy combined with laser or cryotherapy in the treatment of Coats' disease in children [848–851].

In addition to VEGF, it was reported that the levels of pro-inflammation cytokines such as IL-6, IL-8, MCP-1, MIP-1α, IP-10, VCAM-1, and ICAM-1 in the aqueous humor of children with Coats' disease were significantly higher than that of the control group. Moreover, MCP-1 levels were related to the severity of retinal exudation ($r = 0.966$, $p < 0.001$) [852, 853]. In adult patients with Coats' disease, the concentrations of IL-6 and IL-1β were significantly higher than those in the control group ($P = 0.012$, $P = 0.005$), and the concentration of IL-6 was significantly positively correlated with the extent of exudative retinal detachment [847]. Correspondingly, the administration of anti-inflammatory medicines through intravitreal injection, such as the sustained-release agent dexamethasone (Ozurdex) or triamcinolone acetonide (IVTA), has been demonstrated to be successful in treating Coats' illness in both children and adults [854–856].

Examination of concentrations of cytokines in the aqueous humor help precisely guide the treatment of refractory macular edema in Coats' disease: despite the multiple intravitreal injections of anti-VEGF drug, two cases with adult-onset Coats' disease suffered from recurrence of macular edema. Lab examination showed that the aqueous humor level of VEGF was low and the level of IL-8, IL-6, and VACM increased; therefore treatment strategy changed to intravitreal injection of steroids, and the macular thickness dropped remarkably with improvement of vision and without any further recurrence of edema during 3 months [857]. There was a study from other group of authors showed that intravitreal injection of anti-VEGF antibody treatment was ineffective in patients with adult patients with Coats' disease improved significantly after IVTA treatment [854]. Therefore, utilizing intraocular fluid detection can aid in the clinical diagnosis of Coats' illness, particularly in adults exhibiting atypical clinical signs of the condition. Additionally, intraocular fluid tests can be utilized to direct the drug treatment plan for Coats' disease. To choose the appropriate treatment, one might consider the levels of VEGF and inflammatory components in the intraocular fluid and opt for either anti-VEGF medications or anti-inflammatory therapies such glucocorticoids.

6.2.3.6 Management

The conventional treatment for Coats' disease involves the use of photocoagulation and cryotherapy techniques. These methods work by eliminating aberrant blood vessels and ischemic retinal tissue, hence reducing exudation. If there is substantial exudation or retinal detachment, surgery is the primary course of action [817, 858]. The primary objective of treating mild Coats' disease is to eliminate the abnormal retinal blood vessels, maintain visual acuity, and prevent progression to retinal detachment. Laser photocoagulation and cryotherapy have long been the main treatment options for mild to moderate stages of the disease [859–863]. In cases of advanced diseases characterized by extensive telangiectasias, retinal detachment, and widespread exudation, laser photocoagulation and cryotherapy can still be employed. However, vitreoretinal surgery may offer greater efficacy. In severe instances, enucleation or observation, depending on the level of pain, may be required [854, 863].

Recent evidence has demonstrated the efficacy of intravitreal triamcinolone as an adjunctive treatment for Coats' disease [854, 864–867]. Othman et al. conducted a study where they observed an enhancement in visual acuity, as well as the absorption of subretinal fluid and macular exudates, in 15 consecutive patients who were treated with intravitreal triamcinolone along with other treatment methods like laser photocoagulation and/or cryotherapy [867, 868]. Coats' disease treatment has been further improved with the utilization of anti-vascular endothelial growth factor (anti-VEGF) medications. The results of anti-VEGF intravitreal injections have been recorded in a limited number of case reports and small case series [848, 869–872]. Kaul et al. propose it as a possible supplementary treatment in conjunction with current drugs, as it seems to reduce ME and exudates, enhance or preserve visual acuity, and promote the regression of dilated aberrant arteries [872, 873]. The use of bevacizumab should be approached cautiously due to the presence of vitreoretinal fibrosis and the potential risk of traction retinal detachment. These complications were observed in patients who got bevacizumab in combination with conventional therapy, but not in patients who received standard measures alone [872, 874]. It is important to emphasize that anti-VEGF drugs should only be given if the diagnosis of Coats' disease has been confirmed and retinoblastoma has been ruled out, as intraocular injections may cause the spread of cancer cells outside the eye in certain cases of retinoblastoma [875].

Coats' disease follows a natural course that leads to blindness and tissue degeneration. The disease progresses more rapidly and has a poorer visual prognosis when it starts at a younger age [876]. The prognosis of the disease is contingent upon the stage when the patient presents; however, the overall visual prognosis is unfavorable. Patients diagnosed with stage 1 generally have a favorable visual prognosis. The prognosis of patients with stage 2 or stage 3 retinal detachment depends on the extent of the detachment and if the fovea is affected [827].

6.2.4 Age-Related Macular Degeneration

6.2.4.1 Brief Introduction

Age-related macular degeneration (AMD) is a prevalent ocular condition that is responsible for a significant proportion of visual impairment in the senior population, therefore posing a substantial burden on both affected individuals and society as a whole [877]. AMD is distinguished by pathological changes occurring in the deeper retinal layers of the macula, as well as the surrounding vasculature. These modifications ultimately lead to the loss of central vision. The accumulation of retinal deposits, referred to as drusen, is a characteristic clinical manifestation observed in AMD and may serve as an initial sign of the disease's "dry" stage. The morphologic variant that occurs most frequently is dry AMD, which has the potential to progress to "wet" or neovascular AMD. In neovascular AMD, the development of central choroidal neovascular membranes (CNV) can lead to retinal hemorrhage, exudation, and substantial impairment of vision. The formation of these membranes is attributed to the aberrant growth of blood vessels, known as angiogenesis, which is driven by the synthesis of vascular endothelial growth factor (VEGF) [878].

Polypoidal choroidal vasculopathy (PCV) is a distinct form of AMD that was initially characterized by Yannuzzi et al. This condition is characterized by an anomalous vascular network consisting of dilated polyp-like structures located at the terminal ends of the choroidal artery branches. There appears to be a higher incidence of this phenomenon among individuals of Asian and African descent compared to those of Caucasian descent [879–882]. The classification of PCV as a distinct subtype of neovascular AMD continues to be a subject of debate. Multiple papers have posited that PCV can be classified as a subtype of CNV, with certain ophthalmologists contending that PCV is a kind of CNV resulting from AMD [883]. Several publications have indicated that people diagnosed with PCV exhibit distinct angiographic features, genetic backgrounds, prognoses, and treatment responses in comparison to individuals with neovascular AMD [884, 885].

6.2.4.2 Epidemiology

AMD is a prominent etiological factor contributing to the occurrence of central visual impairment in developed nations. In Saudi Arabia, AMD constitutes 3.3% of the primary etiologies contributing to visual impairment among those aged 50 years and above [886]. It impacts approximately 10% of individuals aged 65 and above, and its prevalence increases to over 25% among those aged 75 and above [877]. The aging population indicates that these numbers will continue to increase at an exponential rate. In 2020, the global incidence of new cases amounted to 196 million, with projections indicating an anticipated increase to 288 million by 2024. In the United States, a significant number of individuals, specifically two million, are affected by advanced AMD, while more than eight million individuals have an intermediate form of this ailment [887]. China experiences an annual incidence of around 31 million new cases [888].

Age, racial background, and hypertension are all identified as risk factors for AMD, and the process of aging constitutes a substantial risk factor for the development of AMD. Various systemic diseases, including cardiovascular disease, hypertension, and atherosclerosis, have been identified as factors that can elevate the susceptibility to AMD [889–892]. The risk of AMD in diabetic individuals is heightened by the presence of diabetic retinopathy (DR), high-density lipoprotein (HDL), obesity, and elevated systolic blood pressure [893, 894]. Researches indicated that the habits of smoking and excessive alcohol consumption are associated with an elevated likelihood of developing AMD [895]. Lutein and zeaxanthin have been shown to potentially mitigate the risk of AMD, whereas vitamin C, vitamin E, vitamin D, and zinc oxide have been suggested as potential preventive measures against the development of AMD [896, 897]. The etiology of AMD has been significantly influenced by genetic factors, with a total of 103 genes or loci associated with AMD having been found. The CFH and HTRA1 loci have been identified as the primary genetic loci associated with AMD [898].

6.2.4.3 Clinical Manifestation

Early and intermediate AMD is often characterized by the presence of small and medium-sized drusen in the macula, with minimal or absent symptoms. Patients may exhibit slight changes such as metamorphopsia (distortion); increased blurring at close distances, particularly during reading; and reduced contrast sensitivity. The occurrence of neovascular AMD frequently leads to heightened and prompt vision impairments, which can manifest as either acute or gradually worsening conditions. The presence of retinal hemorrhage and fluid accumulation gives rise to symptoms characterized by pronounced distortion and/or the development of a significant central scotoma, also known as a blind spot. Patients may experience difficulties in recognizing and distinguishing faces. Individuals diagnosed with geographic atrophy may exhibit additional ocular manifestations such as visual distortion and the presence of a central scotoma [878].

The presence and absence of atrophic lesions known as geographic atrophy (GA) and aberrant CNV proliferation are two morphologic markers utilized to further identify AMD. Loss of outer retinal tissue and the accompanying vascular network, especially the RPE layer, Bruch membrane, and choriocapillaris, leads to atrophic changes. It is theorized that inflammatory and degenerative attacks on photoreceptors generate advanced dry AMD.

Dry AMD is characterized by the presence of drusen inside the posterior pole, exhibiting variability in their forms, sizes, and distribution. Additionally, there is a notable level of symmetry between the two eyes of an affected individual [899]. Pseudodrusen exhibit clear differentiation from conventional drusen. The drusenoid deposits are situated in the subretinal area, positioned above the RPE [900]. Pseudodrusen have been found to be correlated with advanced AMD [901]. The individuals can be categorized into three distinct categories according to their morphological characteristics, namely dot, reticular, and confluent pseudodrusen [902]. The study demonstrated that the occurrence of ribbon-dominant (confluent)-type pseudodrusen, large soft drusen, and female gender was shown to be correlated with the prevalence of geographic atrophy (GA) [903]. Pigmentary irregularities, characterized by localized increases or decreases in pigmentation, are frequently observed in AMD. Progressive well-defined atrophic patches of the retinal pigment epithelium (RPE) may arise in the perifoveal area. The aforementioned atrophic regions progressively enlarge and perhaps coalesce, resulting in the development of geographic atrophy (GA) [904]. Wet AMD can manifest with the presence of drusen, pigment epithelial detachment (PED), intraretinal hemorrhages, and choroidal neovascularization (CNV), which is characterized by a distinct delineated grayish region on the retina [905].

It is vital to comprehend that various forms of dry AMD carry a probability ranging from 10% to 15% of transitioning into the wet form of AMD at some stage during the progression of the disease [906]. Wet or neovascular age-related macular degeneration (AMD) has the potential to result in the development of geographic atrophy, and conversely, geographic atrophy may also contribute to the occurrence of wet or neovascular AMD [907].

6.2.4.4 Diagnosis

Individuals diagnosed with AMD often present with frequent reports of either abrupt or gradual deterioration in visual acuity in one or both eyes, often accompanied by distorted vision (metamorphopsia), which is indicative of macular degeneration [908]. A comprehensive diagnostic assessment of age-related macular degeneration (AMD) necessitates the inclusion of various ophthalmological procedures. These procedures encompass measuring best corrected visual acuity; conducting a funduscopic evaluation with dilated pupils; employing imaging techniques such as fluorescein angiography (FA), indocyanine green angiography (ICGA), optical coherence tomography (OCT), optical coherence tomography angiography (OCTA); and utilizing artificial intelligence (AI) [908].

In the context of PCV, it has been observed that serous pigment epithelial detachment (PED) or atypical serous PED is more frequently encountered as compared to CNV [909]. In the case of CNV, the neovascularization network observed under ICGA did not exhibit any polypoid structure. However, in the case of PCV, the aberrant arteries were found to be more pronounced, presenting terminal polypoid or aneurysmal clusters with intense fluorescence [884]. According to OCT imaging, individuals with wet AMD have a greater choroid thickness compared to individuals without the condition. Conversely, individuals with dry AMD demonstrate a lesser choroid thickness in comparison to those without the condition [910]. The utilization of a combination of structural optical coherence tomography (OCT) and OCT angiography (OCTA) has been found to be effective in the screening of polypoidal choroidal vasculopathy (PCV), with a sensitivity of 82.6% and specificity of 100% [911]. Patients diagnosed with dry AMD exhibit significantly reduced levels of superficial and deep vascular density in comparison to individuals without the condition. Individuals diagnosed with wet AMD exhibited a notable reduction in the presence of deep choroid arteries and villi muscle. Patients diagnosed with CNV had reduced perfusion in the chorionic capillaries and a more pronounced depth in the choroid [912].

Furthermore, the rapid progress in artificial intelligence (AI) technology has generated significant potential for the field of eye illness diagnosis. Kermany et al. conducted a study wherein they established that the neural network resume model's classification efficacy in relation to AMD and diabetic macular edema is comparable to that of human specialists [913]. In a similar vein, Treder et al. utilized deep learning techniques to train and validate a dataset consisting of 1112 SD-OCT pictures of age-related macular degeneration (AMD), with the objective of distinguishing between exudative and normal macula. The classifier model that was created yielded favorable outcomes, as evidenced by the training and validation accuracy rates of 100%. Additionally, the average score of the experimental and control groups for AMD exceeded 0.9 [914].

6.2.4.5 Examination of Intraocular Fluids

VEGF has garnered much attention as a cytokine of particular significance, as evidenced by the seminal research conducted by Aiello et al. [694]. Patients with AMD have shown a noteworthy association between the levels of VEGF in the aqueous humor and vitreous humor [915, 916]. Tatsuya observed a significant elevation in the levels of VEGF, sVEGFR-1, sVEGFR-2, as well as inflammatory factors (MCP-1, IL-6, and IL-8) in the AMD group compared to the cataract group ($p = 0.05$ for all variables). In contrast, there was no statistically significant disparity observed between the two cohorts in terms of the levels of PGF, tumor necrosis factor-**α**, sICAM-1, IL-12 (p70), and IL-13 in the aqueous humor. Several inflammatory markers, namely, PGF, sICAM-1, MCP-1, IL-6, and IL-8, exhibited significant correlations with the levels of sVEGFR-1 or sVEGFR-2 [917].

The presence of persistent CNV despite treatment with anti-vascular endothelial growth factor (VEGF) agents suggests deficiencies in the underlying biological processes, namely, related to inflammation and chemokine signaling. SDF-1, often referred to as CXCL12, is a chemokine that exhibits chemotactic properties toward hematopoietic progenitor cells. It is synthesized in response to tissue ischemia and possesses angiogenic capabilities [918, 919]. Sakamoto and colleagues made the observation that the levels of SDF-1 in the aqueous humor were significantly higher in individuals with neovascular AMD compared to a control group. Furthermore, they found that the concentration of SDF-1 decreased significantly after two intravitreal injections of anti-VEGF therapy in patients with AMD [920]. It was anticipated that the administration of anti-VEGF medications would result in a reduction of inflammation through the inhibition of VEGF signaling and VEGF-induced chemotaxis [920]. In their study, Zhou et al. investigated the levels of various angiogenic and inflammatory cytokines in patients with neovascular age-related macular degeneration (AMD), polypoidal choroidal vasculopathy (PCV), and cataracts. The researchers observed that the concentrations of VEGF-A and SDF1–1 were significantly elevated in the eyes of individuals with neovascular AMD and PCV compared to the control group. VEGF and SDF-1 are potentially influential factors in the pathogenesis of clinically active CNV [920].

The development of CCR2 on monocytes with systemic pro-inflammatory properties and the presence of elevated levels of CCL2 in the aqueous humor of patients with wet AMD indicate the significance of this chemokine pathway in the pathogenesis of age-related ocular diseases [921, 922]. Significantly higher concentrations of various biomarkers, including epithelial growth factor (EGF) ($p = 0.017$), human growth factor (HGF) ($p = 0.048$), intercellular adhesion molecule-1 (ICAM-1) ($p = 0.028$), interleukin 12p40 (IL-12p40) ($p = 0.009$), interleukin 1a2 (IL-1a2) ($p = 0.01$), interleukin 3 (IL-3) ($p = 0.02$), interleukin 6 (IL-6) ($p = 0.006$), interleukin 8 (IL-8) ($p = 0.02$), monocyte chemoattractant protein-1 (MCP-1) ($p = 0.048$), monokine induced by interferon-gamma (MIG) ($p = 0.016$), matrix metalloproteinase 9 (MMP-9) ($p = 0.004$), and plasminogen activator inhibitor 1 (PAI-1) ($p = 0.006$), were observed in individuals with exudative age-related macular degeneration (AMD). The results of this study indicate a substantial correlation between macular thickness and the amounts of various biomarkers, including EGF ($p = 0.001$), HGF ($p = 0.02$), ICAM-1 ($p = 0.001$), IL-12p40 ($p = 0.006$), IL-1a2 ($p = 0.002$), MIG ($p = 0.001$), MMP9 ($p < 0.001$), and PAI1 ($p = 0.01$). The height of retinal pigment epithelium detachment demonstrated strong relationships with IL-6 and MCP-1 [921].

6.2.4.6 Management

The basic therapeutic approach for wet AMD involves the prevention of neovascularization, which is achieved through intraocular injection of anti-vascular endothelial growth factor (anti-VEGF) agents [923, 924]. The administration of anti-vascular medicine has been observed to result in a reduction in both blindness and choroidal capillary density in affected people [925, 926]. The primary authorized pharmaceutical agents encompass pegaptanib, ranibizumab, bevacizumab, aflibercept, and conbercept. In the context of neovascular age-related macular degeneration (AMD), there are currently four distinct dosing regimens for anti-vascular endothelial growth factor (anti-VEGF) treatment that are being employed in clinical practice. These regimens include a fixed schedule involving monthly or biweekly injections, a pro re nata (PRN) method, a treat-and-extend approach, and an observe-and-plan regimen [927].

Despite the purported benefits, laser treatment has not been widely considered as an optimal approach for the treatment of subfoveal lesions [928]. Presently, the utilization of laser photocoagulation for the management of wet age-related macular degeneration (AMD) is constrained by several challenges, including a notable propensity for reoccurrence; the potential risk of inducing visual impairment, particularly in cases involving subfoveal membranes; and a restricted potential for enhancing visual acuity [929]. Photodynamic therapy (PDT) involves the administration of a photosensitizing dye called verteporfin via intravenous injection. This dye circulates throughout the body and selectively accumulates in choroidal neovascularization (CNV). By subjecting the accumulated dye to a longer wavelength infrared laser, PDT can induce the closure of CNV lesions. Photodynamic therapy (PDT) continues to be employed as an adjunct in situations where anti-vascular endothelial growth factor (anti-VEGF) treatment alone proves to be ineffective [930, 931].

In the context of dry AMD, both RPE transplantation and stem cell therapy have demonstrated efficacy in achieving sustained visual stability as part of the treatment regimen [932, 933]. In 2012, researchers initially documented the transplantation of retinal pigment epithelium (RPE) cells derived from human embryonic stem cells (hESC) into older people diagnosed with dry age-related macular degeneration (AMD) [933]. Viral vector gene therapy emerges as a promising therapeutic approach for both wet and dry AMD. The results from research involving ADVM-022, RGX-314, GT-005, and HMR59 have the potential to significantly impact the treatment strategies employed for wet and dry AMD [934, 935].

Numerous investigations have been undertaken to ascertain the pharmacodynamics of intravitreal injection of anti-vascular endothelial growth factor (anti-VEGF) antibodies, as well as to refine the timing of injections for maximal therapeutic efficacy [936–941]. Certain individuals diagnosed with wet age-related macular degeneration (AMD), however, have exhibited a lack of therapeutic response, despite receiving injections of anti-vascular endothelial growth factor (anti-VEGF) medicine. These particular patients are commonly referred to as non-responders [942]. It is worth noting that even undergoing a series of anti-vascular endothelial growth factor (anti-VEGF) injections over an extended period, individuals who do not have a positive response to this treatment continue to experience persistent macular edema [943]. Quantification and swift assessment of intraocular cytokines can be conducted in outpatient settings, enabling ophthalmologists to effectively monitor and manage patients who do not respond to initial treatment. By employing alternative treatment protocols such as different anti-VEGF drugs, anti-PDGF drugs, or photodynamic therapy, ophthalmologists can intervene promptly to prevent vision loss.

6.3 Masquerade Syndrome

6.3.1 Intraocular Lymphoma

6.3.1.1 Brief Introduction

Intraocular lymphoma, a rare lymphocytic malignancy, includes primary intraocular lymphoma (PIOL) and secondary lymphoma. It can masquerade as infectious retinitis [944–946], vasculitis [947], Vogt-Koyanagi-Harada disease-like change [948, 949], or other types of uveitis; therefore it is one of the main causes of masquerade syndrome [950]. Primary intraocular lymphoma was first described by Cooper and Riker in 1951 [951], and it was described as uveal malignant lymphoma by Givner in 1955 [952].

Primary intraocular lymphoma is regarded as a subtype of primary central nervous system lymphoma [953, 954], but it only occurs in the eye and without evidence that the brain or cerebrospinal fluid is involved; otherwise it cannot be named as primary intraocular lymphoma [955–957]. Secondary intraocular lymphoma originates from outside the central nervous system and metastasizes into the eye [958, 959]. There are predominantly of B-cell origin, extranodal non-Hodgkin, mainly diffuse large B-cell lymphoma [960–966], and rarely mucosal-associated lymphoid tissue lymphoma (MALT) [967, 968]; however, there are also rare T-cell variants [954].

6.3.1.2 Epidemiology

Primary vitreoretinal lymphoma (PVRL), a rare high-grade extranodal non-Hodgkin lymphoma [969], is the main type of primary intraocular lymphoma [954] and a subtype of primary central nervous system lymphoma [970]. The incidence rate is about 0.047/100,000 population every year[971], and the patients are usually 50–60 years old [972–974], but there are also a few cases that occur in childhood and adolescence, especially in people with low immunity, such as HIV-infected people [972, 975, 976]. Generally, there is no significant ethnic difference in this disease [972]. A few reports showed that women may be more susceptible than men, with a proportion of about 2:1 or higher [974, 977–980]. The pooling results indicated PIOL patients were female, elderly, binocular and B cell-type dominated [981].

Intraocular lymphoma accounts for 1.86% of ocular malignant tumors [954]. About one-third of patients with intraocular lymphoma have concurrent central nervous system lymphoma at presentation, and 42–92% of patients with intraocular lymphoma will have central nervous system lymphoma in the next 8–29 months on average [957]. It accounts for 4–6% of primary brain tumors and 1–2% of extranodal lymphoma [957, 965, 982].

6.3.1.3 Clinical Manifestation

The median age of this disease is about 50–60 years [954, 983]. About 64–83% of patients with intraocular lymphoma encountered bilaterally involved, but initially, the lesions could first appear in one eye [973, 974, 979, 984]. Common symptoms include blurred vision (40–50%), decreased vision (25–30%), and floaters in front of eyes (20–25%) [961, 985, 986]. Visual acuity is usually better than expectation based on the ocular signs. Doctors often judge that the vitreous opacity is very severe, but the patient–s vision is better than expected. This separation of symptoms and signs is a clue to suspect intraocular lymphoma [962, 973, 978].

The anterior segment is often unaffected [974], but sometimes keratic precipitates (KP) and floater cells in the anterior chamber can be observed [956]. In very few patients, there was iris [987, 988], or anterior chamber angle involvement [957] (lymphocytes accumulate on the iris surface and angle, leading to iris discoloration or secondary angle closure) [986], or pseudohypopyon [989–991].

Vitritis is the main manifestation of posterior segment involvement, with mild to moderate opacity [979, 984, 992, 993] (Fig. 6.53). Vitreous cells of intraocular lymphoma are larger than those of vitreous inflammation cells of other uveitis, and they usually do not gather in clusters but are evenly distributed (Fig. 6.54), or leading to "aurora borealis" appearance due to the lining of cells along the vitreous fibrils [985, 986]. Subretinal cells can grow locally and form a translucent gray spot, which is uniform on optical coherence tomography (OCT). The common fundus manifestations in the late stage are multiple, small, well-defined, round or oval, yellowish-white, creamy, and dome-shaped masses under pigment epithelium [974, 984, 992–995] (Fig. 6.55). The lesion will produce a typical "leopard-spot" pigmentation, covering the mass [994]. Sometimes exudative retinal detachment may occur [974]. It can also cause optic nerve infiltration [996, 997]. In late stage or after

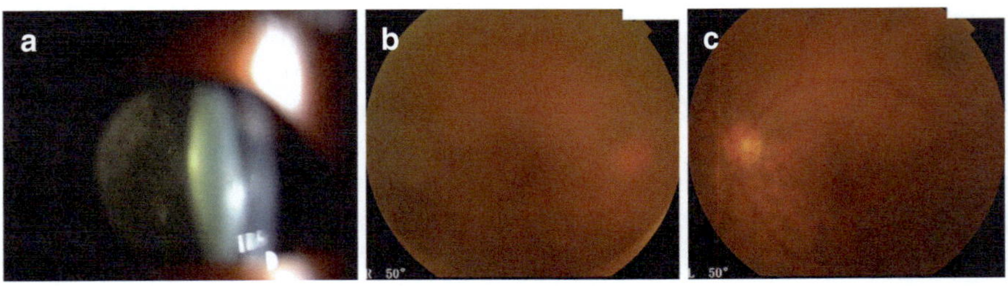

Fig. 6.53 The photography of anterior segment (**a**) and fundus (**b** and **c**) of a 61-year-old female with complaint of bilateral blurred vision and history of central nervous system lymphoma which was pathologically confirmed as diffuse large B-cell lymphoma. Diffused vitreous floater cells (**a**), remarkable vitreous opacity in the right eye (**b**) and mild vitreous opacity in the left eye (**c**) can be observed

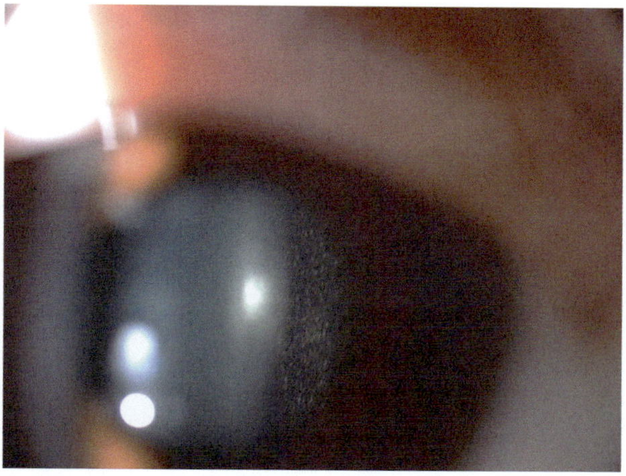

Fig. 6.54 The photograph of the anterior segment of the right eye of a 38-year-old female with vitreoretinal lymphoma, intracranial lesions which appeared 6 months later, and subsequent breast lymph node metastasis. Pathology examination confirmed that it was diffuse large B-cell lymphoma. Diffuse and evenly distributed white granules, larger than ordinary inflammatory cells in the vitreous can be observed

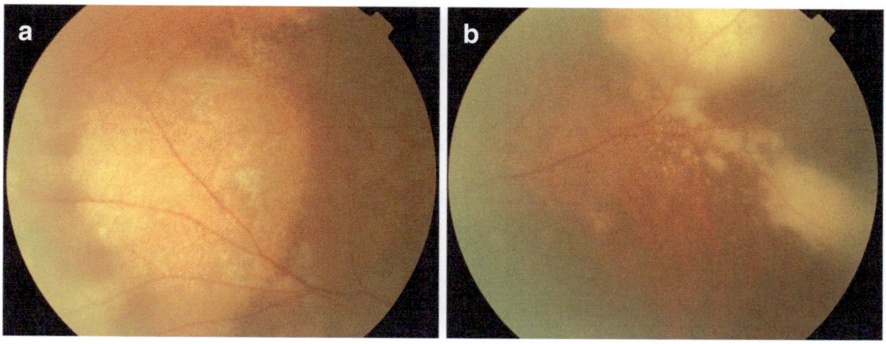

Fig. 6.55 The fundus photography of a 40-year-old female with central nervous system lymphoma and bilateral vitreoretinal lymphoma. The dome-like, yellowish and white lesions (**a**) and the creamy lesions (**b**) beneath the retina can be observed

treatment, choroidal lymphoma lesions became atrophy and formed local depigmented lesions (Fig. 6.56).

Corresponding to the white dot lesions on the fundus, fluorescent angiography showed that the small round cluster like low fluorescence lesions with a diameter of 50–250 μm at the choroidal level in patients with early lymphoma could be located at the posterior pole, peripheral or diffuse (Fig. 6.57). The fundus spontaneous fluorescence shows a slight granular pattern of low spontaneous fluorescence and high spontaneous fluorescence rings (Fig. 6.57) [998]. Nodular hyper-reflective lesions at the retinal pigment epithelium layer are shown on OCT (Fig. 6.58) [999].

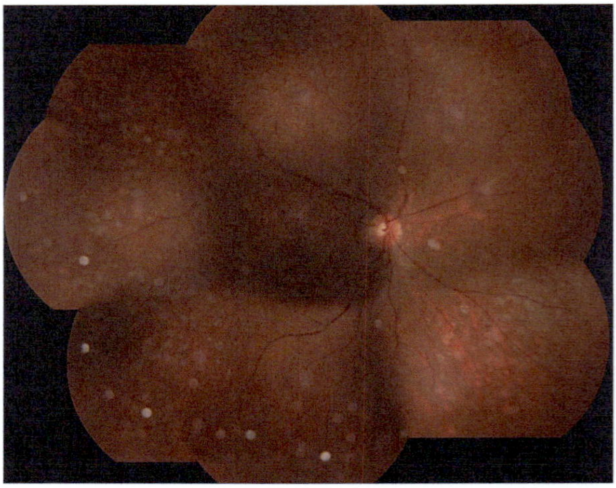

Fig. 6.56 The fundus photography of the right eye of a 61-year-old male with chronic vitreoretinal lymphoma. Diffuse depigmentation scars beneath the equatorial and peripheral retina which were corresponding to the multiple choroidal lymphoma lesions can be observed

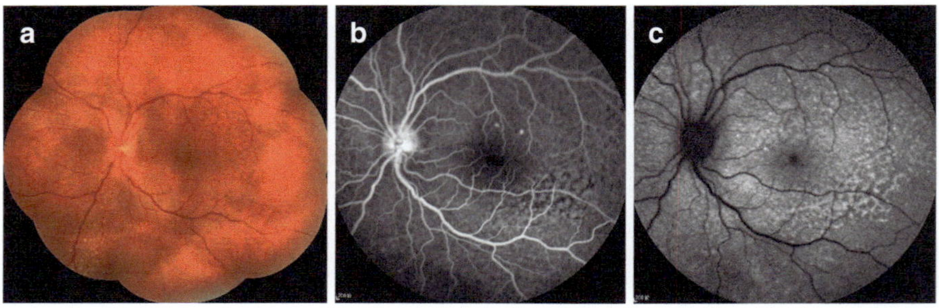

Fig. 6.57 The fundus photograph (**a**), fluorescein angiography (**b**), and autofluorescence imaging (**c**) of the left eye of a 38-year-old male with vitreoretinal lymphoma. Corresponding to diffuse subretinal yellow and white punctate lesions (**a**), small cluster-like hypofluorescence lesions at choroidal level (**b**) on fundus fluorescein angiography, and mosaic pattern of low autofluorescence and high autofluorescence rings on autofluorescence imaging (**c**) can be observed

B-ultrasound examination is helpful to detect vitreous opacity, choroidal thickening, retinal detachment and optic nerve widening [979].

As one kind of masquerading syndrome, the manifestations of intraocular lymphoma are puzzling. Intraocular lymphoma responds well to glucocorticoids at the initial stage of treatment, similar to other types of noninfectious uveitis [957], but it is dose-dependent at the later stage and eventually develops into hormone resistance [1000]. The most common ultrasonographic findings in patients with primary central nervous system lymphoma with ocular involvement included vitreous debris, choroidal-scleral thickening, and widening of the optic nerve; besides, elevated chorioretinal lesions and retinal detachment may also be found [1001].

Intraocular lymphoma caused by T cells has different clinical manifestations, and vitritis is the most frequent clinical sign, followed by anterior uveitis and serous retinal detachment [1002]. It can be clinically manifested as retinal vasculitis [1003]

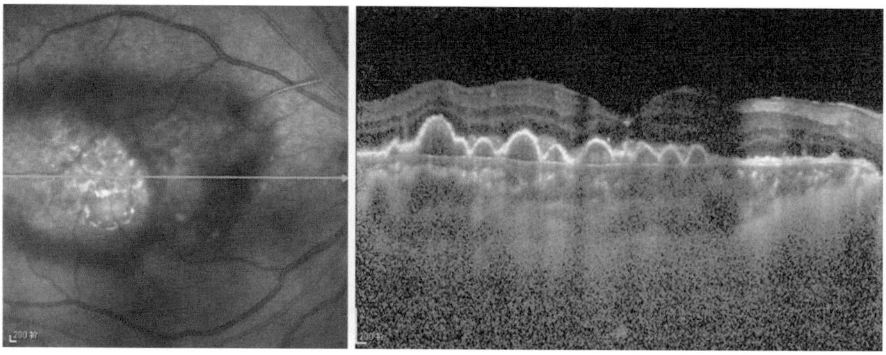

Fig. 6.58 Optic coherence tomography image of the right eye of a 65-year-old woman with vitreoretinal lymphoma which showed multiple nodular hyper-reflective lesions in the retinal pigment epithelium

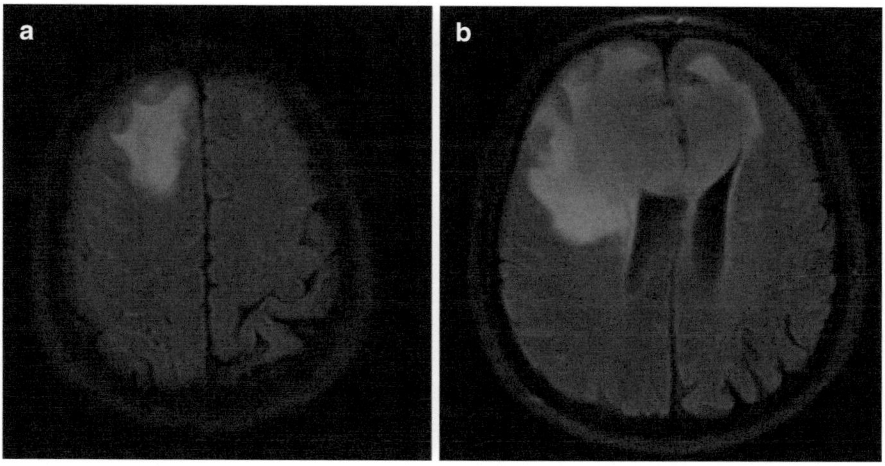

Fig. 6.59 Cranial magnetic resonance imaging (MRI) of the patient of Fig. 6.57 who suffered from failing memory, and slurring of talk and then aggravated to consciousness disorder and lethargy at 7 months after seeing the doctor for ocular diseases. In T2-weighted imaging, occupied frontal lobe (**a**) and compressed ventricles (**b**) can be observed

or disguised as infectious endophthalmitis [1004], and it can present with concomitant systemic involvement such as breast, cutaneous, and central nervous system involvement [1005, 1006].

Central nervous system lymphoma may occur before, after, or together with vitreoretinal lymphoma. Central nervous system lesions can be detected in 62% of patients with primary vitreoretinal lymphoma [991]. Primary vitreoretinal lymphoma patients are diagnosed with intracranial lymphoma within a mean interval of 8–29 months [986]. Central nervous system lymphoma can be focal and/or diffuse, usually observed in the frontal lobe (Fig. 6.59), leading to behavioral changes, even new seizures [957, 961, 985, 1007].

6.3.1.4 Diagnosis

Diagnosis of primary vitreoretinal lymphoma and central nervous system lymphoma is challenging and often delayed. The delayed diagnosis rate was 85%, and it takes an average of 6–13.9 months from onset of ocular symptoms to the final diagnosis [957, 985, 1008, 1009]. The misdiagnosed rate was 64% [981]. Due to the malignant tumor nature, once the clinical manifestations of this disease implied presumed intraocular lymphoma, relevant histological examination should be carried out to confirm or exclude the diagnosis. Aqueous humor test and cranial MRI should be routinely conducted to prompt the need for further invasive procedures to make timely diagnosis and treatment. The diagnosis of intraocular lymphoma is based on the identification of intraocular atypical lymphoid cells [966]; however, cytological examination of the vitreous often results in a low success rate due to the small quantity and poor quality of tissues and cells in the sample [1010]. Holding corticosteroids before diagnostic procedures if possible is recommended [1011]. One should be noticed about the heterogeneity of laboratory examinations of lymphoma among different centers. Poor cytologic preservation, low cellularity, and spurious occurrence of clonal or pseudoclonal PCR result in an unsatisfactory high frequency of false-negative and occasional false-positive results in vitreous body aspirates, often leading to significant delays in diagnosis and commencement of therapy [1012–1014].

Vitreous biopsy plays a pivotal role, and it is still the gold standard for determining the diagnosis of primary vitreoretinal lymphoma [1015, 1016]. The use of genetic sequencing in particular offers the hope of faster diagnosis [1017], and the trend starts to emphasize molecular diagnostic tests [1017, 1018]. However, if there is any difficulty in diagnosis, chorioretinal biopsy or subretinal aspiration can be performed in the meantime or at a later stage [957, 986]. The positive rate of chorioretinal biopsy and brain biopsy was the highest (100%, Table 6.4), followed by vitrectomy to obtain vitreous fluid for cytological examination (61.9–93%, Table 6.4).

6.3.1.5 Examination of Intraocular Fluids

As mentioned above, vitreous biopsy, even chorioretinal biopsy, is still the gold standard for determining the diagnosis of primary vitreoretinal lymphoma. However, a contradiction often encountered in clinical practice is that when the eye is examined histologically, there are large trauma and complications. As for doctors, they bear great psychological pressure. Due to the fact that intraocular lymphoma is suspected only on the basis of clinical signs, invasive surgery with potential severe

Table 6.4 Comparison of positive rate of laboratory examination of intraocular lymphoma by collecting samples in different ways [1009, 1019–1021]

Items	Vitrectomy	Vitreous paracentesis	Aqueous paracentesis	Cerebrospinal fluid puncture	Biopsy of chorioretinal tissue	Brain biopsy
Sensitivity (%)	61.9–93	50	25–100	31.6	100	100

complications is adventurous. It is practically difficult to persuade patients and their families to accept surgery forcefully, and if the result is negative, the patients and their families will have serious doubts. Therefore, it is very useful to measure the level of IL-6 and IL-10 in aqueous humor, which is minimally invasive with sensitivity of 89% and specificity of 93% [1022]. Hereby, the detection of intraocular IL-6 and IL-10 may serve as a screening test before further invasive tests are performed. IL-10 is a cytokine required for the growth and differentiation of malignant B lymphocytes [1023]. The expression of it increases when there are malignant B lymphocytes in the eyes of patients with primary intraocular lymphoma/primary vitreoretinal lymphoma, while the expression of IL-6 increases in the inflammatory state [1024–1026]. The concentration of IL-10 in undiluted aqueous humor/vitreous humor is higher than 150 pg/mL, or the concentration in diluted aqueous humor or vitreous humor is higher than 50 pg/mL, which helps clinical consideration of diagnosis of intraocular B-cell lymphoma [1027]. The sensitivity and specificity of aqueous humor IL-10 titer higher than 50 pg/mL for the diagnosis of intraocular lymphoma were 89% and 93%, respectively, and those of vitreous IL-10 titer higher than 400 pg/mL were 99% and 80%, respectively [1022] (Table 6.5). It was recommended that aqueous humor examination should be regarded as first-line and routine diagnostic technique [981].

Among multiple diagnostic techniques including aqueous humor or vitreous IL-10 > 50 pg/mL, IL-10/IL-6 > 1, flow cytometry, IgH/TCR gene rearrangement, and cytological examinations, pooling results showed that the one with the highest positive rate (98%) was aqueous IL-10/IL-6 > 1 [981]. Whether the ratio of IL-10/IL-6 in intraocular fluid is greater than 1 is widely used for auxiliary diagnosis [1014, 1025, 1026, 1034–1036]. With the development of detection methods over time, the sensitivity and specificity of intraocular fluid IL-10 and IL-6 detection for

Table 6.5 Comparison of cellular and molecular diagnostic tests for intraocular lymphoma [981, 1019, 1020, 1022, 1028–1033]

Items	Cutoff	Sensitivity (%)	Specificity (%)
Cytology		55.4–92.0	100
Flow cytometry		62.5–83.3	70–100
Aqueous IL-10 level	>50 pg/mL	89	93
Vitreous IL-10 level	>400 pg/mL	99	80
IL-10/IL-6	>1	74–93	75–85
Aqueous humor ISOLD[a] (interleukin score for intraocular lymphoma diagnosis)	>−5.76	78.3%	93.8%
Immunoglobulin heavy chain (IgH) rearrangement		63.0–95.5	84.6–100
Myeloid differentiation primary response 88 (MYD88) L265P mutation		75	100

[a]For aqueous humor, the ISOLD formula is: $-12.871 + 5.533 \times \log(\text{IL-10} + 1) - 1.614 \times \log(\text{IL-6} + 1)$. For vitreous, the ISOLD formula is $-12.208 + 4.648 \times \log(\text{IL-10} + 1) - 1.669 \times \log(\text{IL-6} + 1)$ [1029, 1030]

the diagnosis of diffuse large B lymphoma in the eye have been continuously improved: in 2003, Wolf et al. reported that 35 patients with primary intraocular lymphoma and 64 patients with uveitis were studied and found that the sensitivity of IL-10: IL-6 ratio for the diagnosis was 74% and the specificity was 75.0% [1035]; in 2011, Wang et al. studied 80 patients and found that its sensitivity was 88% and specificity was 85% [1014]; in 2017, Kuo DE et al. showed that the prediction accuracy of simultaneous detection of IL-6 and IL-10 in vitreous fluid could reach 95% ± 5% [1037]; and pooling study showed that the sensitivity of IL-10/IL-6 > 1 was higher as 93%[981]. In addition, the ratio IL-10/IFN-γ has also been reported to assist in the diagnosis of intraocular lymphoma [1038].

If more than 100,000 cells can be obtained in a saline suspension, flow cytometry can been employed [1021]. If the cytological analysis of vitreous fluid is properly performed, enough diagnostic evidence can also be obtained to avoid further chorioretinal biopsy: Ranty ML et al. [1039] optimized the method of cytological diagnosis of retinal lymphoma. Vitreous samples were collected in the medium containing RPMI-1640 medium—fetal bovine serum and gentamicin. Transport and technical operations are carried out at 4 °C. May-Grünwald-Giemsa staining, immunocytochemistry (mainly anti-CD3, anti-CD20 and anti-CD68 antibodies), B-cell clonality, flow cytometry, and interleukin-10/IL-6 ratio were used to determine the value. Results of the 38 vitreous cytological samples of 32 patients, except 1 case, and other cases (97.4%) could be finally diagnosed, and biopsy was avoided. If hundreds of cells in one cell block can be harvested, immunohistochemistry can be considered [1021].

Molecular technology combined with microdissection and PCR to detect the clonal and amplified lymphocyte population is an important auxiliary means for the diagnosis of vitreoretinal lymphoma [991, 1040]. Immunoglobulin heavy chains (IgH; FR2, FR3, and/or CDR3 primers) are molecular diagnostic markers of B-cell lymphoma, and T-cell receptor gene rearrangement (TCR-γ) is a molecular diagnostic marker of T-cell lymphoma [1014, 1041]. Wang Y et al. [1014] showed that among 115 patients with positive IgH gene rearrangement, 114 were B-cell lymphoma patients, and only one was other-type uveitis patients; all the 85 other-type uveitis patients showed negative IgH gene rearrangement. According to the calculation, the diagnostic sensitivity of gene rearrangement for intraocular lymphoma is 1.0, the specificity is 0.99, the positive predictive value is 0.99, the negative predictive value is 1.0, and the detection efficiency is 0.995. If microdissection is not performed to select a relatively pure lymphoma cell population, the sensitivity and specificity of molecular detection will decrease [991, 1040]. For example, the positive rate of IgH gene rearrangement detection in the Japanese Intraocular Lymphoma Research Group is 80.6% [1042]. It should be noted that few cells isolated from samples may result in false-positive results [991, 1011, 1014].

Since a high frequency of MYD88 mutations (mostly L265P, rarely codon 103 and 143) was found in as much as 75% of primary central nervous system lymphoma [1012, 1043–1045], MYD88 L265P mutation detection on intraocular cell samples is used to assist the diagnosis of vitreoretinal lymphoma [1036, 1046–1048]. In patients with primary vitreoretinal lymphoma, 69–86.7% of them had this gene mutation [1012, 1046]. The advantage of MYD88 gene mutation as an auxiliary diagnostic tool is that it can serve as a reminder at the early stage of the disease course [1046]. Many patients have undergone glucocorticoid treatment because of vitreous inflammation, which can cause the lysis of lymphoma cells, thus causing difficulties in histopathological diagnosis [1049], while gene mutation detection is not affected. For patients with systemic diffuse large B lymphoma, patients with MYD88 L265P mutation have worse prognosis: shorter survival period [1050]. However, the mutation rate of MYD 88 was significantly lower in young patients than in elderly ones (50% vs. 91.3%; $P = 0.016$) [1051].

Besides MYD88 L265P, the detection of CD79BY196 in vitreous DNA was also suggested to assist in confirming the diagnosis of vitreoretinal lymphoma. Using direct sequencing and allele-specific polymerase chain reaction, Yonese I et al. analyzed the mutation of CD79BY196 and MYD88L265P in vitreous fluid DNA extracted from 17 patients with PVRL at the time of diagnosis. Six patients (35%) had CD79BY196 mutations, 12 (71%) had MYD88L265P mutations, and 6 samples from patients with benign uveitis were negative for both mutations. Patients with CD79BY196 mutations developed CNS diseases 16.5 months earlier than other patients [1052].

Recently, it was reported that metagenomic deep sequencing takes advantages in detection of numerous lymphoma-associated mutations because it is able to utilize minute volume samples and works with whole host cells or even cell-free nucleic acid, so is well-suited for ocular tissues, which may offer an additional tool in the future with which to diagnose vitreoretinal lymphoma [1053].

The positive rate of examinations of collected vitreous fluid by diagnostic vitrectomy reported in different regions/hospitals varied remarkably (Table 6.6, 14.2%–83.3%), which fully shows that the diagnostic value of the above-mentioned intraocular fluid detection method for intraocular lymphoma is related to sample processing, analysis ability, personnel experience, and other factors. In general, as

Table 6.6 Comparison of the profitability of diagnostic vitrectomy for the diagnosis of intraocular lymphoma between varied centers

Author	Country/area	Publication year	Total benefits Number of positive cases/ number of total cases	Proportion (%)
Akpek et al. [993]	Boston, USA	1999	11/34	32.4
Coupland et al. [1054]	Berlin, Germany	2003	12/84	14.2
Zaldivar et al. [1055]	Atlanta, USA	2004	9/14	64.3
Davis et al. [1019]	Miami, USA	2005	48/78	61.5
Yeh et al. [1056]	Bethesda, USA	2010	8/12	67
Kanavi et al. [1057]	Tehran, Iran	2014	12/15	83.3%

the years of publication go by, the technology continues to improve, and the overall yield is improving.

6.3.1.6 Management

The treatment of intraocular lymphoma requires the cooperation of ophthalmologists and physicians. A retrospective study found that the treatment strategies of 72 patients with vitreoretinal lymphoma varied: 13% patients who underwent local pharmaceutical treatment including intravitreal injection of rituximab, methotrexate, glucocorticoid, and rituximab combined with methotrexate, and 14% patients who underwent local radiotherapy, 20% patients who took systemic chemical therapy regimen with high-dose systemic methotrexate as main drug, 10% patients who took MTR regimen (high-dose methotrexate, temozolomide, and rituximab), and 15% patients who took CHOP regimen (cyclophosphamide, doxorubicin, vincristine, and prednisone) with or without rituximab [1036]. According to the guidelines from the European Association for Neuro-Oncology, the CHOP (cyclophosphamide, doxorubicin, vincristine, prednisolone) regimen commonly used for systemic non-Hodgkin lymphomas induces short-lasting responses in primary central nervous system lymphomas (PCNSL) which may attribute to that phosphoramide mustard and doxorubicin are not able to cross the blood-brain barrier [1058]. High-dose intravenous methotrexate is considered the most important and beneficial single agent [1058]. Typically, 3–3.5 g/m^2 MTX is well tolerated and efficacious in patients with sufficient hydration and alkalinity when followed by leucovorin rescue [1059].

The 2011 PCNSL Collaboration Conference formulated the treatment principles for primary intraocular lymphoma [985, 1000] as follows: for the cases without central nervous system (CNS) or systemic involvement: (a) use local therapy if only one eye is affected. It remains debatable whether local intravitreal methotrexate and rituximab should be administered alone or in conjunction with 30–35 Gy of external-beam radiotherapy (EBRT). (b) If both eyes are affected, local therapy is still preferred, but systemic treatment should not be ruled out. Consider the inclusion of intravitreal chemotherapeutic agents to systemic treatment; and for the cases with CNS involvement, (a) high-dose methotrexate-based therapy (possibly with systemic rituximab) in conjunction with local therapy is recommended due to the limited penetration of systemic compounds into the vitreous cavity. (b) Those who have failed systemic therapy and are too debilitated or do not meet the criteria for more aggressive therapies such as autologous stem cell transplantation (ASCT) should be considered for whole-brain radiotherapy in conjunction with ocular radiotherapy.

The dose of methotrexate injected into vitreous cavity was 0.4 mg/0.1 mL [1060–1063]. Smith et al. [1064] reported to use intravitreally injected methotrexate in three phases: induction (twice weekly for 1 month), consolidation (weekly for 1–2 months), and maintenance (monthly for 9–12 months), which is similar to the following treatment scheme raised by Frankel S et al. [998]: inject twice a week for 4 consecutive weeks, and then inject once a week for 8 consecutive weeks and then once a month for 9 consecutive months: totally 25 injections being performed. The most common complications of this scheme are keratitis and cataract [1000]. Rituximab is a chimeric mouse/human monoclonal antibody, and the target cells are

CD20 + B cells. Application of intravitreal injection of rituximab can reduce the number of injections of methotrexate, and it is also a good treatment scheme for methotrexate resistant patients [985]. The injection regimen is 1.0 mg/0.1 mL [999]. At present, there is no unified drug frequency scheme, and the complications of intravitreal chemotherapy include cataract, high intraocular pressure, vitreous hemorrhage, and retinal detachment [1000]. Clinicians should consider how to precisely use methotrexate and rituximab for intraocular injection, reduce the adverse effects of multiple injections, and prevent superfluous patient visits. The clinical response or the IL-10 level in the aqueous humor helps to decrease the number of intravitreal injections [969, 1065–1067]. Once intraocular lymphoma is diagnosed, the level of IL-10 in intraocular fluid can be continuously monitored to assess disease activity and treatment response [970].

Overall, intravitreal injection of chemotherapy drug plus systemic chemotherapy (IV + CT) could achieve satisfactory prognosis, and the combination of local radiotherapy (RT) could further decrease the recurrent and death rate [981]. PIOL patients with CNS involvement had significantly worse prognosis. A recent published pooling results of 87 studies involving 1484 patients showed the incidence of 2-year and 5-year survival rate, and 1-year and 2-year progression-free survival were 82%, 70%, 88%, and 70%, respectively [981].

6.3.2 Malignant Melanoma

6.3.2.1 Brief Introduction

Malignant melanoma, commonly known as uveal melanoma (UM) or choroidal melanomas, is the predominant form of primary intraocular cancer observed among the adult population. Ocular melanoma comprises 80% of total instances of melanoma affecting the eye and represents 3–5% of all reported cases of melanoma [1068, 1069]. The choroid is accountable for roughly 80% of uveal melanomas [1068, 1070]. Choroidal melanomas are infrequent before to reaching maturity and exhibit a maximum occurrence rate at 55 years of age [1071, 1072]. Around 50% of choroidal melanomas are located at a distance of 3 mm from either the fovea or the optic disc [1073].

Most cases of melanoma display a nodular growth pattern characterized by different levels of pigmentation. Based on findings from the Collaborative Ocular Melanoma Study group (COMS), it has been observed that a majority of tumors, specifically over 90%, exhibit development beyond Bruch's membrane and extend into the subretinal region. Additionally, approximately 49% of tumor cells infiltrate the retina, while 25.2% demonstrate growth within the vitreous [1074]. The presence of intrascleral melanoma cells has been observed in a range of 51–64% of cases. Additionally, episcleral extension has been reported in 8–13% of cases, while intravascular tumor cell in growth has been documented in 17–20% of instances [1073].

6.3.2.2 Epidemiology

The choroid is responsible for the majority of occurrences, comprising approximately 90% of cases, with the ciliary body (7%) and the iris (3%) also contributing

[1075]. The prevalence of uveal melanoma (UM) in the United States and Europe is estimated to be between five and six cases per million individuals, whereas in Australia, it is approximately seven cases per million. These rates have exhibited a consistent pattern over the past three decades [1076–1079]. In the regions of Asia and Africa, the incidence rate is seen to be merely 0.2 to 0.3 occurrences per million individuals annually [1080].

The phenomenon of presentation typically manifests at the stage of adulthood, with a notable apex around the age of 60. An equal proportion of males and females are impacted. Risk factors include fair complexion, light-colored irides, congenital ocular melanocytosis, melanocytoma, the BAP1 cancer predisposition syndrome, an autosomal dominant disorder that also causes kidney cancer, mesothelioma, and other melanocytic tumors [1081].

6.3.2.3 Clinical Manifestation

Common symptoms include blurred vision, metamorphopsia (distorted vision), and photopsia (perception of flashes of light) [1076]. The prevalence of asymptomatic tumors is increasing due to advancements in community examination practices [1076]. Proptosis, painful neovascular glaucoma, and uveitis are infrequently observed clinical manifestations.

In large tumors, a patchy fluorescent pattern shown by fluorescein angiography and the internal tumor vascularization known as "double circulation pattern" mainly shown by ICG may be observed (Figs. 6.60 and 6.61) [1082, 1083].

Ocular echography stands out as the most efficient diagnostic tool available to clinicians. Melanomas exhibit a diminished internal reflectivity and possess an

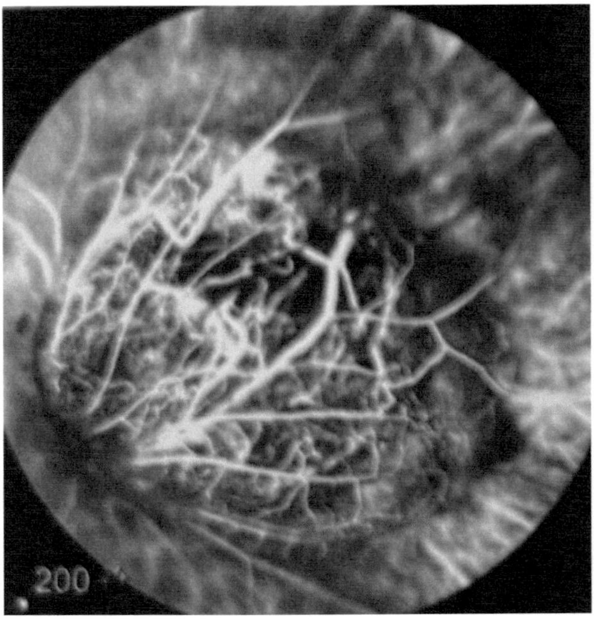

Fig. 6.60 The indocyanine green angiography of a case with choroidal melanoma retinoblastoma. The internal tumor vascularization known as "double circulation pattern" can be observed. (Courtesy of Prof. Hongjian Liang of Department of Ophthalmology, People's Hospital, Peking University, Beijing, China)

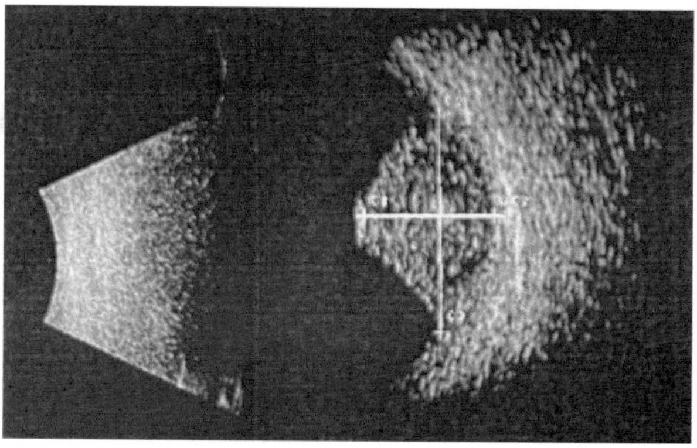

Fig. 6.61 B-scan ultrasound showing a large mushroom-shaped mass lesion in a patient with clinical presumed diagnosis of choroidal melanoma. (Courtesy of Prof. Hongjian Liang of Department of Ophthalmology, People's Hospital, Peking University, Beijing, China)

inherent acoustic quiet zone when visualized using ultrasonography. The majority of melanomas exhibit a dome-shaped morphology; however, those presenting with a collar stud or mushroom configuration are highly indicative of malignancy [1084]. The manifestation arises subsequent to a disturbance in Bruch's membrane, a structural component of the retina. There is a positive correlation between the size of the apical and basal diameters and the likelihood of the lesion being malignant. Several studies suggest a correlation between the thickness of tumors and the probability of distant metastasis. The consensus among experts is that a lesion exhibiting an apical height over 3 mm is highly indicative of a melanoma [1085].

6.3.2.4 Diagnosis

The clinical diagnosis of uveal melanoma relies on a comprehensive evaluation involving the use of the slit lamp and indirect ophthalmoscope, in conjunction with ocular ultrasonography [1086]. The necessity for a clinical biopsy to definitively establish the diagnosis of uveal melanoma is infrequent. The Collaborative Ocular Melanoma Study demonstrated a diagnostic accuracy of over 99% for enucleated eyes exhibiting typical characteristics [1087]. In certain instances, a diagnostic biopsy may be deemed required, particularly when the lesion exhibits characteristics of being amelanotic or presents challenges in identification due to the presence of vitreous hemorrhage or debris. The procedure of fine-needle aspiration can be performed, however under the guidance of a proficient cytologist who possesses expertise in ocular pathology [1088].

Small melanomas may exhibit clinical similarities to ordinary nevi, rendering them difficult to differentiate. The indicators of malignancy in this case include the observation of lipofuscin clusters on the tumor surface, the presence of serous retinal detachment, a tumor thickness above 2 mm, and documented evidence of tumor progression. Various imaging techniques, including autofluorescence imaging, optical coherence tomography, and ultrasonography, are employed to identify and discern these clinical traits. In cases where there is ambiguity, the process of diagnosing a condition may necessitate a protracted period of several months or even years of rigorous testing. Histologic and genetic examination can also be conducted on the tumor by a biopsy procedure. The histological characteristics commonly associated with malignancy encompass spindle-B or epithelioid cytomorphology, characterized by enlarged nuclei, prominent nucleoli, abundant cytoplasm, and the presence of mitoses. However, the utilization of microscopy techniques may provide challenges or render it impossible to differentiate between nevi and low-grade melanomas [1089]. Both of these tumors exhibit mutations in the GNAQ and GNA11 genes [1090, 1091]. However, it is projected that only melanomas exhibit characteristics such as chromosome 3 loss (known as "monosomy 3"), chromosome 8q gain, chromosome 6p gain, a class 2 gene expression profile, and mutations in genes such as BAP1, EIF1AX, and SF3B1. In cases when the biopsy yields conclusive results about the presence or absence of cancer, the patient should be afforded the opportunity to make an informed decision between two options: observation and therapy. It is crucial for the patient to carefully examine any adverse effects, such as sight loss or other forms of morbidity, that may arise from the chosen treatment approach [1092].

6.3.2.5 Examination of Intraocular Fluids

A previous study revealed a significant increase in the levels of vitreal concentrations of many cytokines and chemokines, including IL-6, IL-8, IP-10, MCP-1, MIP-1α, MIP-1β, TNF-α, and RANTES of eyes affected by uveal melanoma [1093]. IL-8 is a chemokine that is generated by a range of cell types and is used to activate and attract polymorph nuclear leukocytes during acute and chronic inflammatory processes. Previous research by Lattanzio et al. suggested that the UM microenvironment might promote IL-8 signaling as an alternate pro-angiogenic route to VEGF [1094].

In addition to tumor cells, normal cells produce cytokines such as IL-6, IL-10, TGFb, MIF, GM-CSF, and VEGF, which have a role in immune responses [1095]. A positive correlation was seen between augmented Treg infiltration and elevated concentrations of IL-6 and IP-10 [1093]. Macrophages exhibiting a high density in uveal melanoma (UM) display an "inflammatory phenotype," a characteristic often observed alongside elevated microvascular density and the presence of epithelioid cells [1096]. Macrophages undergo differentiation into the M2 phenotype upon exposure to IL-6 and IL-10, both of which are associated with tumor promotion and unfavorable prognostic outcomes [1097].

A recent study has established a notable elevation in the levels of MCP-1, a chemokine that has been identified as being connected with tumor-associated macrophages in UM [1098]. MCP-1 has the capacity to induce angiogenesis, in addition to its role in facilitating the chemotaxis of tumor-associated macrophages. In the context of a murine model, the inhibition of MCP-1 led to a notable reduction in both angiogenesis and tumor growth [1099]. The presence of the epidermal growth factor receptor (EGFR) has been detected in various types of malignancies, suggesting its involvement in the process of tumor formation. The expression of EGFR has been observed in a range of 12.5% to 29.2% among patients with UM. Additionally, elevated levels of EGF in the vitreous have been detected in specific subsets of UM patients [1100, 1101]. As previously reported, the expression of EGFR and EGF was found to be associated with the mitotic rate and scleral invasion, respectively. This observation implies that the EGF-EGFR signal could serve as a promising therapeutic target for uveal melanoma [1101]. In addition, the expression of NGF-R was detected in both primary and metastatic melanoma lesions, and a correlation was established between its presence and an unfavorable prognosis [1102–1105].

Previous study also found that levels of vascular endothelial growth factor (VEGF) were detected in the aqueous humor of patients with uveal melanoma (UM). Specifically, the concentration of VEGF-A in the aqueous humor was found to be correlated with the highest basal tumor diameter and tumor height [1106, 1107]. Another pro-angiogenic cytokine, basic fibroblast growth factor (bFGF), was expressed by most uveal melanoma tumour cells (89%) [1108].

The presence of cytokines in the aqueous humor or vitreous fluid has a strong correlation with the genomic profile of tumor tissue, surpassing the efficacy of blood tests. Consequently, this method holds significant promise for the diagnosis, detection, and prognostic evaluation of UM in ocular tissues. Nevertheless, whereas the aqueous humor of eyes containing UM exhibited signs of inflammation, there is currently no evidence indicating that any specific cytokines had diagnostic or prognostic value [1097].

The S-100 protein is a calcium-binding protein with an acidic nature, weighing around 21,000 daltons. It is found in ocular melanomas as well as certain normal ocular tissues. The concentrations of S-100 protein in the vitreous samples were obtained from three eyes harboring melanoma, three eyes undergoing tractional retinal detachment repair, and six healthy eyes exhibited ranging from 10,000 to 11,000 ng/mL, 500 to 1600 ng/mL, and 2 to 120 ng/mL, respectively. Additionally, soluble human leukocyte antigen (sHLA) was measured in the aqueous humor of uveal melanoma patients, and metastases were observed at a higher rate in the sHLA-positive group, where 68% had metastases, compared to 41% in the negative group ($P = 0.0291$). The melanoma-related survival was significantly worse in the sHLA-positive group ($P = 0.025$) [1109]. Compared to healthy controls, 32 miRNAs in the vitreous humor were found to be differentially expressed in UM patients, and miR-146a could be considered a potential circulating marker of UM [1110]. These methodologies offer novel perspectives on the interplay between ocular tumors and the surrounding ocular fluids and have the potential to be utilized for diagnostic purposes with the incorporation of more targeted tumor markers [1111].

6.3.2.6 Management

Patients with ocular lesions displaying ambiguous findings that do not exhibit typical characteristics of melanoma should have regular monitoring by an ophthalmologist. This monitoring is necessary to identify definitive symptoms such as rapid growth or the presence of subretinal fluid. In cases when the patient's condition is deemed too delicate to undergo surgical intervention for the purpose of enucleation or the placement of a radionuclide plaque, surveillance may be advised as the preferred approach.

Before initiating eye therapy, it is imperative to do a comprehensive systemic evaluation to confirm the lack of distant metastases. Once this has been established, attention can be directed on local ophthalmic treatment targeting the underlying tumor. At the time of initial ocular presentation, 5% of people experience distant metastases. In cases where a patient exhibits symptoms of distant disease, it may be advisable to delay local eye therapy in favor of systemic treatment. However, the decision to pursue this approach should be contingent upon the specific ocular symptomatology of the individual.

The utilization of diode laser treatment, i.e., transpupillary thermotherapy, is generally well tolerated; however, its application is constrained by the notable occurrence of local recurrence rates, which can reach up to 20% [1112]. The efficacy of laser treatment in achieving tumor control exhibits a direct correlation with the size of the tumor. Therefore, it is most appropriate for small tumors measuring 3 mm in thickness that originate at a distance from the macula and optic nerve. This approach is commonly utilized as a supplementary treatment subsequent to radiotherapy.

Focal radiation therapy is frequently employed by ocular oncologists as a means to preserve the integrity of the eye. The Collaborative Ocular Melanoma Study conducted a randomized trial with persons who had medium-sized tumors with apical heights ranging from 2.5 to 10.0 mm. These participants were assigned to either receive primary brachytherapy using iodine-125 plaques or undergo enucleation. The experiment did not yield any statistically significant disparity in melanoma-related mortality between the two groups. The user did not provide any text to rewrite. Subsequently, ocular brachytherapy has emerged as the predominant technique for preserving the integrity of the eye in cases with cancers that meet these specified requirements. This approach can be employed for the treatment of patients diagnosed with melanomas exhibiting an apical height over 10.0 mm. However, it is important to note that such patients are at a higher risk of experiencing severe radiation retinopathy and subsequent vision impairment. Iodine-125 is the most often employed isotope in the United States. Additionally, many other radioisotopes are utilized for this purpose. Notably, ruthenium-106 is the prevailing isotope in numerous European facilities [1113]. If charged-particle, proton-beam radiation is accessible, it can serve as a substitute for brachytherapy. The consensus among medical professionals is that both modalities exhibit favorable rates of local tumor control, with certain studies documenting rates as high as 98% [1114].

Enucleation, the surgical procedure involving the removal of the eyeball, continues to be a feasible alternative for persons afflicted with large tumors and those who are likely to experience major ocular and visual complications as a result of radiation therapy. In the majority of instances, the surgical placement of an orbital implant results in favorable cosmetic outcomes. Vitrectomy, a surgical procedure involving the excision of chosen tumors while preserving the integrity of the eye globe, is most suitable for the treatment of small anterior ocular malignancies, such as iris melanomas. The utilization of adjuvant plaque irradiation has the potential to reduce the occurrence of ocular recurrence in individuals who are undergoing selective choroidal excision of melanomas [1115]. Surgical intervention facilitates a comprehensive histopathological assessment, hence enabling the confirmation of microscopic expansion beyond the ocular region. The presence of microvascular loops and the epithelioid cell phenotype have been found to be associated with an unfavorable prognosis [1116]. Exenteration, a surgical procedure involving the removal of the globe and accompanying orbital contents, is typically employed in cases of extensive involvement of the orbital region and in patients who are undergoing palliative treatment.

Almost 50% of patients develop metastatic disease, which usually involves the liver and is usually fatal within 1 year [1117, 1118]. The prognosis of uveal melanoma can be estimated by clinical, histopathological, cytogenetic, and transcriptomic markers [1119–1121]. Tumor sample for genetic testing is either obtained from enucleation specimen or intraoperatively by fine needle aspiration biopsy. It is imperative to distinguish between diagnostic biopsy and prognostic biopsy, wherein the former is conducted to determine the kind of a tumor, while the latter involves assessing the genetic characteristics of the tumor and its potential for future spread [1085]. Chromosome 3 loss, 8p loss, 8q gain, 1p loss, and 6q loss are associated with poor prognosis [1118–1121].

6.3.3 Retinoblastoma

6.3.3.1 Brief Introduction

Retinoblastoma (RB) is the prevailing primary intraocular malignancy in pediatric patients, characterized by the formation of malignant tumors in the developing retina [1122]. Tumor initiation frequently occurs as a result of a mutation in both alleles of the RB1 tumor suppressor gene, leading to subsequent genetic anomalies that correspond to the clinical stage and pathological characteristics of the tumor [1123, 1124]. Knudson's two-hit hypothesis was developed subsequent to an investigation of both sporadic and heritable RB [1125]. Epigenetic investigations have unveiled that the rapid growth of RB following the inactivation of the RB1 gene can be attributed to epigenetic alterations [1126].

A large proportion of RB patients are identified at an advanced stage and still require enucleation to limit the risk of metastasis. The most severe kind could present in developing nations. The primary prognostic factor hinges upon the timely identification of the tumor and the subsequent implementation of treatment for the child through a multidisciplinary team-based approach. The survival rate of RB has witnessed a significant increase over the past two decades as a result of notable breakthroughs in treatment modalities. Nevertheless, it is imperative to conduct extended monitoring of retinoblastoma (RB) survivors due to the potential occurrence of further cancers throughout their later years [1127]. Effective genetic screening and counseling can provide valuable support to parents and patients, aiding them in their comprehension and awareness of the disease [1128].

6.3.3.2 Epidemiology

Retinoblastoma is the most common tumor of the eye in children, accounting for 2.5% to 4% of all pediatric malignancies and 11% of cancers diagnosed within the first year of life [1126]. In the United States and Europe, the typical age-adjusted incidence rate of RB is 2 to 5 per million children (about 1 in 14,000 to 18,000 live births) [1125, 1129].

The occurrence of RB can be classified into two categories: unilateral, which accounts for 60% of cases, and bilateral, which accounts for the remaining 40% of cases [1130]. Bilateral cases are invariably heritable, and the typical age at which the condition is identified is 1 year. The heritability of unilateral cases is not prevalent, with the majority being nonheritable. However, approximately 15% of unilateral cases do exhibit heritability. Additionally, the median age at which these cases are often presented is 2 years. Moreover, RB is identified in children during the early stages of their development, with approximately two-thirds of cases being diagnosed before the age of two, and a staggering 95% of cases being found before the age of 5 [1131].

6.3.3.3 Clinical Manifestation

Leukocoria (white pupil) (60%) is the most prevalent clinical indication of RB, followed by strabismus (misaligned eyes) (20%) [1132]. Any size RB can cause leukocoria, despite that leukocoria is more common in bigger tumors. This white pupillary reflex is caused by light reflection from the retrolental white mass [1132, 1133]. Depending on the stage of the disease at the time of diagnosis, the clinical signs of RB differ [1134]. A tiny RB, defined as less than 2 mm in basal dimension, presents ophthalmoscopically as a mild, transparent, or slightly translucent lesion in the sensory retina in its early clinical stage. Dilated retinal blood vessels are observed in the presence of larger tumors, facilitating both the nourishment and elimination of metabolic waste from the tumor. Certain bigger tumors exhibit calcification foci resembling the texture and appearance of cottage cheese (Fig. 6.62).

The development patterns of retinoblastoma can be classified into three categories: intraretinal, endophytic, and exophytic. Intraretinal tumors are neoplasms that are confined to the anatomical boundaries of the retina (Fig. 6.62). Endophytic RB refers to a specific subtype of RB that originates from the retina and extends into the vitreous cavity. Consequently, it exhibits a discernible white, cloudy formation that causes the retinal blood vessels to be obscured (Fig. 6.63). Due to its characteristic

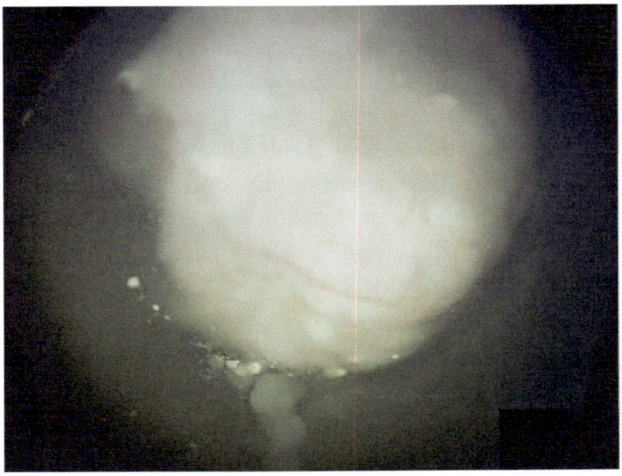

Fig. 6.62 The fundus photography of a child with retinoblastoma. A big tumor with calcification resembling the texture and appearance of cottage cheese located in the posterior pole of fundus. (Courtesy of Prof. Jianmin Ma of Department of Ophthalmology, Tongren Hospital, Capital Medical University, Beijing, China)

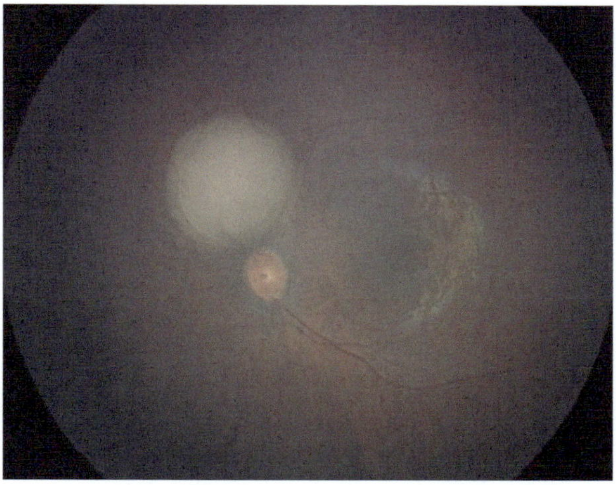

Fig. 6.63 The fundus photography of a child with retinoblastoma. A round and white intraretinal tumor can be observed superior to the optic disc. (Courtesy of Prof. Jianmin Ma of Department of Ophthalmology, Tongren Hospital, Capital Medical University, Beijing, China)

friability, an endophytic tumor has the potential to disseminate throughout the vitreous cavity and anterior chamber, so mimicking the symptoms of endophthalmitis. This resemblance is particularly notable in cases of toxocariasis, a parasitic infection that frequently affects young children. Exophytic RB is a subtype of RB characterized by the growth of tumor cells originating from the retina and extending into the subretinal region. These neoplasms induce a progressive separation of the retina, often resulting in its displacement toward the anterior region, positioned posterior to a transparent lens. Clinically, exophytic RB has the potential to resemble Coats' disease or other forms of exudative retinal detachment. RB has been shown to exhibit a diffuse infiltrating pattern on occasion, characterized by the presence of tumor cells entering the retina in a generally flat manner, without any noticeable bulk. The diagnosis in these patients may present further difficulty, as this particular pattern has the potential to resemble symptoms of uveitis or endophthalmitis. Less common presenting characteristics include pseudohypopyon associated with tumor seeding in the anterior chamber, hyphema resulting from iris neovascularization, vitreous bleeding, or symptoms indicative of orbital cellulitis [1135].

6.3.3.4 Diagnosis

In most cases, RB may be diagnosed and differentiated using conventional clinical characteristics with indirect ophthalmoscopy with the pupil pharmacologically dilated, ultrasonography, CT (Fig. 6.64), MRI, and RetCam fundus imaging. The characteristic CT finding is a partly calcified intravitreous mass lesion mostly confined within the eyeball [1136]. Ocular ultrasonography (B-scan) can reveal calcifications that are diagnostic of RB; however, MRI is required to evaluate optic nerve invasion and the existence of trilateral RB [1137, 1138]. Changes in the color of the iris and larger eyes due to increased ocular pressure are common in advanced disease [1132]. To minimize the spread of the illness outside the eye and the likelihood of increasing the danger of extraocular metastasis, direct biopsy of RB has been avoided [1139–1141]. Therefore, the monitoring of RB and the tiny number of

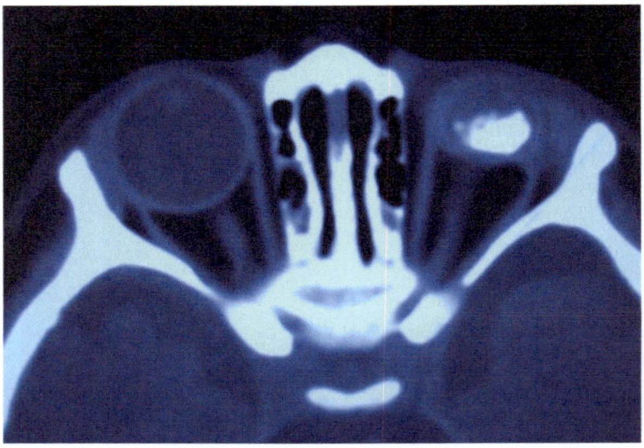

Fig. 6.64 Ocular CT (computed tomography) reveals calcification of an intraocular mass that assist diagnosis of retinoblastoma in the left eye. (Courtesy of Prof. Jianmin Ma of Department of Ophthalmology, Tongren Hospital, Capital Medical University, Beijing, China)

atypical RB suffers from a lack of objective and quantitative specificity. This not only impedes research into the biological activity of RB, impacts disease progression and treatment response monitoring, and inhibits the development of tailored, ocular-specific therapy regimens for individuals.

In addition, it is worth noting that the majority of tumors arise due to the loss of both copies of the RB1 tumor suppressor gene, which plays a crucial role in regulating the cell cycle. However, a small subset of tumors (approximately 2%) is attributed to the amplification of the neuroblastoma-derived myelocytomatosisviral oncogene homolog gene. In such cases, conventional ocular preservation therapy tends to be ineffective. The removal of the eye, known as enucleation, is deemed required in this particular instance, and currently, there is a lack of definitive and unbiased methods to identify this specific subtype during the first diagnosis [1142, 1143].

6.3.3.5 Examination of Intraocular Fluids

Previous research has identified molecular markers associated with RB in peripheral blood. However, the blood-retinal barrier poses a challenge as it limits the amount of tumor-related genetic material present in peripheral blood. Consequently, the detection efficiency is compromised, particularly in cases where RB affects both eyes in children [1141].

Dias et al. were the first to investigate the aqueous humor (AH) in enucleated eyes from children with RB and discovered that a rise in lactic acid dehydrogenase (LDH) activity linked with disease activity; the authors speculated that this may assist in diagnosis [1144]. Shehata et al. conducted high-quality studies that established the prognostic consequences of AH survivin and TGF-β, and the excellent sensitivity, specificity, and accuracy of serum and AH survivin and TGF-β make them attractive markers for early diagnosis and follow-up of RB patients [1145, 1146]. Comoy et al. discovered that repeated AH neuron-specific enolase measurements may play an important role in diagnosing tumor status in RB patients, and future research may further clinically validate the use of this tumor marker [1147, 1148]. Furthermore, Hadjistilianou et al. found that treatment with specific intra-arterial chemotherapy resulted in considerably lower protein concentrations in the eyes [1149]. Furthermore, these scientists advised that PEDF and STRA6 be studied further for future prospects in RB-targeted treatment [1150]. The remaining biochemical markers studied previously, such as xanthine and uric acid, have shown diagnostic utility; however, more research is needed to elucidate their significant clinical utility, including prognostic, clinicopathological, and therapeutic implications.

Berry et al. proposed for the first time the feasibility of using aqueous humor for liquid biopsy of RB, which provides the possibility for the diagnosis of RB and the monitoring of prognostic biomarkers [1141]. They demonstrated that the DNA in the AH is consistent with expectations for RB DNA, exhibiting similar known chromosomal changes, including a gain of 1q, 2p, and 6p and a loss of 16q [1141]. The further study of the same team showed that gain of chromosome 6p was the most common somatic chromosomal copy number alterations (SCNAs) (77% of enucleated eyes versus 25% of salvaged eyes, $P = 0.0092$) and associated with a tenfold increased odds of enucleation (OR = 10). The median amplitude of 6p gain was 1.47 in enucleated versus 1.07 in salvaged eyes ($p = 0.001$) [1151]. Through more investigation, this innovative approach holds the potential to assist medical practitioners in diagnosing retinoblastoma (RB) when faced with diagnostic uncertainties. Furthermore, it may enable the identification of potential correlations between specific chromosomal copy number variation profile features or RB1 mutations and prognosis or therapeutic efficacy.

Despite that the clinical use of AH evaluation for RB patients is not currently implemented, additional investigation into distinct biochemical and genetic indicators and their correlations with treatment response and potential as targets for therapy holds the promise of transforming RB management.

6.3.3.6 Management

The primary objective of therapeutic intervention in retinoblastoma (RB) is to eradicate the tumor while minimizing adverse effects on adjacent organs [1152]. The prioritization of therapy follows a specific order, namely, (1) preservation of life, (2) preservation of the eye, and (3) preservation of vision. The selection of treatment is based on several factors, including the stage of the tumor, the presence of tumor foci (such as unifocal, unilateral multifocal, or bilateral), the location and size of the tumor within the eye, the presence of vitreous seeding, and the age of the child [1153].

The selection of therapy procedures may vary based on the specific stage of the disease. Local therapies, including laser, photocoagulation, cryotherapy, transpupillary thermotherapy, and brachytherapy, are commonly employed alongside systemic chemotherapy. Regrettably, in cases of the disease that are more serious in nature, the necessity arises for the surgical extraction of the entire ocular globe and its intraocular contents, a procedure known as enucleation [1154].

The administration of drugs via intravitreal injection for the treatment of RB was initially reported in 1995. However, its widespread adoption was not achieved until the publication of Munier et al.'s safety-enhanced protocol in 2012. This protocol proposed an initial paracentesis procedure to withdraw aqueous humor (AH) in order to reduce intraocular pressure and thereby prevent the reflux of tumor cells to the injection site in the pars plana [1155, 1156]. The administration of melphalan via intravitreal injection has significantly transformed the management of vitreous seeding and is presently considered the established therapeutic approach for patients with RB in both the United States and globally [1157–1159]. The procedure is widely regarded as being both safe and efficacious in eliminating seeds. The safety-enhanced treatment, which involved an initial paracentesis, was subjected to a thorough examination, revealing no occurrences of tumor metastasis. Consequently, the surgical procedure not only provided an effective treatment for vitreous seeding but also facilitated secure entry into the intraocular space, namely, the anterior chamber in RB eyes. The process disproved the notion that the globe was impenetrable in RB eyes [1141].

In order to mitigate the long-term probability of experiencing repeated occurrences of malignant neoplasms, individuals diagnosed with heritable RB (H1) are advised to refrain from exposure to radiation (such as X-rays, CT scans, and external beam radiation) as well as substances that have the potential to cause DNA damage (such as nicotine and UV light), whenever possible [1160]. Cancer risks in these people might be decreased by reducing their exposure to chemotherapy [1161]. Molecular genetic testing may be performed if the pathogenic variant in the family is known, which can reduce the need for expensive screening procedures in family members who have not inherited the pathogenic variant or eye examinations by an ophthalmologist experienced in the treatment of RB if the pathogenic variant is unknown for early identification of asymptomatic at-risk children [1162, 1163].

Gene therapy and continuous drug release platforms are two novel therapeutic approaches that are now gaining momentum in the field of medicine. The utilization of intravitreal injections of an adenovirus vector encoding the herpes simplex thymidine kinase gene was employed in individuals diagnosed with bilateral retinoblastoma accompanied by vitreous seeds [1164]. A novel sustained-release episcleral exoplant has been developed for the purpose of targeted delivery of medication within the intraocular region [1165]. Major discoveries in understanding the molecular biology of tumors and the development of tailored treatment have increased survival in affluent nations to 97% [1166].

6.4 Other Ocular Diseases

6.4.1 Glaucoma

Several research have assessed the components in aqueous humor from patients with glaucoma and observed significant variations in these components across different kinds of glaucoma. For instance, the concentration of TGFβ2 in aqueous humor of primary open-angle glaucoma patients but not chronic angle-closure glaucoma, primary angle-closure suspects, or acute angle-closure glaucoma patients, was significantly higher than control eyes. The proteome of the aqueous humor in patients with primary open-angle glaucoma exhibits significant activation of the immune system [1167]. Furthermore, significantly negative correlation between SFRP1 and IOP existed in the primary open-angle glaucoma group [1168]. In addition, compared with cataract patients, patients with acute angle closure glaucoma have elevated levels of MCP-3, MDC, and VEGF in aqueous humor, while MCP-1 and MIP-1β levels decrease. However, the levels of G-CSF, IL-6, and IL-8 were similar between the two groups [1169]. The levels of most cytokines in the aqueous humor of patients with primary congenital glaucoma were found to be lower compared to those with primary open-angle glaucoma and healthy individuals. Statistically significant differences were found in the levels of IL-1ra, IL-2, IL-5, IL-7, IL-8, IL-10, IL-12, IL-15, IL-17A, eotaxin, FGF basic, G-CSF, GM-CSF, IFN-γ, MIP-1α, PDGF-bb, MIP-1β, RANTES, TNF-α, and VEGF [1170]. Quantile regression analysis revealed variations in the quantile of selenium content in aqueous humor among patients with open-angle glaucoma of different ages and genders [1171].

Additionally, aqueous humor levels of TGF-β2 were correlated with the severity of glaucomatous neuropathy in primary open-angle glaucoma patients [1172]. The analysis of aqueous humor holds significant importance in assessing the effectiveness of glaucoma surgery. Most of the primary open-angle glaucoma eyes with favorable filtering bleb development after trabeculectomy had normal TGF-β2 levels [1173]. Glaucoma surgery prognosis worsens as the aqueous humor levels of IL-6 and TNF-α increase [1174].

6.4.2 Chronic Ocular Surface Diseases

It is well-known that chronic ocular surface diseases such as corneal lesions may result in anterior chamber immune reaction, even hypopyon. Aqueous humor of patients with chronic ocular surface diseases including scar pemphigoid, chemical burns, thermal burns, Stevens-Johnson syndrome, and exposed keratitis was studied. Compared with cataract control, the aqueous levels of IL-6 (1696 ± 804 pg/mL vs. 6.36 ± 0.94 pg/mL, $P = 0.001$), IL-10 (4.0 ± 1.0 pg/mL vs. 1.68 ± 0.04 pg/mL, $P = 0.0006$), IL-17A (24.3 ± 9.8 pg/mL vs. 3.7 ± 0.2 pg/mL, $P = 0.008$), the levels of GM-CSF (26.0 ± 18.3 pg/mL vs. 2.7 ± 0.3 pg/mL, $P = 0.007$), E-selectin (5150 ± 1232 pg/mL vs. 2093 ± 37 pg/mL, $P = 0.0001$), P-selectin (13,122 ± 7219 pg/mL vs. 3658 ± 137 pg/mL, $P = 0.0001$), and s-ICAM (7914 ± 2813 pg/mL vs. 1397 ± 119, $P = 0.008$) significantly increased. In comparison to patients with corneal scars, individuals with active ocular surface disorders exhibited notably elevated levels of IL-6 (44.1 ± 15.0 pg/mL, $P = 0.0077$), IL-17A (4.1 ± 0.7 pg/mL, $P = 0.034$), E-selectin (2439 ± 302 pg/mL, $P = 0.039$), and P-selectin (5673 ± 1553 pg/mL, $P = 0.017$) in the aqueous humor [1175]. This study offers a comprehensive explanation for the anterior chamber reaction triggered by ocular surface lesions. It also highlights the importance of doing a thorough evaluation of the ocular surface while collecting aqueous humor from the control group in clinical practice.

6.4.3 Femtosecond Laser-Assisted Cataract Surgery

Patients who underwent femtosecond laser-assisted cataract surgery underwent cytokine testing in aqueous humor during surgery, and the results showed that its value was significantly higher than that of the conventional cataract group. The average values of IL-1β, IL-6, and PGE2 in the two groups were 25.6, 24.6, 64.2 pg/mL, and 17.1, 15.2, 45.7 pg/mL, respectively; *P* values are all <0.01). This may be the reason why femtosecond laser-assisted cataract surgery is more prone to pupil narrowing during surgery.

During femtosecond laser-aided cataract surgery, patients underwent cytokine testing in the aqueous humor. The results revealed a significantly greater value compared to the traditional cataract group. The mean concentrations of IL-1β, IL-6, and PGE2 in the two groups were 25.6 pg/mL vs. 17.1 pg/mL, 15.2 pg/mL vs. 24.6 pg/mL, and 64.2 pg/mL vs. 45.7 pg/mL, respectively ($P < 0.01$ for all comparisons). This could explain why femtosecond laser-assisted cataract surgery is more susceptible to pupil constriction during the procedure [1176].

6.4.4 Cataract Progression After Pars Plana Vitrectomy

Metabolomic analysis of aqueous humor in patients with cataracts after vitrectomy revealed significant differences in regulatory molecules involved in oxidative stress and inflammatory responses, such as glutaric acid and pelargonic acid [1177].

References

1. Takase H, Kubono R, Terada Y, Imai A, Fukuda S, Tomita M, Miyanaga M, Kamoi K, Sugita S, Miyata K, et al. Comparison of the ocular characteristics of anterior uveitis caused by herpes simplex virus, varicella-zoster virus, and cytomegalovirus. Jpn J Ophthalmol. 2014a;58(6):473–82.
2. Neumann R, Barequet D, Rosenblatt A, Amer R, Ben-Arie-Weintrob Y, Hareuveni-Blum T, Vishnevskia-Dai V, Raskin E, Blumenfeld O, Shulman S, et al. Herpetic anterior uveitis—analysis of presumed and PCR proven cases. Ocul Immunol Inflamm. 2019a;27(2):211–8.
3. Keorochana N, Treesit I, Funarunart P. Characteristics and clinical outcomes of hypertensive anterior uveitis. Ocul Immunol Inflamm. 2020;28(4):538–48.
4. Chan NS, Chee SP, Caspers L, Bodaghi B. Clinical features of CMV-associated anterior uveitis. Ocul Immunol Inflamm. 2018a;26(1):107–15.
5. Accorinti M, Gilardi M, Pirraglia MP, Amorelli GM, Nardella C, Abicca I, Pesci FR. Cytomegalovirus anterior uveitis: long-term follow-up of immunocompetent patients. Graefes Arch Clin Exp Ophthalmol. 2014;252(11):1817–24.
6. Antoun J, Willermain F, Makhoul D, Motulsky E, Caspers L, Relvas LJ. Topical Ganciclovir in cytomegalovirus anterior uveitis. J Ocul Pharmacol Ther. 2017a;33(4):313–8.
7. Chee SP, Jap A. Cytomegalovirus anterior uveitis: outcome of treatment. Br J Ophthalmol. 2010;94(12):1648–52.
8. Sira M, Murray PI. Treatment of cytomegalovirus anterior uveitis with oral valaciclovir. Ocul Immunol Inflamm. 2007;15(1):31–2.
9. Wong MOM, Yu AHY, Chan CKM. Efficacy and safety of oral valganciclovir in cytomegalovirus anterior uveitis with uncontrolled intraocular pressure. Br J Ophthalmol. 2020;105:1666–71.
10. Relvas LJM, Antoun J, de Groot-Mijnes JDF, Motulsky E, Ten Dam-Van Loon NH, Makhoul D, Willermain F, Caspers L. Diagnosis of cytomegalovirus anterior uveitis in two European Referral Centers. Ocul Immunol Inflamm. 2018a;26(1):116–21.

11. Harada Y, Fukuda K, Nakahira A, Tada K, Sumi T, Fukushima A. Requirement of longer term antiviral therapy in patients with cytomegalovirus anterior uveitis with corneal endothelial cell damage. Clin Ophthalmol. 2018;12:1311–6.
12. Standardization of Uveitis Nomenclature Working Group. Classification criteria for cytomegalovirus anterior uveitis. Am J Ophthalmol. 2021a;228:89–95.
13. Rao VG, Janani MK, Biswas J. Real-time polymerase chain reaction in recurrent cytomegalovirus anterior uveitis. Am J Ophthalmol Case Rep. 2019;15:100470.
14. Shirahama S, Kaburaki T, Takada S, Nakahara H, Tanaka R, Komae K, Fujino Y, Kawashima H, Aihara M. Comparison of visual field defect progression in secondary glaucoma due to anterior uveitis caused by three types of herpes viruses. Graefes Arch Clin Exp Ophthalmol. 2020;258(3):639–45.
15. Terada Y, Kaburaki T, Takase H, Goto H, Nakano S, Inoue Y, Maruyama K, Miyata K, Namba K, Sonoda KH, et al. Distinguishing features of anterior uveitis caused by herpes simplex virus, varicella-zoster virus, and cytomegalovirus. Am J Ophthalmol. 2021;227:191–200.
16. Chee SP, Bacsal K, Jap A, Se-Thoe SY, Cheng CL, Tan BH. Clinical features of cytomegalovirus anterior uveitis in immunocompetent patients. Am J Ophthalmol. 2008a;145(5):834–40.
17. Tsubota Y, Fujino Y, Ohtomo K, Ueda K, Yoshida J, Miyai T, Kaburaki T, Mayama C. Severe cytomegalovirus anterior uveitis and corneal endotheliitis after use of topical tacrolimus. Int J Ophthalmol. 2021;14(3):468–71.
18. Siak J, Chee SP. Cytomegalovirus anterior uveitis following topical cyclosporine a. Ocul Immunol Inflamm. 2018;26(1):90–3.
19. Babu K, Murthy GJ. Cytomegalovirus anterior uveitis in immunocompetent individuals following topical prostaglandin analogues. J Ophthalmic Inflamm Infect. 2013;3(1):55.
20. Hsiao YT, Kuo MT, Chiang WY, Chao TL, Kuo HK. Epidemiology and clinical features of viral anterior uveitis in southern Taiwan-diagnosis with polymerase chain reaction. BMC Ophthalmol. 2019;19(1):87.
21. Papasavvas I, Herbort CP Jr. Cytomegalovirus anterior uveitis from the perspective of the common practitioner: missed diagnosis can be at the origin of severe functional loss - a scenario to be avoided. Klin Monbl Augenheilkd. 2021;238(4):448–53.
22. Choi JA, Kim JE, Noh SJ, Kyoung Kim E, Park CK, Paik SY. Enhanced cytomegalovirus infection in human trabecular meshwork cells and its implication in glaucoma pathogenesis. Sci Rep. 2017;7:43349.
23. de Schryver I, Rozenberg F, Cassoux N, Michelson S, Kestelyn P, Lehoang P, Davis JL, Bodaghi B. Diagnosis and treatment of cytomegalovirus iridocyclitis without retinal necrosis. Br J Ophthalmol. 2006;90(7):852–5.
24. Nguyen M, Siak J, Chee SP, Diem VQH. The spectrum of uveitis in southern Vietnam. Ocul Immunol Inflamm. 2017a;25(sup1):S100–6.
25. Kongyai N, Sirirungsi W, Pathanapitoon K, Tananuvat N, Kunavisarut P, Leechanachai P, de Groot-Mijnes JD, Rothova A. Viral causes of unexplained anterior uveitis in Thailand. Eye (Lond). 2012a;26(4):529–34.
26. Park SW, Yu HG. Association of cytomegalovirus with idiopathic chronic anterior uveitis with ocular hypertension in Korean patients. Ocul Immunol Inflamm. 2013;21(3):192–6.
27. Anwar Z, Galor A, Albini TA, Miller D, Perez V, Davis JL. The diagnostic utility of anterior chamber paracentesis with polymerase chain reaction in anterior uveitis. Am J Ophthalmol. 2013;155(5):781–6.
28. Wong JX, Agrawal R, Wong EP, Teoh SC. Efficacy and safety of topical ganciclovir in the management of cytomegalovirus (CMV)-related anterior uveitis. J Ophthalmic Inflamm Infect. 2016;6(1):10.
29. Choi JA, Kim KS, Jung Y, Park HY, Park CK. Cytomegalovirus as a cause of hypertensive anterior uveitis in immunocompetent patients. J Ophthalmic Inflamm Infect. 2016;6(1):32.
30. Khieu C, Kongyai N, Pathanapitoon K, Van Der Eijk AA, Rothova A. Causes of hypertensive anterior uveitis in Thailand. Ocul Immunol Inflamm. 2020;28(4):559–65.

31. Martin Ramirez A, Cardenoso Domingo L, Gonzalez Guijarro JJ. PCR multiplex for CMV detection in patients with anterior uveitis. Ocul Immunol Inflamm. 2019;27(2):197–202.
32. Altan C, Basarir B. Aetiology and clinical characteristics of uveitic glaucoma in Turkish patients. Int Ophthalmol. 2021;41(6):2225–34.
33. Teoh SB, Thean L, Koay E. Cytomegalovirus in aetiology of Posner-Schlossman syndrome: evidence from quantitative polymerase chain reaction. Eye (Lond). 2005;19(12):1338–40.
34. van Boxtel LA, van der Lelij A, van der Meer J, Los LI. Cytomegalovirus as a cause of anterior uveitis in immunocompetent patients. Ophthalmology. 2007;114(7):1358–62.
35. Markomichelakis NN, Canakis C, Zafirakis P, Marakis T, Mallias I, Theodossiadis G. Cytomegalovirus as a cause of anterior uveitis with sectoral iris atrophy. Ophthalmology. 2002;109(5):879–82.
36. Yoshida A, Obata H, Kawashima H. Cytomegalovirus uveitis with Hypopyon mimicking bacterial Endophthalmitis. Case Rep Ophthalmol Med. 2015;2015:489813.
37. Babu K, Parameswarappa DC, Sudheer B. Tonic pupil in cytomegalovirus anterior uveitis in an immunocompetent adult male—a case report. Ocul Immunol Inflamm. 2018;26(1):104–6.
38. Leleu I, Jhanji V, Touhami S, Westcott M, Angi M, Titah C, Rousseau A, Hamard P, Brasnu E, Manicom T, et al. Clinical features and diagnosis of anterior segment inflammation related to cytomegalovirus in Immunocompetent African, Asian, and Caucasian patients. Ocul Immunol Inflamm. 2021;29(1):160–8.
39. Tanyildiz B, Kaymak NZ, Oklar M, Goktas E. Peripapillary retinal nerve fiber layer and ganglion cell-inner plexiform layer changes on optical coherence tomography in patients with unilateral hypertensive cytomegalovirus anterior uveitis. Photodiagnosis Photodyn Ther. 2021;33:102132.
40. Hwang YS, Shen CR, Chang SH, Lai CC, Liu CL, Chen KJ, Lin KK, Chen TL, Hsiao CH. The validity of clinical feature profiles for cytomegaloviral anterior segment infection. Graefes Arch Clin Exp Ophthalmol. 2011;249(1):103–10.
41. Sakai JI, Usui Y, Suzuki J, Kezuka T, Goto H. Clinical features of anterior uveitis caused by three different herpes viruses. Int Ophthalmol. 2019;39(12):2785–95.
42. Kam KW, Wong CH, Ho M, Sze RKH, Chan PKS, Young AL. Iris depigmentation in the prediction of cytomegalovirus anterior uveitis. Ocul Immunol Inflamm. 2022;30:1775–80.
43. Woo JH, Lim WK, Ho SL, Teoh SC. Characteristics of cytomegalovirus uveitis in immunocompetent patients. Ocul Immunol Inflamm. 2015;23(5):378–83.
44. Pohlmann D, Pahlitzsch M, Schlickeiser S, Metzner S, Lenglinger M, Bertelmann E, Maier AB, Winterhalter S, Pleyer U. Virus-associated anterior uveitis and secondary glaucoma: diagnostics, clinical characteristics, and surgical options. PLoS One. 2020;15(2):e0229260.
45. De Simone L, Belloni L, Aldigeri R, Zerbini A, Mastrofilippo V, Sangiovanni A, Parmeggiani M, Fontana L, Cimino L. Aqueous tap and rapid diagnosis of cytomegalovirus anterior uveitis: the Reggio Emilia experience. Graefes Arch Clin Exp Ophthalmol. 2019;257(1):181–6.
46. Miyazaki D, Shimizu D, Shimizu Y, Inoue Y, Inoue T, Higaki S, Ueta M, Sugita S. Real-time PCRfocisg: diagnostic efficacy of real-time PCR for ocular cytomegalovirus infections. Graefes Arch Clin Exp Ophthalmol. 2018;256(12):2413–20.
47. Touhami S, Qu L, Angi M, Bojanova M, Touitou V, Lehoang P, Rozenberg F, Bodaghi B. Cytomegalovirus anterior uveitis: clinical characteristics and long-term outcomes in a French series. Am J Ophthalmol. 2018a;194:134–42.
48. Kandori M, Miyazaki D, Yakura K, Komatsu N, Touge C, Ishikura R, Inoue Y. Relationship between the number of cytomegalovirus in anterior chamber and severity of anterior segment inflammation. Jpn J Ophthalmol. 2013;57(6):497–502.
49. Miyanaga M, Sugita S, Shimizu N, Morio T, Miyata K, Maruyama K, Kinoshita S, Mochizuki M. A significant association of viral loads with corneal endothelial cell damage in cytomegalovirus anterior uveitis. Br J Ophthalmol. 2010;94(3):336–40.
50. Xi L, Zhang L, Fei W. Cytomegalovirus-related uncontrolled glaucoma in an immunocompetent patient: a case report and systematic review. BMC Ophthalmol. 2018;18(1):259.

51. Bhoopat T, Takhar JS, Oldenburg CE, Keenan JD, Gonzales JA, Margolis TP. Treatment of cytomegalovirus anterior uveitis at a north American Tertiary Center with oral Valganciclovir. Cornea. 2020;39(5):584–9.
52. Tendolkar S, Murthy SI, Bhatia P, Senthil S. Cytomegalovirus endotheliitis with recurrent anterior uveitis and secondary glaucoma misdiagnosed as HLA-B27 uveitis. BMJ Case Rep. 2021;14(2):e240061.
53. Carmichael A. Cytomegalovirus and the eye. Eye (Lond). 2012;26(2):237–40.
54. Tsui E, Gonzales JA, Shantha JG, Acharya N, Doan T. Letermovir for the management of cytomegalovirus-associated uveitis. Ocul Immunol Inflamm. 2021a;29(1):169–74.
55. Hwang YS, Lin KK, Lee JS, Chang SH, Chen KJ, Lai CC, Huang JC, Kuo YH, Hsiao CH. Intravitreal loading injection of ganciclovir with or without adjunctive oral valganciclovir for cytomegalovirus anterior uveitis. Graefes Arch Clin Exp Ophthalmol. 2010;248(2):263–9.
56. Zandi S, Bodaghi B, Garweg JG. Review for disease of the year: treatment of viral anterior uveitis: a perspective. Ocul Immunol Inflamm. 2018;26(7):1135–42.
57. Delwig A, Keenan JD, Margolis TP. Topical Valganciclovir for the treatment of hypertensive anterior uveitis. Cornea. 2015;34(11):1513–5.
58. Chen PJ, Lin IH, Chi YC, Lai CC, Hung JH, Tseng SH, Huang YH. Long-term outcome of treatment with 2% topical Ganciclovir solution in cytomegalovirus anterior uveitis and corneal Endotheliitis. Infect Drug Resist. 2022;15:3395–403.
59. Takhar JS, Joye AS, Somkijrungroj T, Laovirojjanakul W, Lin CP, Lietman TM, Porco TC, Keenan JD, Gebreegziabher EA, Seitzman GD, et al. A double masked randomised 4-week, placebo-controlled study in the USA, Thailand and Taiwan to compare the efficacy of oral valganciclovir and topical 2% ganciclovir in the treatment of cytomegalovirus anterior uveitis: study protocol. BMJ Open. 2019;9(12):e033175.
60. Pahlitzsch M, Torun N, Gonnermann J, Maier AK, Pleyer U, Bertelmann E, Joussen A, Klamann MK. Trabeculectomy ab interno (trabectome): yet another possibility in the treatment of uncontrolled glaucomatocyclitic crisis under systemic valganciclovir therapy? Eye (Lond). 2015;29(10):1335–9.
61. Cunningham ET Jr. Diagnosing and treating herpetic anterior uveitis. Ophthalmology. 2000;107(12):2129–30.
62. Gaynor BD, Margolis TP, Cunningham ET Jr. Advances in diagnosis and management of herpetic uveitis. Int Ophthalmol Clin. 2000;40(2):85–109.
63. Tabbara KF, Chavis PS. Herpes simplex anterior uveitis. Int Ophthalmol Clin. 1998;38(4):137–47.
64. Liesegang TJ. Classification of herpes simplex virus keratitis and anterior uveitis. Cornea. 1999a;18(2):127–43.
65. The Herpetic Eye Disease Study Group. A controlled trial of oral acyclovir for iridocyclitis caused by herpes simplex virus. Arch Ophthalmol. 1996;114(9):1065–72.
66. The Herpetic Eye Disease Study Group. A controlled trial of oral acyclovir for the prevention of stromal keratitis or iritis in patients with herpes simplex virus epithelial keratitis. The epithelial keratitis trial. Arch Ophthalmol. 1997;115(6):703–12.
67. Liesegang TJ. Varicella-zoster virus eye disease. Cornea. 1999b;18(5):511–31.
68. Kianersi F, Taghdiri MH, Kianersi H, Bagi A, Naderi Beni A. Reactivation of varicella-zoster virus anterior uveitis after YAG peripheral Iridotomy. Ocul Immunol Inflamm. 2020;28(6):956–7.
69. Wensing B, Mochizuki M, De Boer JH. Clinical characteristics of herpes simplex virus associated anterior uveitis. Ocul Immunol Inflamm. 2018;26(3):333–7.
70. Van der Lelij A, Ooijman FM, Kijlstra A, Rothova A. Anterior uveitis with sectoral iris atrophy in the absence of keratitis: a distinct clinical entity among herpetic eye diseases. Ophthalmology. 2000;107(6):1164–70.
71. Tugal-Tutkun I, Otuk-Yasar B, Altinkurt E. Clinical features and prognosis of herpetic anterior uveitis: a retrospective study of 111 cases. Int Ophthalmol. 2010;30(5):559–65.

72. Falcon MG, Williams HP. Herpes simplex kerato-uveitis and glaucoma. Trans Ophthalmol Soc Aust. 1978;98(1):101–4.
73. Harding SP, Lipton JR, Wells JC. Natural history of herpes zoster ophthalmicus: predictors of postherpetic neuralgia and ocular involvement. Br J Ophthalmol. 1987;71(5):353–8.
74. Womack LW, Liesegang TJ. Complications of herpes zoster ophthalmicus. Arch Ophthalmol. 1983;101(1):42–5.
75. Buchi ER, Herbort CP, Ruffieux C. Oral acyclovir in the treatment of acute herpes zoster ophthalmicus. Am J Ophthalmol. 1986;102(4):531–2.
76. Siverio Junior CD, Imai Y, Cunningham ET Jr. Diagnosis and management of herpetic anterior uveitis. Int Ophthalmol Clin. 2002;42(1):43–8.
77. Kazokoglu H, Onal S, Tugal-Tutkun I, Mirza E, Akova Y, Ozyazgan Y, Soylu M, Batioglu F, Apaydin C. Demographic and clinical features of uveitis in tertiary centers in Turkey. Ophthalmic Epidemiol. 2008;15(5):285–93.
78. Keorochana N. Pattern and outcome of uveitis in a Tertiary Military Hospital in Thailand. Ocul Immunol Inflamm. 2020;28(3):424–32.
79. Nalcacioglu-Yuksekkaya P, Ozdal PC, Teke MY, Kara C, Ozturk F. Presumed herpetic anterior uveitis: a study with retrospective analysis of 79 cases. Eur J Ophthalmol. 2014;24(1):14–20.
80. Thygeson P, Hogan MJ, Kimura SJ. Observations on uveitis associated with viral disease. Trans Am Ophthalmol Soc. 1957;55:333–49; discussion 349–352.
81. Kimura SJ. Herpes simplex uveitis: a clinical and experimental study. Trans Am Ophthalmol Soc. 1962;60:440–70.
82. Miserocchi E, Fogliato G, Bianchi I, Bandello F, Modorati G. Clinical features of ocular herpetic infection in an italian referral center. Cornea. 2014;33(6):565–70.
83. Schwab IR. Herpes zoster sine herpete. A potential cause of iridoplegic granulomatous iridocyclitis. Ophthalmology. 1997;104(9):1421–5.
84. Gueudry J, Muraine M. Anterior uveitis. J Fr Ophtalmol. 2018;41(1):e11–21.
85. Hoeksema L, Jansonius NM, Los LI. Risk factors for secondary glaucoma in herpetic anterior uveitis. Am J Ophthalmol. 2017;181:55–60.
86. Ozer MD, Batur M, Seven E, Tekin S, Kebapci F. In vivo analysis and comparison of anterior segment structures of both eyes in unilateral herpetic anterior uveitis. Ocul Immunol Inflamm. 2020a;29:1438–44.
87. Knoll AB, Postole AS, Auffarth GU, Mackensen F. Frequency of dendritiform inflammatory cells in the cornea in herpetic anterior uveitis without clinical keratitis and Fuchs uveitis. J Ophthalmic Inflamm Infect. 2014;4:31.
88. Invernizzi A, Mameli C, Giacomet V, Chiari P, Zuccotti GV. Herpetic acute anterior uveitis complicated by retinal vasculitis in an immunocompetent child. Can J Ophthalmol. 2013;48(6):e171–2.
89. Qian Z, Fan H, Tao Y, Li W, Gu W. Herpetic anterior uveitis in a Chinese referral Center: clinical manifestations and laboratory test results. Ocul Immunol Inflamm. 2020;28(5):758–63.
90. Lenglinger M, Pohlmann D, Pleyer U. Anterior viral uveitis: clinical aspects, diagnostic procedure and treatment options. Ophthalmologe. 2020;117(1):83–92.
91. Korra AE, Mourad AS. el-Sahn ME: isolation of herpes simplex virus from the aqueous humour in herpetic kerato-iritis. Bull Ophthalmol Soc Egypt. 1976;69(73):89–93.
92. Bock J, Fanta D, Soltz-Szots J, Zehetbauer G, Gebhart W. Isolation of herpes simplex virus from the aqueous humour of an eye affected by relapsing iridocyclitis. Albrecht Von Graefes Arch Klin Exp Ophthalmol. 1972;185(4):349–53.
93. Kieselbach G, Romani N, Gottinger W, Miller K. Electron microscopy diagnosis of intraocular herpes infection with a case demonstration. Klin Monbl Augenheilkd. 1986;188(1):55–6.
94. Schacher S, Garweg JG, Russ C, Bohnke M. Diagnosis of herpetic uveitis and keratouveitis. Klin Monbl Augenheilkd. 1998;212(5):359–62.

95. Yamamoto S, Tada R, Shimomura Y, Pavan-Langston D, Dunkel EC, Tano Y. Detecting varicella-zoster virus DNA in iridocyclitis using polymerase chain reaction: a case of zoster sine herpete. Arch Ophthalmol. 1995;113(11):1358–9.
96. Yamamoto S, Pavan-Langston D, Kinoshita S, Nishida K, Shimomura Y, Tano Y. Detecting herpesvirus DNA in uveitis using the polymerase chain reaction. Br J Ophthalmol. 1996;80(5):465–8.
97. Uchoa UB, Rezende RA, Carrasco MA, Rapuano CJ, Laibson PR, Cohen EJ. Long-term acyclovir use to prevent recurrent ocular herpes simplex virus infection. Arch Ophthalmol. 2003;121(12):1702–4.
98. Sudesh S, Laibson PR. The impact of the herpetic eye disease studies on the management of herpes simplex virus ocular infections. Curr Opin Ophthalmol. 1999;10(4):230–3.
99. Young RC, Hodge DO, Liesegang TJ, Baratz KH. Incidence, recurrence, and outcomes of herpes simplex virus eye disease in Olmsted County, Minnesota, 1976–2007: the effect of oral antiviral prophylaxis. Arch Ophthalmol. 2010;128(9):1178–83.
100. Wilhelmus KR, Falcon MG, Jones BR. Herpetic iridocyclitis. Int Ophthalmol. 1982;4(3):143–50.
101. Krwawicz T. The use of low temperature in the treatment of iridocyclitis and of herpetic infections of the cornea. Trans Ophthalmol Soc Aust. 1969;88:137–52.
102. Gierczynska A. Low temperature used in treatment of uveitis (author's transl). Klin Oczna. 1979;81(4):275.
103. Bate SL, Dollard SC, Cannon MJ. Cytomegalovirus seroprevalence in the United States: the national health and nutrition examination surveys, 1988–2004. Clin Infect Dis. 2010;50(11):1439–47.
104. Cannon MJ, Schmid DS, Hyde TB. Review of cytomegalovirus seroprevalence and demographic characteristics associated with infection. Rev Med Virol. 2010;20(4):202–13.
105. Korndewal MJ, Mollema L, Tcherniaeva I, van der Klis F, Kroes AC, Oudesluys-Murphy AM, Vossen AC, de Melker HE. Cytomegalovirus infection in the Netherlands: seroprevalence, risk factors, and implications. J Clin Virol. 2015;63:53–8.
106. Staras SA, Dollard SC, Radford KW, Flanders WD, Pass RF, Cannon MJ. Seroprevalence of cytomegalovirus infection in the United States, 1988-1994. Clin Infect Dis. 2006;43(9):1143–51.
107. Jin Q, Su J, Wu S. Cytomegalovirus infection among pregnant women in Beijing: seroepidemiological survey and intrauterine transmissions. J Microbiol Biotechnol. 2017;27(5):1005–9.
108. Sun HY, Peng XY, Li D, Mao FF, You QS, Jonas JB. Cytomegalovirus retinitis in patients with AIDS before and after introduction of HAART in China. Eur J Ophthalmol. 2014a;24(2):209–15.
109. Shi Y, Lu H, He T, Yang Y, Liu L, Zhang R, Zheng Y, Shen Y, Zhang Y, Zhang Z. Prevalence and clinical management of cytomegalovirus retinitis in AIDS patients in Shanghai, China. BMC Infect Dis. 2011;11:326.
110. Port AD, Orlin A, Kiss S, Patel S, D'Amico DJ, Gupta MP. Cytomegalovirus retinitis: a review. J Ocul Pharmacol Ther. 2017;33(4):224–34.
111. Zhang C, Wang YE, Miao H, Hou J. Efficacy and safety of aqueous Interleukin-8-guided treatment in cytomegalovirus retinitis after bone marrow hematopoietic stem cell transplantation. Ocul Immunol Inflamm. 2022;30:758–65.
112. Cugley DR, Darby J, Lim LL. Tofacitinib-associated cytomegalovirus retinitis. Rheumatology (Oxford). 2020;59(9):e35–7.
113. Deliege PG, Bastien J, Mokri L, Guyot-Colosio C, Arndt C, Rieu P. Belatacept associated—cytomegalovirus retinitis in a kidney transplant recipient: a case report and review of the literature. BMC Ophthalmol. 2020;20(1):468.
114. Reddy S, Tyagi M, Behera S, Pappuru RR. Cytomegalovirus retinitis in a patient of granulomatosis with polyangiitis on long-term immunosuppressants. BMJ Case Rep. 2021;14(2):e236632.

115. Khochtali S, Mahjoub A, Dridi T, Ksiaa I, Abroug N, Khairallah M. Cytomegalovirus retinitis following corticosteroid overdose for Vogt-Koyanagi-Harada disease. Indian J Ophthalmol. 2020;68(9):2012–4.
116. Witmer MT, Connolly BP. Cytomegalovirus retinitis after an intravitreal dexamethasone implant in an immunocompetent patient. Retin Cases Brief Rep. 2021;15(6):670–2.
117. Vannozzi L, Bacherini D, Sodi A, Beccastrini E, Emmi G, Giorni A, Menchini U. Cytomegalovirus retinitis following intravitreal dexamethasone implant in a patient with central retinal vein occlusion. Acta Ophthalmol. 2016;94(2):e158–60.
118. Dogra M, Rohilla V, Dogra M, Singh R. Macular cytomegalovirus retinitis following dexamethasone intravitreal implant combined with phacoemulsification. Indian J Ophthalmol. 2018a;66(9):1361–3.
119. Delyfer MN, Rougier MB, Hubschman JP, Aouizerate F, Korobelnik JF. Cytomegalovirus retinitis following intravitreal injection of triamcinolone: report of two cases. Acta Ophthalmol Scand. 2007;85(6):681–3.
120. Tetsuju S, Iida T, Kaneko H, Saito M. Cytomegalovirus retinitis after intravitreal triamcinolone acetonide in an immunocompetent patient. Jpn J Ophthalmol. 2008;52(5):414–6.
121. Jabs DA, Green WR, Fox R, Polk BF, Bartlett JG. Ocular manifestations of acquired immune deficiency syndrome. Ophthalmology. 1989;96(7):1092–9.
122. Palestine AG, Rodrigues MM, Macher AM, Chan CC, Lane HC, Fauci AS, Masur H, Longo D, Reichert CM, Steis R, et al. Ophthalmic involvement in acquired immunodeficiency syndrome. Ophthalmology. 1984;91(9):1092–9.
123. Jabs DA. Ocular manifestations of HIV infection. Trans Am Ophthalmol Soc. 1995;93:623–83.
124. Teoh SC, Wang PX, Wong EP. The epidemiology and incidence of cytomegalovirus retinitis in the HIV population in Singapore over 6 years. Invest Ophthalmol Vis Sci. 2012;53(12):7546–52.
125. Schwarcz L, Chen MJ, Vittinghoff E, Hsu L, Schwarcz S. Declining incidence of AIDS-defining opportunistic illnesses: results from 16 years of population-based AIDS surveillance. AIDS. 2013;27(4):597–605.
126. Pollard RB, Egbert PR, Gallagher JG, Merigan TC. Cytomegalovirus retinitis in immunosuppressed hosts. I. Natural history and effects of treatment with adenine arabinoside. Ann Intern Med. 1980;93(5):655–64.
127. Wren SM, Fielder AR, Bethell D, Lyall EG, Tudor-Williams G, Cocker KD, Mitchell SM. Cytomegalovirus retinitis in infancy. Eye (Lond). 2004;18(4):389–92.
128. Sadik MT, Aksu Ceylan N, Cebeci Z, Kir N, Oray M, Tugal-Tutkun I. Patterns of cytomegalovirus retinitis at a tertiary referral center in Turkey. Int Ophthalmol. 2021;41(9):2981–92.
129. Iu LP, Fan MC, Lau JK, Chan TS, Kwong YL, Wong IY. Long-term follow-up of cytomegalovirus retinitis in non-HIV immunocompromised patients: clinical features and visual prognosis. Am J Ophthalmol. 2016;165:145–53.
130. Shapira Y, Mimouni M, Vishnevskia-Dai V. Cytomegalovirus retinitis in HIV-negative patients—associated conditions, clinical presentation, diagnostic methods and treatment strategy. Acta Ophthalmol. 2018;96(7):e761–7.
131. Kingkosol P, Pooprasert P, Choopong P, Hunchangsith B, Laksanaphuk V, Tantibundhit C. Automated cytomegalovirus retinitis screening in fundus images. Annu Int Conf IEEE Eng Med Biol Soc. 2020;2020:1996–2002.
132. Standardization of Uveitis Nomenclature Working Group. Classification criteria for Cytomegalovirus retinitis. Am J Ophthalmol. 2021b;228:245–54.
133. Pathanapitoon K, Ausayakhun S, Kunavisarut P, Pungrasame A, Sirirungsi W. Detection of cytomegalovirus in vitreous, aqueous and conjunctiva by polymerase chain reaction (PCR). J Med Assoc Thai. 2005;88(2):228–32.
134. Vishnevskia-Dai V, Shapira Y, Rahav G, Shimoni A, Somech R, Moisseiev J. Cytomegalovirus retinitis in HIV-negative patients: a practical management approach. Ophthalmology. 2015;122(4):866–868 e863.

135. Kijlstra A, van den Horn GJ, Luyendijk L, Baarsma GS, Schweitzer CM, Zaal MJ, Timmerman Z, Beintema M, Rothova A. Laboratory tests in uveitis. New developments in the analysis of local antibody production. Doc Ophthalmol. 1990a;75(3-4):225–31.
136. Abe T, Tsuchida K, Tamai M. A comparative study of the polymerase chain reaction and local antibody production in acute retinal necrosis syndrome and cytomegalovirus retinitis. Graefes Arch Clin Exp Ophthalmol. 1996a;234(7):419–24.
137. Doornenbal P, Seerp Baarsma G, Quint WG, Kijlstra A, Rothbarth PH, Niesters HG. Diagnostic assays in cytomegalovirus retinitis: detection of herpesvirus by simultaneous application of the polymerase chain reaction and local antibody analysis on ocular fluid. Br J Ophthalmol. 1996;80(3):235–40.
138. Iyer JV, Agrawal R, Yeo TK, Gunasekeran DV, Balne PK, Lee B, Au VB, Connolly J, Teoh SC. Aqueous humor immune factors and cytomegalovirus (CMV) levels in CMV retinitis through treatment—the CRIGSS study. Cytokine. 2016;84:56–62.
139. Wang B, Tian B, Tao Y, Hou J, Zhao XT, Li XX. Continued decline of aqueous interleukin-8 after multiple intravitreal injections of ganciclovir for cytomegalovirus retinitis. J Ocul Pharmacol Ther. 2014a;30(7):587–92.
140. Qian Z, Fan H, Chen X, Tao Y. The predictive value of interleukin-8 in the development of cytomegalovirus retinitis in HIV-negative patients. Ophthalmic Res. 2022a;65:287–92.
141. Zhou Y, Hong F, Wang X, Feng J, Zhu D, Xu Y, Tao Y. Abnormal levels of aqueous humor trace elements in patients with cytomegalovirus retinitis. Eye (Lond). 2019;33(10):1606–12.
142. Munro M, Yadavalli T, Fonteh C, Arfeen S, Lobo-Chan AM. Cytomegalovirus retinitis in HIV and non-HIV individuals. Microorganisms. 2019;8(1):55.
143. Kaplan JE, Benson C, Holmes KK, Brooks JT, Pau A, Masur H, Centers for Disease C, Prevention, National Institutes of H, America HIVMAotIDSo. Guidelines for prevention and treatment of opportunistic infections in HIV-infected adults and adolescents: recommendations from CDC, the National Institutes of Health, and the HIV Medicine Association of the Infectious Diseases Society of America. MMWR Recomm Rep. 2009;58(RR-4):1–207; quiz CE201-204.
144. Jabs DA, Bolton SG, Dunn JP, Palestine AG. Discontinuing anticytomegalovirus therapy in patients with immune reconstitution after combination antiretroviral therapy. Am J Ophthalmol. 1998;126(6):817–22.
145. Macdonald JC, Karavellas MP, Torriani FJ, Morse LS, Smith IL, Reed JB, Freeman WR. Highly active antiretroviral therapy-related immune recovery in AIDS patients with cytomegalovirus retinitis. Ophthalmology. 2000;107(5):877–81; discussion 881-873.
146. Jabs DA, Ahuja A, Van Natta ML, Lyon AT, Yeh S, Danis R, Studies of the Ocular Complications of ARG. Long-term outcomes of cytomegalovirus retinitis in the era of modern antiretroviral therapy: results from a United States Cohort. Ophthalmology. 2015;122(7):1452–63.
147. Song WK, Min YH, Kim YR, Lee SC. Cytomegalovirus retinitis after hematopoietic stem cell transplantation with alemtuzumab. Ophthalmology. 2008;115(10):1766–70.
148. Miao H, Tao Y, Jiang YR, Li XX. Multiple intravitreal injections of ganciclovir for cytomegalovirus retinitis after stem-cell transplantation. Graefes Arch Clin Exp Ophthalmol. 2013;251(7):1829–33.
149. Singh R, Singh R, Trehan A, Jain R, Bhalekar S. Cytomegalovirus retinitis in an ALL child on exclusive chemotherapy treated successfully with intravitreal ganciclovir alone. J Pediatr Hematol Oncol. 2013;35(3):e118–9.
150. Yutthitham K, Ruamviboonsuk P. The high-dose, alternate-week intravitreal ganciclovir injections for cytomegalovirus retinitis in acquired immune deficiency syndrome patients on highly active antiretroviral therapy. J Med Assoc Thai. 2005;88(Suppl 9):S63–8.
151. Hodge WG, Lalonde RG, Sampalis J, Deschenes J. Once-weekly intraocular injections of ganciclovir for maintenance therapy of cytomegalovirus retinitis: clinical and ocular outcome. J Infect Dis. 1996;174(2):393–6.

152. Arevalo JF, Garcia RA, Mendoza AJ. High-dose (5000-microg) intravitreal ganciclovir combined with highly active antiretroviral therapy for cytomegalovirus retinitis in HIV-infected patients in Venezuela. Eur J Ophthalmol. 2005;15(5):610–8.
153. Young SH, Morlet N, Heery S, Hollows FC, Coroneo MT. High dose intravitreal ganciclovir in the treatment of cytomegalovirus retinitis. Med J Aust. 1992;157(6):370–3.
154. Cochereau-Massin I, Lehoang P, Lautier-Frau M, Zazoun L, Marcel P, Robinet M, Matheron S, Katlama C, Gharakhanian S, Rozenbaum W, et al. Efficacy and tolerance of intravitreal ganciclovir in cytomegalovirus retinitis in acquired immune deficiency syndrome. Ophthalmology. 1991;98(9):1348–53, discussion 1353-1345.
155. Fan JJ, Tao Y, Hwang DK. Comparison of intravitreal ganciclovir monotherapy and combination with foscarnet as initial therapy for cytomegalovirus retinitis. Int J Ophthalmol. 2018;11(10):1638–42.
156. Chen WB, Long Z, Hou J, Miao H, Zhao MW. Continuous high-dose (6 mg) vs. low-dose (3 mg) intravitreal Ganciclovir for cytomegalovirus retinitis after haploidentical hematopoietic stem cell transplantation: a randomized controlled study. Front Med (Lausanne). 2021a;8:750760.
157. Jeon S, Lee WK. Cytomegalovirus retinitis in a human immunodeficiency virus-negative cohort: long-term management and complications. Ocul Immunol Inflamm. 2015;23(5):392–9.
158. Qian Z, Chen X, Tao Y, Li W, Gu W. Prognostic factors of cytomegalovirus infection associated retinitis in HIV-negative patients: a retrospective cohort study. Ocul Immunol Inflamm. 2021;29(1):154–9.
159. Tajunisah I, Reddy SC, Tan LH. Acute retinal necrosis by cytomegalovirus in an immunocompetent adult: case report and review of the literature. Int Ophthalmol. 2009;29(2):85–90.
160. Culbertson WW, Blumenkranz MS, Haines H, Gass DM, Mitchell KB, Norton EW. The acute retinal necrosis syndrome. Part 2: Histopathology and etiology. Ophthalmology. 1982;89(12):1317–25.
161. Culbertson WW, Blumenkranz MS, Pepose JS, Stewart JA, Curtin VT. Varicella zoster virus is a cause of the acute retinal necrosis syndrome. Ophthalmology. 1986;93(5):559–69.
162. Matsuo T, Nakayama T, Koyama T, Matsuo N. Cytological and immunological study of the aqueous humor in acute retinal necrosis syndrome. Ophthalmologica. 1987;195(1):38–44.
163. Lewis ML, Culbertson WW, Post JD, Miller D, Kokame GT, Dix RD. Herpes simplex virus type 1. A cause of the acute retinal necrosis syndrome. Ophthalmology. 1989;96(6):875–8.
164. Nishi M, Hanashiro R, Mori S, Masuda K, Mochizuki M, Hondo R. Polymerase chain reaction for the detection of the varicella-zoster genome in ocular samples from patients with acute retinal necrosis. Am J Ophthalmol. 1992;114(5):603–9.
165. de Boer JH, Luyendijk L, Rothova A, Baarsma GS, de Jong PT, Bollemeijer JG, Rademakers AJ, Van der Lelij A, Zaal MJ, Kijlstra A. Detection of intraocular antibody production to herpesviruses in acute retinal necrosis syndrome. Am J Ophthalmol. 1994;117(2):201–10.
166. Chan EW, Sun V, Eldeeb M, Kapusta MA. Epstein-Barr virus acute retinal necrosis in an immunocompetent host. Retin Cases Brief Rep. 2021;15(4):412–6.
167. Zhang ZY, Liu XY, Jiang T. Acute retinal necrosis following dexamethasone intravitreal implant (Ozurdex(R)) administration in an immunocompetent adult with a history of HSV encephalitis: a case report. BMC Ophthalmol. 2020;20(1):247.
168. Cheraqpour K, Ahmadraji A, Rashidinia A, Irannejad M, Shahriari M. Acute retinal necrosis caused by co-infection with multiple viruses in a natalizumab-treated patient: a case report and brief review of literature. BMC Ophthalmol. 2021;21(1):337.
169. van Kempen ZLE, van Rossum JA, Hoogervorst E, Strijbis E, Toorop A, Bosscha MI, Frequin S, Dam-van Loon NT, Wattjes MP, Murk JL, et al. Varicella zoster-associated acute retinal necrosis and central nervous system complications in natalizumab treated MS patients. Mult Scler Relat Disord. 2021;50:102838.
170. Menghini M, Raja V, Raiter J, Balaratnasingam C, Constable IJ. Acute retinal necrosis associated with Herpes Zoster vaccination. Retin Cases Brief Rep. 2021;15(2):166–8.

171. Mairot K, Ramtohul P, Gascon P, Beylerian M, Denis D. Bilateral acute retinal necrosis with encephalitis in a premature infant. Eur J Ophthalmol. 2022;32(1):NP185–6.
172. Shahi SK. Acute retinal necrosis results in low vision in a young patient with a history of herpes simplex virus encephalitis. Clin Exp Optom. 2017;100(3):208–13.
173. Okafor K, Lu J, Thinda S, Schwab I, Morse LS, Park SS, Moshiri A. Acute retinal necrosis presenting in developmentally-delayed patients with neonatal encephalitis: a case series and literature review. Ocul Immunol Inflamm. 2017;25(4):563–8.
174. Tran TH, Stanescu D, Caspers-Velu L, Rozenberg F, Liesnard C, Gaudric A, Lehoang P, Bodaghi B. Clinical characteristics of acute HSV-2 retinal necrosis. Am J Ophthalmol. 2004;137(5):872–9.
175. Muthiah MN, Michaelides M, Child CS, Mitchell SM. Acute retinal necrosis: a national population-based study to assess the incidence, methods of diagnosis, treatment strategies and outcomes in the UK. Br J Ophthalmol. 2007;91(11):1452–5.
176. Cochrane TF, Silvestri G, McDowell C, Foot B, McAvoy CE. Acute retinal necrosis in the United Kingdom: results of a prospective surveillance study. Eye (Lond). 2012;26(3):370–7; quiz 378.
177. Todokoro D, Kamei S, Goto H, Ikeda Y, Koyama H, Akiyama H. Acute retinal necrosis following herpes simplex encephalitis: a nationwide survey in Japan. Jpn J Ophthalmol. 2019;63(4):304–9.
178. Costa de Andrade G, Marchesi Mello LG, Martines GC, Maia A. Optical coherence tomography angiography findings in acute retinal necrosis. Retin Cases Brief Rep. 2021;15(3):256–60.
179. Fisher JP, Lewis ML, Blumenkranz M, Culbertson WW, Flynn HW Jr, Clarkson JG, Gass JD, Norton EW. The acute retinal necrosis syndrome. Part 1: Clinical manifestations. Ophthalmology. 1982;89(12):1309–16.
180. Okunuki Y, Usui Y, Kezuka T, Takeuchi M, Goto H. Four cases of bilateral acute retinal necrosis with a long interval after the initial onset. Br J Ophthalmol. 2011;95(9):1251–4.
181. Lei B, Jiang R, Wang Z, Xu G, Wu X, Zhou M. Bilateral acute retinal necrosis: a case series. Retina. 2020;40(1):145–53.
182. Witmer MT, Pavan PR, Fouraker BD, Levy-Clarke GA. Acute retinal necrosis associated optic neuropathy. Acta Ophthalmol. 2011;89(7):599–607.
183. Zhao XY, Meng LH, Zhang WF, Wang DY, Chen YX. Retinal detachment after acute retinal necrosis and the efficacies of different interventions: a systematic review and metaanalysis. Retina. 2021;41(5):965–78.
184. Perhiar BA, Siddiqui MR, Ibrahim S. Acute retinal necrosis with exudative retinal detachment in a child. BMJ Case Rep. 2021;14(12):e245984.
185. Holland GN. Standard diagnostic criteria for the acute retinal necrosis syndrome. Executive Committee of the American Uveitis Society. Am J Ophthalmol. 1994a;117(5):663–7.
186. Takase H, Okada AA, Goto H, Mizuki N, Namba K, Ohguro N, Sonoda KH, Tomita M, Keino H, Kezuka T, et al. Development and validation of new diagnostic criteria for acute retinal necrosis. Jpn J Ophthalmol. 2015;59(1):14–20.
187. Schoenberger SD, Kim SJ, Thorne JE, Mruthyunjaya P, Yeh S, Bakri SJ, Ehlers JP. Diagnosis and treatment of acute retinal necrosis: a report by the American Academy of Ophthalmology. Ophthalmology. 2017;124(3):382–92.
188. Standardization of Uveitis Nomenclature Working Group. Classification criteria for acute retinal necrosis syndrome. Am J Ophthalmol. 2021c;228:237–44.
189. Itoh N, Matsumura N, Ogi A, Nishide T, Imai Y, Kanai H, Ohno S. High prevalence of herpes simplex virus type 2 in acute retinal necrosis syndrome associated with herpes simplex virus in Japan. Am J Ophthalmol. 2000;129(3):404–5.
190. Lau CH, Missotten T, Salzmann J, Lightman SL. Acute retinal necrosis features, management, and outcomes. Ophthalmology. 2007;114(4):756–62.
191. Sugita S, Shimizu N, Watanabe K, Mizukami M, Morio T, Sugamoto Y, Mochizuki M. Use of multiplex PCR and real-time PCR to detect human herpes virus genome in ocular fluids of patients with uveitis. Br J Ophthalmol. 2008;92(7):928–32.

192. Hillenkamp J, Nolle B, Bruns C, Rautenberg P, Fickenscher H, Roider J. Acute retinal necrosis: clinical features, early vitrectomy, and outcomes. Ophthalmology. 2009;116(10):1971–1975e1972.
193. Wong R, Pavesio CE, Laidlaw DA, Williamson TH, Graham EM, Stanford MR. Acute retinal necrosis: the effects of intravitreal foscarnet and virus type on outcome. Ophthalmology. 2010;117(3):556–60.
194. Zhao C, Yi J, Dong F, Dai R, Min H, Zheng L, Chen Y, Ye J, Zhao Y, Wang N, et al. Intraocular detection of Herpes viruses by xTAG Liquid Chip Technology in patients with acute retinal necrosis. Ocul Immunol Inflamm. 2018;26(8):1271–7.
195. Hedayatfar A, Ebrahimiadib N, Zarei M, Ashraf Khorasani M, Mahbod M, Asgari S, Sedaghat A. Acute retinal necrosis: clinical manifestation and long-term visual outcomes in a series of polymerase chain reaction-positive patients. Eur J Ophthalmol. 2021;31(4):1961–9.
196. Botsford BW, Nguyen VQ, Eller AW. Acute retinal necrosis: difference in outcome by viral type and options for antiviral therapy. Retina. 2021;41(7):1547–52.
197. Bernheim D, Germi R, Labetoulle M, Romanet JP, Morand P, Chiquet C. Time profile of viral DNA in aqueous humor samples of patients treated for varicella-zoster virus acute retinal necrosis by use of quantitative real-time PCR. J Clin Microbiol. 2013;51(7):2160–6.
198. Calvo CM, Khan MA, Mehta S, Garg SJ, Dunn JP. Correlation of clinical outcomes with quantitative polymerase chain reaction DNA copy number in patients with acute retinal necrosis. Ocul Immunol Inflamm. 2017;25(2):246–52.
199. Kang H, Wei Y, Liu M, Yu D, Tao Y. Flow cytometric analysis of T lymphocytes and cytokines in aqueous humor of patients with varicella zoster virus-mediated acute retinal necrosis. BMC Ophthalmol. 2021;21(1):193.
200. de Visser L, de Boer J, Rijkers G, Wiertz K, van den Ham HJ, de Boer R, van Loon A, Rothova A, de Groot-Mijnes JD. Cytokines and chemokines involved in acute retinal necrosis. Invest Ophthalmol Vis Sci. 2017;58(4):2139–51.
201. Sato M, Abe T, Tamai M. Expression of the Varicella Zoster virus thymidine kinase and cytokines in patients with acute retinal necrosis syndrome. Jpn J Ophthalmol. 2000;44(6):693.
202. Blumenkranz MS, Culbertson WW, Clarkson JG, Dix R. Treatment of the acute retinal necrosis syndrome with intravenous acyclovir. Ophthalmology. 1986;93(3):296–300.
203. Shantha JG, Weissman HM, Debiec MR, Albini TA, Yeh S. Advances in the management of acute retinal necrosis. Int Ophthalmol Clin. 2015;55(3):1–13.
204. Palay DA, Sternberg P Jr, Davis J, Lewis H, Holland GN, Mieler WF, Jabs DA, Drews C. Decrease in the risk of bilateral acute retinal necrosis by acyclovir therapy. Am J Ophthalmol. 1991;112(3):250–5.
205. Kawaguchi T, Spencer DB, Mochizuki M. Therapy for acute retinal necrosis. Semin Ophthalmol. 2008;23(4):285–90.
206. Fletcher C, Bean B. Evaluation of oral acyclovir therapy. Drug Intell Clin Pharm. 1985;19(7-8):518–24.
207. Wang LH, Schultz M, Weller S, Smiley ML, Blum MR. Pharmacokinetics and safety of multiple-dose valaciclovir in geriatric volunteers with and without concomitant diuretic therapy. Antimicrob Agents Chemother. 1996;40(1):80–5.
208. !!! INVALID CITATION !!!. p. 52–54.
209. Flaxel CJ, Yeh S, Lauer AK. Combination systemic and intravitreal antiviral therapy in the management of acute retinal necrosis syndrome (an American Ophthalmological Society thesis). Trans Am Ophthalmol Soc. 2013;111:133–44.
210. Lee MY, Kim KS, Lee WK. Intravitreal foscarnet for the treatment of acyclovir-resistant acute retinal necrosis caused by varicella zoster virus. Ocul Immunol Inflamm. 2011;19(3):212–3.
211. Roy R, Pal BP, Mathur G, Rao C, Das D, Biswas J. Acute retinal necrosis: clinical features, management and outcomes—a 10 year consecutive case series. Ocul Immunol Inflamm. 2014;22(3):170–4.

212. Hafidi M, Janin-Manificat H, Denis P, Charleux B, Rabilloud M, Boibieux A, Burillon C, Kodjikian L, Frobert E. Acute retinal necrosis: virological features using quantitative polymerase chain reaction, therapeutic management, and clinical outcomes. Am J Ophthalmol. 2019;208:376–86.
213. Ando F, Kato M, Goto S, Kobayashi K, Ichikawa H, Kamiya T. Platelet function in bilateral acute retinal necrosis. Am J Ophthalmol. 1983;96(1):27–32.
214. Austin RB. Progressive outer retinal necrosis syndrome: a comprehensive review of its clinical presentation, relationship to immune system status, and management. Clin Eye Vis Care. 2000;12(3-4):119–29.
215. Forster DJ, Dugel PU, Frangieh GT, Liggett PE, Rao NA. Rapidly progressive outer retinal necrosis in the acquired immunodeficiency syndrome. Am J Ophthalmol. 1990;110(4):341–8.
216. Gunturu M, Gosi SK, Kanduri S, Garla V. Varicella Zoster meningitis, optic neuritis preceding the development of posterior outer retinal necrosis, and central retinal artery occlusion in a HIV patient. Case Rep Med. 2019;2019:4213162.
217. Holland GN. The progressive outer retinal necrosis syndrome. Int Ophthalmol. 1994b;18(3):163–5.
218. Engstrom RE Jr, Holland GN, Margolis TP, Muccioli C, Lindley JI, Belfort R Jr, Holland SP, Johnston WH, Wolitz RA, Kreiger AE. The progressive outer retinal necrosis syndrome. A variant of necrotizing herpetic retinopathy in patients with AIDS. Ophthalmology. 1994;101(9):1488–502.
219. Sfeir M. Cytomegalovirus implicated in a case of progressive outer retinal necrosis (PORN). J Clin Virol. 2015;69:86–90.
220. Biswas J, Choudhry S, Priya K, Gopal L. Detection of cytomegalovirus from vitreous humor in a patient with progressive outer retinal necrosis. Indian J Ophthalmol. 2002;50(4):319–21.
221. Park KH, Bang JH, Park WB, Kim HB, Kim NJ, Ahn JK, Chang KH, Oh MD, Choe KW. Retrobulbar optic neuritis and meningoencephalitis following progressive outer retinal necrosis due to CMV in a patient with AIDS. Infection. 2008;36(5):475–9.
222. Greven CM, Ford J, Stanton C, Shogreen M, Feldman S, Pegram S, Slusher MM. Progressive outer retinal necrosis secondary to varicella zoster virus in acquired immune deficiency syndrome. Retina. 1995;15(1):14–20.
223. Turno-Krecicka A, Tomczyk-Socha M, Zimny A. Progressive outer retinal necrosis syndrome in the course of systemic lupus erythematosus. Lupus. 2016;25(14):1610–4.
224. Feinman MC, Friedberg MA, Schwartz JC, Pilkerton AR, Perman KI, Barth WF, Bunning RD. Central nervous system herpesvirus infection in systemic lupus erythematosus: diagnosis by endoretinal biopsy. J Rheumatol. 1993;20(6):1058–61.
225. Dogra M, Bajgai P, Kumar A, Sharma A. Progressive outer retinal necrosis after rituximab and cyclophosphamide therapy. Indian J Ophthalmol. 2018b;66(4):591–3.
226. Sachan A, Lata S. Unforeseen progressive outer retinal necrosis in a child following bone marrow transplant. BMJ Case Rep. 2021;14(1):e238697.
227. Lewis JM, Nagae Y, Tano Y. Progressive outer retinal necrosis after bone marrow transplantation. Am J Ophthalmol. 1996;122(6):892–5.
228. Van Tassel SH, Gupta MP, Orlin A, Nealon NM, Patel SS. Progressive outer retinal necrosis in a multiple sclerosis patient on natalizumab. Neurology. 2015;84(21):2198–9.
229. Parekh P, Oldfield EC, Marik PE. Progressive outer retinal necrosis: a missed diagnosis and a blind, young woman. BMJ Case Rep. 2013;2013:bcr2013009333.
230. Lo PF, Lim R, Antonakis SN, Almeida GC. Progressive outer retinal necrosis: manifestation of human immunodeficiency virus infection. BMJ Case Rep. 2015;2015:bcr2014207344.
231. Narayanan R, Kuppermann BD. Optical coherence tomography in progressive outer retinal necrosis. Ophthalmic Surg Lasers Imaging. 2006;37(6):506–7.
232. Pavesio CE, Mitchell SM, Barton K, Schwartz SD, Towler HM, Lightman S. Progressive outer retinal necrosis (PORN) in AIDS patients: a different appearance of varicella-zoster retinitis. Eye (Lond). 1995;9(Pt 3):271–6.

233. Walton RC, Byrnes GA, Chan CC, Nussenblatt RB. Fluorescein angiography in the progressive outer retinal necrosis syndrome. Retina. 1996;16(5):393–8.
234. Yiu G, Young LH. Progressive outer retinal necrosis presenting as cherry red spot. Ocul Immunol Inflamm. 2012;20(5):384–6.
235. Blair MP, Goldstein DA, Shapiro MJ. Optical coherence tomography of progressive outer retinal necrosis. Retina. 2007;27(9):1313–4.
236. Wu CY, Garcia P, Rosen RB. Multimodal Imaging of Progressive Outer Retinal Necrosis. Ophthalmol Retina. 2019;3(1):41.
237. Tran PT, Crow RW, Blomquist PH, He YG. Progressive outer retinal necrosis complicated by combined central retinal vein and central retinal artery occlusions. Retin Cases Brief Rep. 2007;1(3):138–40.
238. Coisy S, Ebran JM, Milea D. Progressive outer retinal necrosis and immunosuppressive therapy in myasthenia gravis. Case Rep Ophthalmol. 2014;5(1):132–7.
239. Kashiwase M, Sata T, Yamauchi Y, Minoda H, Usui N, Iwasaki T, Kurata T, Usui M. Progressive outer retinal necrosis caused by herpes simplex virus type 1 in a patient with acquired immunodeficiency syndrome. Ophthalmology. 2000;107(4):790–4.
240. Bartolini CE, Liang MC, Goldberg RA, Goldman DR, Witkin SR, Duker JS. Progressive outer retinal necrosis secondary to Herpes Simplex Virus type 2. Ophthalmic Surg Lasers Imaging Retina. 2014:1–2.
241. Yang CM, Wang WW, Lin CP. Progressive outer retinal necrosis syndrome as an early manifestation of human immunodeficiency virus infection. J Formos Med Assoc. 1999;98(2):141–4.
242. Moharana B, Tekchandani U, Sharma SP, Kumar A, Singh R. Progressive outer retinal necrosis: Dual virus involvement. Indian J Ophthalmol. 2020;68(9):1955–6.
243. Margolis TP, Lowder CY, Holland GN, Spaide RF, Logan AG, Weissman SS, Irvine AR, Josephberg R, Meisler DM, O'Donnell JJ. Varicella-zoster virus retinitis in patients with the acquired immunodeficiency syndrome. Am J Ophthalmol. 1991;112(2):119–31.
244. Galindez OA, Sabates NR, Whitacre MM, Sabates FN. Rapidly progressive outer retinal necrosis caused by varicella zoster virus in a patient infected with human immunodeficiency virus. Clin Infect Dis. 1996;22(1):149–51.
245. Gore DM, Gore SK, Visser L. Progressive outer retinal necrosis: outcomes in the intravitreal era. Arch Ophthalmol. 2012;130(6):700–6.
246. You YS, Lee SJ, Lee SH, Park CH, Kwon OW. Progressive outer retinal necrosis combined with vitreous hemorrhage in a patient with acquired immunodeficiency syndrome. Korean J Ophthalmol. 2007;21(1):51–4.
247. Tran TH, Rozenberg F, Cassoux N, Rao NA, LeHoang P, Bodaghi B. Polymerase chain reaction analysis of aqueous humour samples in necrotising retinitis. Br J Ophthalmol. 2003;87(1):79–83.
248. Turno-Krecicka A, Boratynska M, Tomczyk-Socha M, Mazanowska O. Progressive outer retinal necrosis in immunocompromised kidney allograft recipient. Transpl Infect Dis. 2015;17(3):400–5.
249. Tseng CC, Chen SN, Hwang JF, Lin CJ, Chen HS. Progressive outer retinal necrosis associated with occlusive vasculitis in acquired immunodeficiency syndrome. J Formos Med Assoc. 2015;114(5):469–72.
250. Yeh S, Wong WT, Weichel ED, Lew JC, Chew EY, Nussenblatt RB. Fundus autofluorescence and OCT in the management of progressive outer retinal necrosis. Ophthalmic Surg Lasers Imaging. 2010;9:1–4.
251. Yin PD, Kurup SK, Fischer SH, Rhee HH, Byrnes GA, Levy-Clarke GA, Buggage RR, Nussenblatt RB, Mican JM, Wright ME. Progressive outer retinal necrosis in the era of highly active antiretroviral therapy: successful management with intravitreal injections and monitoring with quantitative PCR. J Clin Virol. 2007;38(3):254–9.
252. Pinnolis MK, Foxworthy D, Kemp B. Treatment of progressive outer retinal necrosis with sorivudine. Am J Ophthalmol. 1995;119(4):516–7.

253. Perez-Blazquez E, Traspas R, Mendez Marin I, Montero M. Intravitreal ganciclovir treatment in progressive outer retinal necrosis. Am J Ophthalmol. 1997;124(3):418–21.
254. Mehrotra N, Khandelwal J, Nagpal M. Surgical management of complications in a case of progressive outer retinal necrosis. Taiwan J Ophthalmol. 2020;10(4):312–4.
255. Spaide RF, Martin DF, Teich SA, Katz A, Toth I. Successful treatment of progressive outer retinal necrosis syndrome. Retina. 1996;16(6):479–87.
256. Keikha M, Ghazvini K, Eslami M, Yousefi B, Casseb J, Yousefi M, Karbalaei M. Molecular targeting of PD-1 signaling pathway as a novel therapeutic approach in HTLV-1 infection. Microb Pathog. 2020;144:104198.
257. Alvarez C, Gotuzzo E, Vandamme AM, Verdonck K. Family Aggregation of Human T-Lymphotropic Virus 1-Associated Diseases: A Systematic Review. Front Microbiol. 2016;7:1674.
258. Kamoi K, Mochizuki M. HTLV infection and the eye. Curr Opin Ophthalmol. 2012a;23(6):557–61.
259. Percher F, Jeannin P, Martin-Latil S, Gessain A, Afonso PV, Vidy-Roche A, Ceccaldi PE. Mother-to-child transmission of HTLV-1 epidemiological aspects, mechanisms and determinants of mother-to-child transmission. Viruses. 2016;8(2):40.
260. Yamaguchi K, Mochizuki M, Watanabe T, Yoshimura K, Shirao M, Araki S, Miyata N, Mori S, Kiyokawa T, Takatsuki K. Human T lymphotropic virus type 1 uveitis after Graves' disease. Br J Ophthalmol. 1994;78(3):163–6.
261. Takahashi T, Takase H, Urano T, Sugita S, Miyata K, Miyata N, Mochizuki M. Clinical features of human T-lymphotropic virus type 1 uveitis: a long-term follow-up. Ocul Immunol Inflamm. 2000;8(4):235–41.
262. Rathsam-Pinheiro RH, Boa-Sorte N, Castro-Lima-Vargens C, Pinheiro CA, Castro-Lima H, Galvao-Castro B. Ocular lesions in HTLV-1 infected patients from Salvador, State of Bahia: the city with the highest prevalence of this infection in Brazil. Rev Soc Bras Med Trop. 2009;42(6):633–7.
263. Bangham CR. HTLV-1 infections. J Clin Pathol. 2000;53(8):581–6.
264. Kamoi K. HTLV-1 in Ophthalmology. Front Microbiol. 2020;11:388.
265. Terada Y, Kamoi K, Komizo T, Miyata K, Mochizuki M. Human T Cell Leukemia Virus Type 1 and Eye Diseases. J Ocul Pharmacol Ther. 2017;33(4):216–23.
266. Nakao K, Ohba N. Clinical features of HTLV-I associated uveitis. Br J Ophthalmol. 1993;77(5):274–9.
267. Willems L, Hasegawa H, Accolla R, Bangham C, Bazarbachi A, Bertazzoni U, Carneiro-Proietti AB, Cheng H, Chieco-Bianchi L, Ciminale V, et al. Reducing the global burden of HTLV-1 infection: An agenda for research and action. Antiviral Res. 2017;137:41–8.
268. Ahmadi Ghezeldasht S, Shirdel A, Assarehzadegan MA, Hassannia T, Rahimi H, Miri R, Rezaee SA. Human T Lymphotropic Virus Type I (HTLV-I) Oncogenesis: Molecular Aspects of Virus and Host Interactions in Pathogenesis of Adult T cell Leukemia/Lymphoma (ATL). Iran J Basic Med Sci. 2013;16(3):179–95.
269. Watanabe T. Current status of HTLV-1 infection. Int J Hematol. 2011;94(5):430–4.
270. Takeda A, Ishibashi T, Sonoda KH. Epidemiology of Uveitis, Caused by HTLV-1, Toxoplasmosis, and Tuberculosis; the Three Leading Causes of Endemic Infectious Uveitis in Japan. Ocul Immunol Inflamm. 2017a;25(sup1):S19–23.
271. Ohguro N, Sonoda KH, Takeuchi M, Matsumura M, Mochizuki M. The 2009 prospective multi-center epidemiologic survey of uveitis in Japan. Jpn J Ophthalmol. 2012;56(5):432–5.
272. Kamoi K, Okayama A, Izumo S, Hamaguchi I, Uchimaru K, Tojo A, Watanabe T, Ohno-Matsui K. Tackling HTLV-1 infection in ophthalmology: a nationwide survey of ophthalmic care in an endemic country, Japan. Br J Ophthalmol. 2020;104(12):1647–51.
273. Carneiro-Proietti AB, Catalan-Soares BC, Castro-Costa CM, Murphy EL, Sabino EC, Hisada M, Galvao-Castro B, Alcantara LC, Remondegui C, Verdonck K, et al. HTLV in the Americas: challenges and perspectives. Rev Panam Salud Publica. 2006;19(1):44–53.

274. Yoshimura K, Mochizuki M, Araki S, Miyata N, Yamaguchi K, Tajima K, Watanabe T. Clinical and immunologic features of human T-cell lymphotropic virus type I uveitis. Am J Ophthalmol. 1993;116(2):156–63.
275. Kamoi K, Mochizuki M. HTLV-1 uveitis. Front Microbiol. 2012b;3:270.
276. Merle H, Cabre P, Olindo S, Merle S, Smadja D. Ocular lesions in 200 patients infected by the human T-cell lymphotropic virus type 1 in martinique (French West Indies). Am J Ophthalmol. 2002;134(2):190–5.
277. Pinheiro SR, Martins-Filho OA, Ribas JG, Catalan-Soares BC, Proietti FA, Namen-Lopes S, Brito-Melo GE, Carneiro-Proietti AB. Giph: Immunologic markers, uveitis, and keratoconjunctivitis sicca associated with human T-cell lymphotropic virus type 1. Am J Ophthalmol. 2006;142(5):811–5.
278. Pinheiro SR, Carneiro-Proietti AB, Lima-Martins MV, Proietti FA, Pereira AA, Orefice F. HTLV-I/II seroprevalence in 55 Brazilian patients with idiopathic uveitis. Rev Soc Bras Med Trop. 1996;29(4):383–4.
279. Kase S, Namba K, Kitaichi N, Iwata D, Ohno S, Ishida S. Clinical features of human T lymphotropic virus type 1-associated uveitis in Hokkaido, Japan. Jpn J Ophthalmol. 2013a;57(4):379–84.
280. Millan-Rodriguez AC, Fernandez-Cid C, Garcia-Campello M, Sevillano C, Fernandez-Vila PC. Intermediate uveitis due to human T-cell lymphotropic virus type 1. Arch Soc Esp Oftalmol. 2012;87(2):44–6.
281. Yukawa E, Urano T, Nakahara M, Miyata K, Matsuura T, Taketani F, Hara Y, Mochizuki M. Pattern-reversal visual evoked potentials in patients with human T-lymphotropic virus type 1 uveitis. Curr Eye Res. 2006;31(1):37–42.
282. Ohba N, Nakao K, Isashiki Y, Kaminagayoshi T, Sonoda S, Yashiki S, Osame M. Clinical features of HTLV-I associated uveitis determined in multicenter collaborative study. Study Group for HTLV-I Associated Ocular Diseases. Jpn J Ophthalmol. 1994;38(2):168–74.
283. Chew R, Henderson T, Aujla J, Whist E, Einsiedel L. Turning a blind eye: HTLV-1-associated uveitis in Indigenous adults from Central Australia. Int Ophthalmol. 2018;38(5):2159–62.
284. Mochizuki M, Watanabe T, Yamaguchi K, Takatsuki K, Yoshimura K, Shirao M, Nakashima S, Mori S, Araki S, Miyata N. HTLV-I uveitis: a distinct clinical entity caused by HTLV-I. Jpn J Cancer Res. 1992a;83(3):236–9.
285. Pineda MV, Bouzas MB, Remesar M, Fridman A, Remondegui C, Mammana L, Altamirano N, Paradiso P, Costantini P, Tadey L, et al. Relevance of HTLV-1 proviral load in asymptomatic and symptomatic patients living in endemic and non-endemic areas of Argentina. PLoS One. 2019;14(11):e0225596.
286. Ono A, Mochizuki M, Yamaguchi K, Miyata N, Watanabe T. Immunologic and virologic characterization of the primary infiltrating cells in the aqueous humor of human T-cell leukemia virus type-1 uveitis. Accumulation of the human T-cell leukemia virus type-1-infected cells and constitutive expression of viral and interleukin-6 messenger ribonucleic acids. Invest Ophthalmol Vis Sci. 1997;38(3):676–89.
287. Mochizuki M, Watanabe T, Yamaguchi K, Tajima K, Yoshimura K, Nakashima S, Shirao M, Araki S, Miyata N, Mori S, et al. Uveitis associated with human T lymphotropic virus type I: seroepidemiologic, clinical, and virologic studies. J Infect Dis. 1992b;166(4):943–4.
288. Mochizuki M, Watanabe T, Yamaguchi K, Yoshimura K, Nakashima S, Shirao M, Araki S, Takatsuki K, Mori S, Miyata N. Uveitis associated with human T-cell lymphotropic virus type I. Am J Ophthalmol. 1992c;114(2):123–9.
289. Sagawa K, Mochizuki M, Katagirl K, Tsuboi I, Sugita S, Mukaida N, Itoh K. In vitro effects of immunosuppressive agents on cytokine production by HTLV-I-infected T cell clones derived from the ocular fluid of patients with HTLV-I uveitis. Microbiol Immunol. 1996;40(5):373–9.
290. Pohlmann D, Schlickeiser S, Metzner S, Lenglinger M, Winterhalter S, Pleyer U. Different composition of intraocular immune mediators in Posner-Schlossman-Syndrome and Fuchs' Uveitis. PLoS One. 2018;13(6):e0199301.

291. Muller A, McGhee CN. Professor Ernst Fuchs (1851-1930): a defining career in ophthalmology. Arch Ophthalmol. 2003;121(6):888–91.
292. Cunningham ET Jr, Baglivo E. Fuchs heterochromic iridocyclitis—syndrome, disease, or both? Am J Ophthalmol. 2009;148(4):479–81.
293. La Hey E, Baarsma GS, De Vries J, Kijlstra A. Clinical analysis of Fuchs' heterochromic cyclitis. Doc Ophthalmol. 1991;78(3-4):225–35.
294. Sun Y, Ji Y. A literature review on Fuchs uveitis syndrome: An update. Surv Ophthalmol. 2020;65(2):133–43.
295. Bloch-Michel E, Nussenblatt RB. International Uveitis Study Group recommendations for the evaluation of intraocular inflammatory disease. Am J Ophthalmol. 1987;103(2):234–5.
296. Tugal-Tutkun I, Guney-Tefekli E, Kamaci-Duman F. Corum I: A cross-sectional and longitudinal study of Fuchs uveitis syndrome in Turkish patients. Am J Ophthalmol. 2009;148(4):510–515 e511.
297. Gregoire MA, Kodjikian L, Varron L, Grange JD, Broussolle C, Seve P. Characteristics of uveitis presenting for the first time in the elderly: analysis of 91 patients in a tertiary center. Ocul Immunol Inflamm. 2011;19(4):219–26.
298. Kardes E, Sezgin Akcay BI, Unlu C, Ergin A. Choroidal Thickness in Eyes with Fuchs Uveitis Syndrome. Ocul Immunol Inflamm. 2017;25(2):259–66.
299. Groen-Hakan F, van de Laar S, van der Eijk-Baltissen AA, Ten Dam-van LN, de Boer J, Rothova A. Clinical Manifestations, Prognosis, and Vaccination Status of Patients With Rubella Virus-Associated Uveitis. Am J Ophthalmol. 2019;202:37–46.
300. Yang P, Fang W, Jin H, Li B, Chen X, Kijlstra A. Clinical features of Chinese patients with Fuchs' syndrome. Ophthalmology. 2006;113(3):473–80.
301. Accorinti M, Spinucci G, Pirraglia MP, Bruschi S, Pesci FR, Iannetti L. Fuchs' Heterochromic Iridocyclitis in an Italian Tertiary Referral Centre: Epidemiology, Clinical Features, and Prognosis. J Ophthalmol. 2016;2016:1458624.
302. Babu K, Adiga M, Govekar SR, Kumar BR, Murthy KR. Associations of Fuchs heterochromic iridocyclitis in a South Indian patient population. J Ophthalmic Inflamm Infect. 2013;3(1):14.
303. Nasrollahi K, Fazel F, Mirjani T, Kianersi F, Fazel M, Pourazizi M. Ultra-Widefield Fundus Fluorescein Angiography Findings in Patients with Fuchs' Uveitis Syndrome. Adv Biomed Res. 2022;11:1.
304. Bagheri M, Ahoor MH, Jafari A, Hashemi HS, Mohammadkhani M. Pattern of Uveitis in Iran: A Systematic Review. J Ophthalmic Vis Res. 2021;16(1):93–102.
305. Brydak-Godowska J, Moskal K, Borkowski PK, Przybys M, Turczynska M, Kecik D. A Retrospective Observational Study of Uveitis in a Single Center in Poland with a Review of Findings in Europe. Med Sci Monit. 2018;24:8734–49.
306. Jakob E, Reuland MS, Mackensen F, Harsch N, Fleckenstein M, Lorenz HM, Max R, Becker MD. Uveitis subtypes in a German Interdisciplinary Uveitis Center—analysis of 1916 patients. J Rheumatol. 2009;36(1):127–36.
307. Hao T, Yang LI, Li B, Chen X, Li D, Liu X. Epidemiology of 2000 Chinese uveitis patients from Northeast China. Br J Ophthalmol. 2021;105(3):317–21.
308. Guney E, Akcay BI, Erdogan G, Unlu C, Akcali G, Bayramlar H. The etiological features of anterior uveitis in a Turkish population. Clin Ophthalmol. 2012;6:845–9.
309. Nalcacioglu P, Cakar Ozdal P, Simsek M. Clinical Characteristics of Fuchs' Uveitis Syndrome. Turk J Ophthalmol. 2016;46(2):52–7.
310. Aziz S, Arya B, Westcott M, Pavesio C. An investigation of the disc hyperfluorescence in Fuchs uveitis syndrome using optical coherence tomography imaging. Ocul Immunol Inflamm. 2015;23(2):152–6.
311. Tappeiner C, Dreesbach J, Roesel M, Heinz C, Heiligenhaus A. Clinical manifestation of Fuchs uveitis syndrome in childhood. Graefes Arch Clin Exp Ophthalmol. 2015;253(7):1169–74.
312. Zarei M, Ebrahimiadib N. Atypical Keratic Precipitates in Fuchs Uveitis. Ocul Immunol Inflamm. 2021;29(7-8):1363–5.

313. Hasler S, Thiel MA, Becht CN. In vivo confocal microscopy of keratic precipitates in fuchs heterochromic uveitis syndrome. Klin Monbl Augenheilkd. 2009;226(4):237–40.
314. Ozer MD, Kebapci F, Batur M, Seven E, Tekin S. In vivo analysis and comparison of anterior segment structures of both eyes in unilateral Fuchs' uveitis syndrome. Graefes Arch Clin Exp Ophthalmol. 2019;257(7):1489–98.
315. Simsek M, Cakar Ozdal P, Cankurtaran M, Ozdemir HB, Elgin U. Analysis of Corneal Densitometry and Endothelial Cell Function in Fuchs Uveitis Syndrome. Eye Contact Lens. 2021;47(4):196–202.
316. Szepessy Z, Toth G, Barsi A, Kranitz K, Nagy ZZ. Anterior Segment Characteristics of Fuchs Uveitis Syndrome. Ocul Immunol Inflamm. 2016;24(5):594–8.
317. Kanavi MR, Soheilian M, Naghshgar N. Confocal scan of keratic precipitates in uveitic eyes of various etiologies. Cornea. 2010;29(6):650–4.
318. Johnson D, Liesegang TJ, Brubaker RF. Aqueous humor dynamics in Fuchs' uveitis syndrome. Am J Ophthalmol. 1983;95(6):783–7.
319. Liu Q, Jia Y, Zhang S, Xie J, Chang X, Hou J, Li G, Koch DD, Wang L. Iris autofluorescence in Fuchs' heterochromic uveitis. Br J Ophthalmol. 2016a;100(10):1397–402.
320. Zarei M, Abdollahi A, Darabeigi S, Ebrahimiadib N, Roohipoor R, Ghassemi H, Moghaddam RS, Fard MA. An investigation on optic nerve head involvement in Fuchs uveitis syndrome using optical coherence tomography and fluorescein angiography. Graefes Arch Clin Exp Ophthalmol. 2018;256(12):2421–7.
321. Zarei M, Darabeigi S, Mehrpour M, Roohipoor R, Ghassemi H, Ebrahimiadib N. Fuchs' Uveitis in Iranian Patients: A Review of 89 Eyes. Ocul Immunol Inflamm. 2019;27(7):1077–85.
322. Aksoy FE, Altan C, Basarir B, Garip D, Pasaoglu I, Perente I, Yigit U, Taskapili M. Analysis of retinal microvasculature in Fuchs' uveitis syndrome. Retinal microvasculature in Fuchs' uveitis. J Fr Ophtalmol. 2020;43(4):324–9.
323. Ozer MD, Batur M, Tekin S, Seven E, Kebapci F. Choroid vascularity index as a parameter for chronicity of Fuchs' uveitis syndrome. Int Ophthalmol. 2020b;40(6):1429–37.
324. Ozcelik-Kose A, Balci S, Turan-Vural E. In vivo analysis of choroidal vascularity index changes in eyes with Fuchs uveitis syndrome. Photodiagnosis Photodyn Ther. 2021;34:102332.
325. Goker YS, Ozdal PC, Erol YO, Kiziltoprak H, Karatepe MS. Evaluation of radial peripapillary capillary density in patients with Fuchs uveitis syndrome. Graefes Arch Clin Exp Ophthalmol. 2019;257(12):2735–42.
326. Cerquaglia A, Iaccheri B, Fiore T, Lupidi M, Torroni G, Fruttini D, Giacalone C, Cagini C. Full-thickness choroidal thinning as a feature of Fuchs uveitis syndrome: quantitative evaluation of the choroid by enhanced depth imaging optical coherence tomography in a cohort of consecutive patients. Graefes Arch Clin Exp Ophthalmol. 2016;254(10):2025–31.
327. Przybys M, Brydak-Godowska J, Kecik D. Subfoveal choroidal thickness and its intereye differences in Fuchs uveitis syndrome evaluated using optical coherent tomography. Ocul Immunol Inflamm. 2021;29(5):896–901.
328. Balci O, Ozsutcu M. Evaluation of retinal and choroidal thickness in Fuchs' uveitis syndrome. J Ophthalmol. 2016;2016:1657078.
329. Moschos MM, Gouliopoulos NS, Kalogeropoulos C. Electrophysiological examination in uveitis: a review of the literature. Clin Ophthalmol. 2014;8:199–214.
330. Yildiz Balci S, Kose AO, Yildiz MB, Ozcaliskan S. Systemic inflammatory biomarkers in patients with Fuchs' uveitis syndrome: neutrophil/lymphocyte ratio and platelet/lymphocyte ratio. J Coll Physicians Surg Pak. 2020;30(7):722–5.
331. Simsek M, Ozdal PC. Inflammatory markers of complete blood count in Fuchs uveitis syndrome. Can J Ophthalmol. 2021;56(3):197–202.
332. Provost J, Labetoulle M, Bouthry E, Haigh O, Leleu I, Kobal A, Mouriaux F, Barreau E, Vauloup-Fellous C, Rousseau A. Rubella virus-associated uveitis: the essentiality of aqueous humor virological analysis. Eur J Ophthalmol. 2022;32:3489.

333. Yang P, Zhang W, Chen Z, Zhang H, Su G, Cao Q, Zhu Y, Zhong Z, Zhou C, Wang Y, et al. Development of revised diagnostic criteria for Fuchs' uveitis syndrome in a Chinese population. Br J Ophthalmol. 2021;106:1678.
334. Standardization of Uveitis Nomenclature Working G. Classification criteria for Fuchs uveitis syndrome. Am J Ophthalmol. 2021;228:262–7.
335. Ruokonen PC, Metzner S, Ucer A, Torun N, Hofmann J, Pleyer U. Intraocular antibody synthesis against rubella virus and other microorganisms in Fuchs' heterochromic cyclitis. Graefes Arch Clin Exp Ophthalmol. 2010;248(4):565–71.
336. de Groot-Mijnes JD, de Visser L, Rothova A, Schuller M, van Loon AM, Weersink AJ. Rubella virus is associated with fuchs heterochromic iridocyclitis. Am J Ophthalmol. 2006;141(1):212–4.
337. Suzuki J, Goto H, Komase K, Abo H, Fujii K, Otsuki N, Okamoto K. Rubella virus as a possible etiological agent of Fuchs heterochromic iridocyclitis. Graefes Arch Clin Exp Ophthalmol. 2010a;248(10):1487–91.
338. Mitchell SM, Phylactou L, Fox JD, Kilpatrick MW, Murray PI. The detection of herpesviral DNA in aqueous fluid samples from patients with Fuchs' heterochromic cyclitis. Ocul Immunol Inflamm. 1996a;4(1):33–8.
339. Chee SP, Jap A. Presumed Fuchs heterochromic iridocyclitis and Posner-Schlossman syndrome: comparison of cytomegalovirus-positive and negative eyes. Am J Ophthalmol. 2008;146(6):883–889 e881.
340. Joye A, Gonzales JA. Ocular manifestations of cytomegalovirus in immunocompetent hosts. Curr Opin Ophthalmol. 2018;29(6):535–42.
341. Mahendradas P, Shetty R, Malathi J, Madhavan HN. Chikungunya virus iridocyclitis in Fuchs' heterochromic iridocyclitis. Indian J Ophthalmol. 2010;58(6):545–7.
342. Babu K, Murthy GJ. Chikungunya virus iridocyclitis in Fuchs' heterochromic iridocyclitis. Indian J Ophthalmol. 2012;60(1):73–4.
343. Toledo de Abreu M, Belfort R Jr, Hirata PS. Fuchs' heterochromic cyclitis and ocular toxoplasmosis. Am J Ophthalmol. 1982;93(6):739–44.
344. Kang H, Bao H, Shi Y, Feng J, Yang W, He Y, Wang H, Hu X, Tao Y. Clinical characteristics and aqueous humor laboratory analysis of Chinese patients with Rubella Virus-associated and cytomegalovirus-associated Fuchs uveitis syndrome. Front Med (Lausanne). 2020;7:610341.
345. Abernathy E, Peairs RR, Chen MH, Icenogle J, Namdari H. Genomic characterization of a persistent rubella virus from a case of Fuch' uveitis syndrome in a 73 year old man. J Clin Virol. 2015;69:104–9.
346. Stunf S, Petrovec M, Zigon N, Hawlina M, Kraut A, de Groot-Mijnes JD, Valentincic NV. High concordance of intraocular antibody synthesis against the rubella virus and Fuchs heterochromic uveitis syndrome in Slovenia. Mol Vis. 2012;18:2909–14.
347. de Visser L, Braakenburg A, Rothova A, de Boer JH. Rubella virus-associated uveitis: clinical manifestations and visual prognosis. Am J Ophthalmol. 2008;146(2):292–7.
348. Fazil Z, Ten Berge JC, Langerak AW, Rothova A, Dik WA. An intraocular inflammatory profile of rubella associated uveitis. Ocul Immunol Inflamm. 2019;27(3):418–23.
349. Murray PI, Hoekzema R, van Haren MA, de Hon FD, Kijlstra A. Aqueous humor interleukin-6 levels in uveitis. Invest Ophthalmol Vis Sci. 1990;31(5):917–20.
350. Suzuki K, Suzuki Y, Matsumoto M, Nakazawa M. Expression profile of intravitreous cytokines, chemokines and growth factors in patients with Fuchs heterochromic iridocyclitis. Case Rep Ophthalmol. 2010b;1(1):5–13.
351. Simsek M, Cakar Ozdal P, Akbiyik F, Citirik M, Berker N, Ozdamar Erol Y, Yilmazbas P. Aqueous humor IL-8, IL-10, and VEGF levels in Fuchs' uveitis syndrome and Behcet's uveitis. Int Ophthalmol. 2019;39(11):2629–36.
352. Wang H, Tao Y. Relationship between the higher inflammatory cytokines level in the aqueous humor of Fuchs uveitis syndrome and the presence of cataract. BMC Ophthalmol. 2021a;21(1):108.

353. Bauer D, Kasper M, Walscheid K, Koch JM, Muther PS, Kirchhof B, Heiligenhaus A, Heinz C. Alteration of MCP-1 and MMP-9 in aqueous humor is associated with secondary glaucoma in Fuchs uveitis syndrome. Ocul Immunol Inflamm. 2020;28(4):688–98.
354. Labalette P, Caillau D, Grutzmacher C, Dessaint JP, Labalette M. Highly focused clonal composition of CD8(+) CD28(neg) T cells in aqueous humor of fuchs heterochromic cyclitis. Exp Eye Res. 2002a;75(3):317–25.
355. Mehta S, Linton MM, Kempen JH. Outcomes of cataract surgery in patients with uveitis: a systematic review and meta-analysis. Am J Ophthalmol. 2014;158(4):676–692 e677.
356. Bhargava R, Kumar P, Sharma SK, Arora Y. Phacoemulsification versus manual small incision cataract surgery in patients with Fuchs heterochromic iridocyclitis. Asia Pac J Ophthalmol (Phila). 2016;5(5):330–4.
357. Bhargava R, Kumar P, Sharma SK, Ranjan S, Kumar M, Godara R. Small-incision cataract surgery in patients with Fuch's heterochromic iridocyclitis. Nepal J Ophthalmol. 2014;6(2):153–61.
358. Estafanous MF, Lowder CY, Meisler DM, Chauhan R. Phacoemulsification cataract extraction and posterior chamber lens implantation in patients with uveitis. Am J Ophthalmol. 2001;131(5):620–5.
359. Budak K, Akova YA, Yalvac I, Somer D, Aslan BS, Duman S. Cataract surgery in patients with Fuchs' heterochromic iridocyclitis. Jpn J Ophthalmol. 1999;43(4):308–11.
360. Waters FM, Goodall K, Jones NP, McLeod D. Vitrectomy for vitreous opacification in Fuchs' heterochromic uveitis. Eye (Lond). 2000;14(Pt 2):216–8.
361. Scott RA, Sullivan PM, Aylward GW, Pavesio CE, Charteris DG. The effect of pars plana vitrectomy in the management of Fuchs heterochromic cyclitis. Retina. 2001;21(4):312–6.
362. Nilforushan N, Yadgari M, Alemzadeh SA. Surgical management of glaucoma in Fuchs uveitis syndrome: trabeculectomy or Ahmed glaucoma valve. J Curr Ophthalmol. 2019;31(1):24–30.
363. Voykov B, Doycheva D, Deuter C, Leitritz MA, Dimopoulos S, William A. Outcomes of Ahmed Glaucoma Valve implantation for Glaucoma Secondary to Fuchs Uveitis syndrome. Ocul Immunol Inflamm. 2017;25(6):760–6.
364. Voykov B, Deuter C, Zierhut M, Leitritz MA, Guenova E, Doycheva D. Is cyclophotocoagulation an option in the management of glaucoma secondary to Fuchs' uveitis syndrome? Graefes Arch Clin Exp Ophthalmol. 2014;252(3):485–9.
365. Kee AR, Gonzalez-Lopez JJ, Al-Hity A, Gupta B, Lee CS, Gunasekeran DV, Jayabalan N, Grant R, Kon OM, Gupta V, et al. Anti-tubercular therapy for intraocular tuberculosis: a systematic review and meta-analysis. Surv Ophthalmol. 2016;61(5):628–53.
366. Agarwal A, Aggarwal K, Gupta V. Infectious uveitis: an Asian perspective. Eye (Lond). 2019a;33(1):50–65.
367. Collaborators GBDT. The global burden of tuberculosis: results from the Global Burden of Disease Study 2015. Lancet Infect Dis. 2018;18(3):261–84.
368. Abdisamadov A, Tursunov O. Ocular tuberculosis epidemiology, clinic features and diagnosis: a brief review. Tuberculosis (Edinb). 2020;124:101963.
369. Helm CJ, Holland GN. Ocular tuberculosis. Surv Ophthalmol. 1993;38(3):229–56.
370. Varma D, Anand S, Reddy AR, Das A, Watson JP, Currie DC, Sutcliffe I, Backhouse OC. Tuberculosis: an under-diagnosed aetiological agent in uveitis with an effective treatment. Eye (Lond). 2006;20(9):1068–73.
371. Gupta V, Gupta A, Rao NA. Intraocular tuberculosis—an update. Surv Ophthalmol. 2007;52(6):561–87.
372. Agrawal R, Testi I, Rousselot A, Chen EJ, Lakshminarayanan R, Singhal A, Bundele M, Hutchison P, Kon OM, Gupta V, et al. Insights into the molecular pathogenesis of ocular tuberculosis. Tuberculosis (Edinb). 2021a;126:102018.
373. Biswas J, Madhavan HN, Gopal L, Badrinath SS. Intraocular tuberculosis.Clinicopathologic study of five cases. Retina. 1995;15(6):461–8.

374. Darian-Smith E, Lin ML, Lim LL, McCluskey P, Hall AJ. The incidence of ocular tuberculosis in Australia over the past 10 years (2006-2015). Ophthalmic Epidemiol. 2017;24(6):406–12.
375. Hermann L, Falcao-Reis F, Figueira L. Epidemiology of uveitis in a Tertiary Care Centre in Portugal. Semin Ophthalmol. 2021;36(1-2):51–7.
376. Rahman Z, Ahsan Z, Rahman NA, Dutta Majumder P. Pattern of uveitis in a Referral Hospital in Bangladesh. Ocul Immunol Inflamm. 2018;26(6):893–6.
377. Al Dhibi HA, Al Shamsi HN, Al-Mahmood AM, Al Taweel HM, Al Shamrani MA, Arevalo JF, Gupta V, The Kkesh Uveitis Survey Study G. Patterns of Uveitis in a Tertiary Care Referral Institute in Saudi Arabia. Ocul Immunol Inflamm. 2017;25(3):388–95.
378. Wakabayashi T, Morimura Y, Miyamoto Y, Okada AA. Changing patterns of intraocular inflammatory disease in Japan. Ocul Immunol Inflamm. 2003;11(4):277–86.
379. Gonzalez Fernandez D, Nascimento H, Nascimento C, Muccioli C, Belfort R Jr. Uveitis in Sao Paulo, Brazil: 1053 new patients in 15 months. Ocul Immunol Inflamm. 2017;25(3):382–7.
380. Dogra M, Singh R, Agarwal A, Sharma A, Singh SR, Gautam N, Yangzes S, Samanta R, Sharma M, Aggarwal K, et al. Epidemiology of uveitis in a Tertiary-Care Referral Institute in North India. Ocul Immunol Inflamm. 2017;25(sup1):S46–53.
381. Bertrand PJ, Jamilloux Y, Ecochard R, Richard-Colmant G, Gerfaud-Valentin M, Guillaud M, Denis P, Kodjikian L, Seve P. Uveitis: autoimmunity... and beyond. Autoimmun Rev. 2019;18(9):102351.
382. Lee JY. Diagnosis and treatment of extrapulmonary tuberculosis. Tuberc Respir Dis (Seoul). 2015;78(2):47–55.
383. Ramirez-Lapausa M, Menendez-Saldana A, Noguerado-Asensio A. Extrapulmonary tuberculosis. Rev Esp Sanid Penit. 2015;17(1):3–11.
384. Mehta S, Mansoor H, Khan S, Saranchuk P, Isaakidis P. Ocular inflammatory disease and ocular tuberculosis in a cohort of patients co-infected with HIV and multidrug-resistant tuberculosis in Mumbai, India: a cross-sectional study. BMC Infect Dis. 2013;13:225.
385. Singh R, Gupta V, Gupta A. Pattern of uveitis in a referral eye clinic in north India. Indian J Ophthalmol. 2004;52(2):121–5.
386. Tsirouki T, Dastiridou A, Symeonidis C, Tounakaki O, Brazitikou I, Kalogeropoulos C, Androudi S. A focus on the epidemiology of uveitis. Ocul Immunol Inflamm. 2018;26(1):2–16.
387. Agrawal R, Gunasekeran DV, Raje D, Agarwal A, Nguyen QD, Kon OM, Pavesio C, Gupta V, Collaborative Ocular Tuberculosis Study G. Global variations and challenges with tubercular uveitis in the Collaborative Ocular Tuberculosis Study. Invest Ophthalmol Vis Sci. 2018;59(10):4162–71.
388. Llorenc V, Mesquida M, de la Maza M, Keller J, Molins B, Espinosa G, Hernandez MV, Gonzalez-Martin J, Adan A. Epidemiology of uveitis in a Western urban multiethnic population. The challenge of globalization. Acta Ophthalmol. 2015;93(6):561–7.
389. Siak J, Kumaradas M, Chee SP. The pattern of uveitis in Sri Lanka. Ocul Immunol Inflamm. 2017a;25(sup1):S63–8.
390. Biswas J, Kharel Sitaula R, Multani P. Changing uveitis patterns in South India—comparison between two decades. Indian J Ophthalmol. 2018;66(4):524–7.
391. Smit RL, Baarsma GS, de Vries J. Classification of 750 consecutive uveitis patients in the Rotterdam Eye Hospital. Int Ophthalmol. 1993;17(2):71–6.
392. Siak J, Jansen A, Waduthantri S, Teoh CS, Jap A, Chee SP. The pattern of uveitis among Chinese, Malays, and Indians in Singapore. Ocul Immunol Inflamm. 2017b;25(sup1):S81–93.
393. Al-Qarni A, Abouammoh MA, Almousa AN, Mousa A, Abu El-Asrar AM. Presumed tuberculous uveitis in a university-based tertiary referral center in Saudi Arabia. Int Ophthalmol. 2019;39(2):317–33.
394. Gargouri S, Kaibi I, Zone I, Khairallah M, Koubaa M, Ben Jemaa M, Feki J. Presumed Tuberculous uveitis: clinical features and management. Tunis Med. 2019;97(1):106–12.

395. Alvarez S, McCabe WR. Extrapulmonary tuberculosis revisited: a review of experience at Boston City and other hospitals. Medicine (Baltimore). 1984;63(1):25–55.
396. Oluleye TS. Tuberculous uveitis. J Multidiscip Healthc. 2013;6:41–3.
397. Arej N, Fadlallah A, Chelala E. Choroidal tuberculoma as a presenting sign of tuberculosis. Int Med Case Rep J. 2016;9:365–8.
398. Mao Y, Peng XY, You QS, Wang H, Zhao M, Jonas JB. Tuberculous uveitis in China. Acta Ophthalmol. 2014;92(5):e393–7.
399. Lardenoye CW, van Kooij B, Rothova A. Impact of macular edema on visual acuity in uveitis. Ophthalmology. 2006;113(8):1446–9.
400. Urzua CA, Lantigua Y, Abuauad S, Liberman P, Berger O, Sabat P, Velasquez V, Castiglione E, Calonge M. Clinical features and prognostic factors in presumed ocular tuberculosis. Curr Eye Res. 2017;42(7):1029–34.
401. Dutta Majumder P, Burugupalli K, Menia NK, Ganesh SK, Biswas J. Pattern of uveitic hypotony in a Tertiary Eye Hospital in India. Ocul Immunol Inflamm. 2018;26(6):924–8.
402. Lou SM, Montgomery PA, Larkin KL, Winthrop K, Zierhut M, Rosenbaum JT, Uveitis Specialists Study G. Diagnosis and treatment for ocular tuberculosis among uveitis specialists: the international perspective. Ocul Immunol Inflamm. 2015;23(1):32–9.
403. Goyal JL, Jain P, Arora R, Dokania P. Ocular manifestations of tuberculosis. Indian J Tuberc. 2015;62(2):66–73.
404. Standardization of Uveitis Nomenclature Working Group. Classification criteria for tubercular uveitis. Am J Ophthalmol. 2021d;228:142–51.
405. Ang M, Htoon HM, Chee SP. Diagnosis of tuberculous uveitis: clinical application of an interferon-gamma release assay. Ophthalmology. 2009;116(7):1391–6.
406. Wroblewski KJ, Hidayat AA, Neafie RC, Rao NA, Zapor M. Ocular tuberculosis: a clinicopathologic and molecular study. Ophthalmology. 2011;118(4):772–7.
407. Rishi E, Rishi P, Therese KL, Ramasubban G, Biswas J, Sharma T, Bhende P, Susvar P, Agarwal M, George AE, et al. Culture and reverse transcriptase polymerase chain reaction (RT-PCR) proven Mycobacterium Tuberculosis endophthalmitis: a case series. Ocul Immunol Inflamm. 2018;26(2):220–7.
408. Ang M, Vasconcelos-Santos DV, Sharma K, Accorinti M, Sharma A, Gupta A, Rao NA, Chee SP. Diagnosis of ocular tuberculosis. Ocul Immunol Inflamm. 2018;26(2):208–16.
409. Aggarwal K, Agarwal A, Sehgal S, Sharma S, Singh N, Sharma K, Samanta R, Invernizzi A, Sharma A, Gupta V. An unusual presentation of intraocular tuberculosis in a monocular patient: clinicopathological correlation. J Ophthalmic Inflamm Infect. 2016;6(1):46.
410. Sudheer B, Lalitha P, Kumar AL, Rathinam S. Polymerase Chain Reaction and its Correlation with Clinical Features and Treatment Response in Tubercular Uveitis. Ocul Immunol Inflamm. 2018;26(6):845–52.
411. Kharel Sitaula R, Janani MK, Madhavan HN, Biswas J. Outcome of polymerase chain reaction (PCR) analysis in 100 suspected cases of infectious uveitis. J Ophthalmic Inflamm Infect. 2018;8(1):2.
412. Barik MR, Rath S, Modi R, Rana R, Reddy MM, Basu S. Normalised quantitative polymerase chain reaction for diagnosis of tuberculosis-associated uveitis. Tuberculosis (Edinb). 2018;110:30–5.
413. Sharma K, Gupta V, Bansal R, Sharma A, Sharma M, Gupta A. Novel multi-targeted polymerase chain reaction for diagnosis of presumed tubercular uveitis. J Ophthalmic Inflamm Infect. 2013;3(1):25.
414. Sharma K, Gupta V, Sharma A, Singh R, Sharma M, Aggarwal K, Bansal R, Fiorella PD, Prakash S, Gupta A. Gene Xpert MTB/RIF assay for the diagnosis of intra-ocular tuberculosis from vitreous fluid samples. Tuberculosis (Edinb). 2017;102:1–2.
415. Sharma K, Gupta A, Sharma M, Sharma A, Bansal R, Sharma SP, Singh RD, Gupta V. The emerging challenge of diagnosing drug-resistant tubercular uveitis: experience of 110 eyes from North India. Ocul Immunol Inflamm. 2021;29(1):107–14.

416. Ludi Z, Sule AA, Samy RP, Putera I, Schrijver B, Hutchinson PE, Gunaratne J, Verma I, Singhal A, Nora RD, et al. Diagnosis and biomarkers for ocular tuberculosis: From the present into the future. Theranostics. 2023;13(7):2088–113.
417. Sharma K, Gupta A, Sharma M, Singh S, Sharma A, Singh R, Gupta V. Detection of viable Mycobacterium tuberculosis in ocular fluids using mRNA-based multiplex polymerase chain reaction. Indian J Med Microbiol. 2022;40(2):254–7.
418. Agarwal A, Agrawal R, Gunasekaran DV, Raje D, Gupta B, Aggarwal K, Murthy SL, Westcott M, Chee SP, McCluskey P, et al. The Collaborative Ocular Tuberculosis Study (COTS)-1 Report 3: polymerase chain reaction in the diagnosis and management of tubercular uveitis: global trends. Ocul Immunol Inflamm. 2019b;27(3):465–73.
419. Mohan N, Balne PK, Panda KG, Sharma S, Basu S. Polymerase chain reaction evaluation of infectious multifocal serpiginoid choroiditis. Ocul Immunol Inflamm. 2014;22(5):384–90.
420. Sharma K, Sharma M, Ayyadurai N, Dogra M, Sharma A, Gupta V, Singh R, Gupta A. Comparative evaluation of GeneXpert MTB/RIF Ultra and GeneXpert MTB/RIF for detecting tuberculosis and identifying Rifampicin resistance in Pars Plana Vitrectomy samples of patients with ocular tuberculosis. Ocul Immunol Inflamm. 2023;31(5):914–20.
421. Sharma RKMS, Gupta VMS, Bansal RMS, Sharma KMD, Gupta AMS, Sachdeva NPD. Immune profiling of T cells infiltrating vitreous humor in tubercular uveitis. Immunol Invest. 2018a;47(6):615–31.
422. Tagirasa R, Parmar S, Barik MR, Devadas S, Basu S. Autoreactive T Cells in immunopathogenesis of TB-associated uveitis. Invest Ophthalmol Vis Sci. 2017;58(13):5682–91.
423. Ang M, Cheung G, Vania M, Chen J, Yang H, Li J, Chee SP. Aqueous cytokine and chemokine analysis in uveitis associated with tuberculosis. Mol Vis. 2012a;18:565–73.
424. Sharma RK, Gupta A, Kamal S, Bansal R, Singh N, Sharma K, Virk S, Sachdeva N. Role of regulatory T cells in tubercular uveitis. Ocul Immunol Inflamm. 2018b;26(1):27–36.
425. Abu El-Asrar AM, Struyf S, Kangave D, Al-Obeidan SA, Opdenakker G, Geboes K, Van Damme J. Cytokine and CXC chemokine expression patterns in aqueous humor of patients with presumed tuberculous uveitis. Cytokine. 2012;59(2):377–81.
426. Chadalawada S, Kathirvel K, Lalitha P, Rathinam SR, Devarajan B. Dysregulated expression of microRNAs in aqueous humor from intraocular tuberculosis patients. Mol Biol Rep. 2022;49(1):97–107.
427. Agrawal R, Testi I, Mahajan S, Yuen YS, Agarwal A, Kon OM, Barisani-Asenbauer T, Kempen JH, Gupta A, Jabs DA, et al. Collaborative Ocular Tuberculosis Study Consensus Guidelines on the Management of Tubercular Uveitis-Report 1: guidelines for initiating antitubercular therapy in tubercular choroiditis. Ophthalmology. 2021b;128(2):266–76.
428. Krassas N, Wells J, Bell C, Woodhead M, Jones N. Presumed tuberculosis-associated uveitis: rising incidence and widening criteria for diagnosis in a non-endemic area. Eye (Lond). 2018;32(1):87–92.
429. Ang M, Hedayatfar A, Wong W, Chee SP. Duration of anti-tubercular therapy in uveitis associated with latent tuberculosis: a case-control study. Br J Ophthalmol. 2012b;96(3):332–6.
430. Wakefield MJ, Kumar P. Liver failure following antituberculosis (ATT) chemotherapy for presumed tuberculous uveitis. Eye (Lond). 2014;28(1):110–1.
431. Souissi S, David T, Beral L. Steroid treatment in ocular tuberculosis: a double-edged sword? J Fr Ophtalmol. 2017;40(2):126–32.
432. Tsui E, Fern CM, Goldberg NR. Treatment of refractory tubercular serpiginous-like choroiditis with intravitreal methotrexate. Retin Cases Brief Rep. 2021b;15(2):169–73.
433. Cimino L, Herbort CP, Aldigeri R, Salvarani C, Boiardi L. Tuberculous uveitis, a resurgent and underdiagnosed disease. Int Ophthalmol. 2009;29(2):67–74.
434. Tomkins-Netzer O, Leong BCS, Zhang X, Lightman S, McCluskey PJ, Sydney-London Latent Ocular TBSG. Effect of antituberculous therapy on uveitis associated with latent tuberculosis. Am J Ophthalmol. 2018;190:164–70.
435. Multani PK, Modi R, Basu S. Pattern of recurrent inflammation following anti-tubercular therapy for ocular tuberculosis. Ocul Immunol Inflamm. 2022;30(1):185–90.

436. Furtado JM, Winthrop KL, Butler NJ, Smith JR. Ocular toxoplasmosis I: parasitology, epidemiology and public health. Clin Exp Ophthalmol. 2013;41(1):82–94.
437. Frenkel JK, Ruiz A, Chinchilla M. Soil survival of toxoplasma oocysts in Kansas and Costa Rica. Am J Trop Med Hyg. 1975;24(3):439–43.
438. Dumetre A, Le Bras C, Baffet M, Meneceur P, Dubey JP, Derouin F, Duguet JP, Joyeux M, Moulin L. Effects of ozone and ultraviolet radiation treatments on the infectivity of Toxoplasma gondii oocysts. Vet Parasitol. 2008;153(3-4):209–13.
439. Kijlstra A, Petersen E. Epidemiology, pathophysiology, and the future of ocular toxoplasmosis. Ocul Immunol Inflamm. 2014;22(2):138–47.
440. Jones LA, Alexander J, Roberts CW. Ocular toxoplasmosis: in the storm of the eye. Parasite Immunol. 2006;28(12):635–42.
441. Smith JR, Ashander LM, Arruda SL, Cordeiro CA, Lie S, Rochet E, Belfort R Jr, Furtado JM. Pathogenesis of ocular toxoplasmosis. Prog Retin Eye Res. 2021;81:100882.
442. Bosch-Driessen LE, Berendschot TT, Ongkosuwito JV, Rothova A. Ocular toxoplasmosis: clinical features and prognosis of 154 patients. Ophthalmology. 2002a;109(5):869–78.
443. Maenz M, Schluter D, Liesenfeld O, Schares G, Gross U, Pleyer U. Ocular toxoplasmosis past, present and new aspects of an old disease. Prog Retin Eye Res. 2014;39:77–106.
444. Pappas G, Roussos N, Falagas ME. Toxoplasmosis snapshots: global status of Toxoplasma gondii seroprevalence and implications for pregnancy and congenital toxoplasmosis. Int J Parasitol. 2009;39(12):1385–94.
445. Ozgonul C, Besirli CG. Recent developments in the diagnosis and treatment of ocular toxoplasmosis. Ophthalmic Res. 2017;57(1):1–12.
446. Dubey JP, Lago EG, Gennari SM, Su C, Jones JL. Toxoplasmosis in humans and animals in Brazil: high prevalence, high burden of disease, and epidemiology. Parasitology. 2012;139(11):1375–424.
447. Kamani J, Mani AU, Egwu GO, Kumshe HA. Seroprevalence of human infection with Toxoplasma gondii and the associated risk factors, in Maiduguri, Borno state, Nigeria. Ann Trop Med Parasitol. 2009;103(4):317–21.
448. Swai ES, Schoonman L. Seroprevalence of Toxoplasma gondii infection amongst residents of Tanga district in north-east Tanzania. Tanzan J Health Res. 2009;11(4):205–9.
449. Hofhuis A, van Pelt W, van Duynhoven YT, Nijhuis CD, Mollema L, van der Klis FR, Havelaar AH, Kortbeek LM. Decreased prevalence and age-specific risk factors for Toxoplasma gondii IgG antibodies in The Netherlands between 1995/1996 and 2006/2007. Epidemiol Infect. 2011;139(4):530–8.
450. Xiao Y, Yin J, Jiang N, Xiang M, Hao L, Lu H, Sang H, Liu X, Xu H, Ankarklev J, et al. Seroepidemiology of human Toxoplasma gondii infection in China. BMC Infect Dis. 2010;10:4.
451. Basavaraju A. Toxoplasmosis in HIV infection: an overview. Tropenmed Parasitol. 2016;6(2):129–35.
452. Nissapatorn V. Toxoplasmosis in HIV/AIDS: a living legacy. Southeast Asian J Trop Med Public Health. 2009;40(6):1158–78.
453. Pereira-Chioccola VL, Vidal JE, Su C. Toxoplasma gondii infection and cerebral toxoplasmosis in HIV-infected patients. Future Microbiol. 2009;4(10):1363–79.
454. Holland GN. Ocular toxoplasmosis: a global reassessment. Part I: epidemiology and course of disease. Am J Ophthalmol. 2003;136(6):973–88.
455. Huang PK, Jianping C, Vasconcelos-Santos DV, Arruda JSD, Dutta Majumder P, Anthony E, Ganesh SK, Biswas J, Ling HS, Teoh SC, et al. Ocular toxoplasmosis in tropical areas: analysis and outcome of 190 patients from a Multicenter Collaborative Study. Ocul Immunol Inflamm. 2018;26(8):1289–96.
456. Das D, Bhattacharjee H, Bhattacharyya PK, Jain L, Panicker MJ, Das K, Deka AC. Pattern of uveitis in North East India: a Tertiary Eye Care Center Study. Indian J Ophthalmol. 2009;57(2):144–6.

457. Souto FMS, Giampietro BV, Takiuti JT, Campos LMA, Hirata CE, Yamamoto JH. Clinical features of paediatric uveitis at a tertiary referral centre in Sao Paulo, SP, Brazil. Br J Ophthalmol. 2018.
458. Gilbert RE, Dunn DT, Lightman S, Murray PI, Pavesio CE, Gormley PD, Masters J, Parker SP, Stanford MR. Incidence of symptomatic toxoplasma eye disease: aetiology and public health implications. Epidemiol Infect. 1999;123(2):283–9.
459. Khan K, Khan W. Congenital toxoplasmosis: an overview of the neurological and ocular manifestations. Parasitol Int. 2018;67(6):715–21.
460. Vasconcelos-Santos DV, Machado Azevedo DO, Campos WR, Orefice F, Queiroz-Andrade GM, Carellos EV, Castro Romanelli RM, Januario JN, Resende LM, Martins-Filho OA, et al. Congenital toxoplasmosis in southeastern Brazil: results of early ophthalmologic examination of a large cohort of neonates. Ophthalmology. 2009;116(11):2199–2205 e2191.
461. Mets MB, Holfels E, Boyer KM, Swisher CN, Roizen N, Stein L, Stein M, Hopkins J, Withers S, Mack D, et al. Eye manifestations of congenital toxoplasmosis. Am J Ophthalmol. 1997;123(1):1–16.
462. Kodjikian L, Wallon M, Fleury J, Denis P, Binquet C, Peyron F, Garweg JG. Ocular manifestations in congenital toxoplasmosis. Graefes Arch Clin Exp Ophthalmol. 2006;244(1):14–21.
463. O'Neill JF. The ocular manifestations of congenital infection: a study of the early effect and long-term outcome of maternally transmitted rubella and toxoplasmosis. Trans Am Ophthalmol Soc. 1998;96:813–79.
464. Rassi A, Todorich B, Faia LJ, Trese M, Drenser K, Capone A Jr. Congenital toxoplasmosis associated with tractional retinal detachment. Retin Cases Brief Rep. 2021;15(3):243–5.
465. Cochereau-Massin I, LeHoang P, Lautier-Frau M, Zerdoun E, Zazoun L, Robinet M, Marcel P, Girard B, Katlama C, Leport C, et al. Ocular toxoplasmosis in human immunodeficiency virus-infected patients. Am J Ophthalmol. 1992;114(2):130–5.
466. Park YH, Nam HW. Clinical features and treatment of ocular toxoplasmosis. Korean J Parasitol. 2013;51(4):393–9.
467. Rothova A. Ocular manifestations of toxoplasmosis. Curr Opin Ophthalmol. 2003;14(6):384–8.
468. Smith JR, Cunningham ET Jr. Atypical presentations of ocular toxoplasmosis. Curr Opin Ophthalmol. 2002;13(6):387–92.
469. Hovakimyan A, Cunningham ET Jr. Ocular toxoplasmosis. Ophthalmol Clin North Am. 2002;15(3):327–32.
470. Fardeau C, Romand S, Rao NA, Cassoux N, Bettembourg O, Thulliez P, Lehoang P. Diagnosis of toxoplasmic retinochoroiditis with atypical clinical features. Am J Ophthalmol. 2002;134(2):196–203.
471. Labalette P, Delhaes L, Margaron F, Fortier B, Rouland JF. Ocular toxoplasmosis after the fifth decade. Am J Ophthalmol. 2002b;133(4):506–15.
472. Schuman JS, Weinberg RS, Ferry AP, Guerry RK. Toxoplasmic scleritis. Ophthalmology. 1988;95(10):1399–403.
473. Harper TW, Miller D, Schiffman JC, Davis JL. Polymerase chain reaction analysis of aqueous and vitreous specimens in the diagnosis of posterior segment infectious uveitis. Am J Ophthalmol. 2009;147(1):140–147 e142.
474. Rothova A, de Boer JH, Ten Dam-van Loon NH, Postma G, de Visser L, Zuurveen SJ, Schuller M, Weersink AJ, van Loon AM, de Groot-Mijnes JD. Usefulness of aqueous humor analysis for the diagnosis of posterior uveitis. Ophthalmology. 2008;115(2):306–11.
475. Mathis T, Beccat S, Seve P, Peyron F, Wallon M, Kodjikian L. Comparison of immunoblotting (IgA and IgG) and the Goldmann-Witmer coefficient for diagnosis of ocular toxoplasmosis in immunocompetent patients. Br J Ophthalmol. 2018;102(10):1454–8.
476. Robert-Gangneux F, Binisti P, Antonetti D, Brezin A, Yera H, Dupouy-Camet J. Usefulness of immunoblotting and Goldmann-Witmer coefficient for biological diagnosis of toxoplasmic retinochoroiditis. Eur J Clin Microbiol Infect Dis. 2004;23(1):34–8.

477. Fekkar A, Bodaghi B, Touafek F, Le Hoang P, Mazier D, Paris L. Comparison of immunoblotting, calculation of the Goldmann-Witmer coefficient, and real-time PCR using aqueous humor samples for diagnosis of ocular toxoplasmosis. J Clin Microbiol. 2008;46(6):1965–7.
478. Talabani H, Asseraf M, Yera H, Delair E, Ancelle T, Thulliez P, Brezin AP, Dupouy-Camet J. Contributions of immunoblotting, real-time PCR, and the Goldmann-Witmer coefficient to diagnosis of atypical toxoplasmic retinochoroiditis. J Clin Microbiol. 2009;47(7):2131–5.
479. Fawzy M, Mahmoud LA, El Gindy AE, Hegab MA, Bahgat MA. Value of estimating intraocular antibody production in diagnosis of typical and atypical lesions of ocular toxoplasmosis. J Egypt Soc Parasitol. 1999;29(3):735–43.
480. De Marco R, Ceccarelli R, Frulio R, Palmero C, Vittone P. Retinochoroiditis associated with congenital toxoplasmosis in children: IgG antibody profiles demonstrating the synthesis of local antibodies. Eur J Ophthalmol. 2003;13(1):74–9.
481. Garweg JG, Garweg SD, Flueckiger F, Jacquier P, Boehnke M. Aqueous humor and serum immunoblotting for immunoglobulin types G, A, M, and E in cases of human ocular toxoplasmosis. J Clin Microbiol. 2004;42(10):4593–8.
482. Ronday MJ, Ongkosuwito JV, Rothova A, Kijlstra A. Intraocular anti-Toxoplasma gondii IgA antibody production in patients with ocular toxoplasmosis. Am J Ophthalmol. 1999;127(3):294–300.
483. Farhadi A, Haniloo A, Fazaeli A, Moradian S, Farhadi M. PCR-based diagnosis of toxoplasma parasite in ocular infections having clinical indications of toxoplasmosis. Iran J Parasitol. 2017;12(1):56–62.
484. Rudzinski M, Arguelles C, Couto C, Oubina JR, Reina S. Immune mediators against toxoplasma gondii during reactivation of toxoplasmic retinochoroiditis. Ocul Immunol Inflamm. 2019;27(6):949–57.
485. Matias M, Gomes A, Marques T, Fonseca AC. Ocular toxoplasmosis: a very rare presentation in an immunocompetent patient. BMJ Case Rep. 2014;2014:bcr2014205846.
486. Accorinti M, Bruscolini A, Pirraglia MP, Liverani M, Caggiano C. Toxoplasmic retinochoroiditis in an Italian referral center. Eur J Ophthalmol. 2009;19(5):824–30.
487. Borkowski PK, Brydak-Godowska J, Basiak W, Switaj K, Zarnowska-Prymek H, Olszynska-Krowicka M, Kajfasz P, Rabczenko D. The impact of short-term, intensive antifolate treatment (with pyrimethamine and sulfadoxine) and antibiotics followed by long-term, secondary antifolate prophylaxis on the rate of toxoplasmic retinochoroiditis recurrence. PLoS Negl Trop Dis. 2016;10(8):e0004892.
488. Bawdekar AC, Jindal A, Shah M, Pathengay A, Shah M. Intravitreal triamcinolone acetonide in management of ocular toxoplasmosis in an HIV patient: a case report. Can J Ophthalmol. 2013;48(4):e94–5.
489. Eyles DE, Coleman N. Synergistic effect of sulfadiazine and daraprim against experimental toxoplasmosis in the mouse. Antibiot Chemother (Northfield). 1953;3(5):483–90.
490. Eyles DE, Coleman N. The effect of metabolites on the antitoxoplasmic action of pyrimethamine and sulfadiazine. Am J Trop Med Hyg. 1960;9:277–83.
491. Bosch-Driessen LH, Verbraak FD, Suttorp-Schulten MS, van Ruyven RL, Klok AM, Hoyng CB, Rothova A. A prospective, randomized trial of pyrimethamine and azithromycin vs pyrimethamine and sulfadiazine for the treatment of ocular toxoplasmosis. Am J Ophthalmol. 2002b;134(1):34–40.
492. Guaraldo L, Villar BBF, Durao NMG, Louro VC, Quintana MSB, Curi ALL, Neves ES. Ocular toxoplasmosis: adverse reactions to treatment in a Brazilian cohort. Trans R Soc Trop Med Hyg. 2018;112(4):188–92.
493. Zhang Y, Lin X, Lu F. Current treatment of ocular toxoplasmosis in immunocompetent patients: a network meta-analysis. Acta Trop. 2018;185:52–62.
494. Ben-Harari RR, Goodwin E, Casoy J. Adverse event profile of pyrimethamine-based therapy in toxoplasmosis: a systematic review. Drugs R D. 2017;17(4):523–44.
495. Jasper S, Vedula SS, John SS, Horo S, Sepah YJ, Nguyen QD. Corticosteroids as adjuvant therapy for ocular toxoplasmosis. Cochrane Database Syst Rev. 2017;1:CD007417.

496. Moreira FV, Iwanusk AM, Amaral ARD, Nobrega MJ, Novelli FJ. Surgical outcomes of rhegmatogenous retinal detachment associated with ocular toxoplasmosis. Arq Bras Oftalmol. 2018;81(4):281–5.
497. Magnaval JF, Bouhsira E, Fillaux J. Therapy and prevention for human toxocariasis. Microorganisms. 2022;10(2):241.
498. Molk R. Ocular toxocariasis: a review of the literature. Ann Ophthalmol. 1983;15(3):216–9, 222-217, 230-211.
499. Schneier AJ, Durand ML. Ocular toxocariasis: advances in diagnosis and treatment. Int Ophthalmol Clin. 2011;51(4):135–44.
500. Hu XF, Feng J, Kang H, Wang H, Liu XH, Tao Y. Clinical characteristics of ocular toxocariasis in adults in north China. Int J Ophthalmol. 2022;15(3):401–6.
501. Stewart JM, Cubillan LD, Cunningham ET Jr. Prevalence, clinical features, and causes of vision loss among patients with ocular toxocariasis. Retina. 2005;25(8):1005–13.
502. Schantz PM. Toxocara larva migrans now. Am J Trop Med Hyg. 1989;41(3 Suppl):21–34.
503. Rahimi M, Oustad M, Ashrafi A. Demographic and clinical features of pediatric uveitis at a Tertiary Referral Center in Iran. Middle East Afr J Ophthalmol. 2016;23(3):237–40.
504. Badri M, Eslahi AV, Olfatifar M, Dalvand S, Houshmand E, Abdoli A, Majidiani H, Eslami A, Zibaei M, Johkool MG, et al. Keys to unlock the enigma of ocular toxocariasis: a systematic review and meta-analysis. Ocul Immunol Inflamm. 2021;29(7-8):1265–76.
505. Chieffi PP, Santos SV, Queiroz ML, Lescano SA. Human toxocariasis: contribution by Brazilian researchers. Rev Inst Med Trop Sao Paulo. 2009;51(6):301–8.
506. Rubinsky-Elefant G, Hirata CE, Yamamoto JH, Ferreira MU. Human toxocariasis: diagnosis, worldwide seroprevalences and clinical expression of the systemic and ocular forms. Ann Trop Med Parasitol. 2010;104(1):3–23.
507. Ahn SJ, Woo SJ, Jin Y, Chang YS, Kim TW, Ahn J, Heo JW, Yu HG, Chung H, Park KH, et al. Clinical features and course of ocular toxocariasis in adults. PLoS Negl Trop Dis. 2014;8(6):e2938.
508. Centers for Disease C, Prevention. Ocular toxocariasis—United States, 2009-2010. MMWR Morb Mortal Wkly Rep. 2011;60(22):734–6.
509. Wang H, Tao Y. Clinical features and prognostic factors in northern Chinese patients with peripheral granuloma type of ocular toxocariasis: a retrospective cohort study. Ocul Immunol Inflamm. 2021b;29(7-8):1259–64.
510. Wan WL, Cano MR, Pince KJ, Green RL. Echographic characteristics of ocular toxocariasis. Ophthalmology. 1991;98(1):28–32.
511. Shields JA. Ocular toxocariasis. A review. Surv Ophthalmol. 1984;28(5):361–81.
512. Woodhall D, Starr MC, Montgomery SP, Jones JL, Lum F, Read RW, Moorthy RS. Ocular toxocariasis: epidemiologic, anatomic, and therapeutic variations based on a survey of ophthalmic subspecialists. Ophthalmology. 2012;119(6):1211–7.
513. Guo X, Liu H, Li M, Fan K, Li S, Lei B. Multimodality image analysis in a cohort of patients with atypical juvenile ocular toxocariasis. J Ophthalmol. 2021;2021:4853531.
514. Despreaux R, Fardeau C, Touhami S, Brasnu E, Champion E, Paris L, Touitou V, Bodaghi B, Lehoang P. Ocular toxocariasis: clinical features and long-term visual outcomes in adult patients. Am J Ophthalmol. 2016;166:162–8.
515. Martinez J, Ivankovich-Escoto G, Wu L. Pediatric ocular toxocariasis in Costa Rica: 1998-2018 experience. Ocul Immunol Inflamm. 2021;29(7-8):1246–51.
516. Kennedy JJ, Defeo E. Ocular toxocariasis demonstrated by ultrasound. Ann Ophthalmol. 1981;13(12):1357–8.
517. Morais FB, Maciel AL, Arantes TE, Muccioli C, Allemann N. Ultrasonographic findings in ocular toxocariasis. Arq Bras Oftalmol. 2012;75(1):43–7.
518. Gupta A, Tripathy K. Ocular Toxocariasis. In: StatPearls. Treasure Island, FL: StatPearls; 2022.
519. Rubinsky-Elefant G, Yamamoto JH, Hirata CE, Prestes-Carneiro LE. Toxocariasis: critical analysis of serology in patients attending a public referral center for ophthalmology in Brazil. Jpn J Ophthalmol. 2018;62(1):77–83.

520. Sowemimo OA, Lee YL, Asaolu SO, Chuang TW, Akinwale OP, Badejoko BO, Gyang VP, Nwafor T, Henry E, Fan CK. Seroepidemiological study and associated risk factors of Toxocara canis infection among preschool children in Osun State, Nigeria. Acta Trop. 2017;173:85–9.
521. Inchauspe S, Echandi LV, Dodds EM. Diagnosis of ocular toxocariasis by detecting antibodies in the vitreous humor. Arch Soc Esp Oftalmol (Engl Ed). 2018;93(5):220–4.
522. Iddawela D, Ehambaram K, Bandara P. Prevalence of Toxocara antibodies among patients clinically suspected to have ocular toxocariasis: a retrospective descriptive study in Sri Lanka. BMC Ophthalmol. 2017;17(1):50.
523. Wang ZJ, Zhou M, Cao WJ, Ji J, Bi YW, Huang X, Xu GZ. Evaluation of the Goldmann-Witmer coefficient in the immunological diagnosis of ocular toxocariasis. Acta Trop. 2016a;158:20–3.
524. Huang L, Sun L, Liu C, Li S, Zhang T, Luo X, Ding X. Diagnosis of ocular toxocariasis by serum and aqueous humor IgG ELISA. Transl Vis Sci Technol. 2021;10(8):33.
525. Alabiad CR, Albini TA, Santos CI, Davis JL. Ocular toxocariasis in a seronegative adult. Ophthalmic surg lasers imaging; 2010. p. 1–3.
526. Tian JX, O'Hagan S. Toxocara polymerase chain reaction on ocular fluids in bilateral granulomatous chorioretinitis. Int Med Case Rep J. 2015;8:107–10.
527. Jee D, Kim KS, Lee WK, Kim W, Jeon S. Clinical features of ocular toxocariasis in adult Korean patients. Ocul Immunol Inflamm. 2016;24(2):207–16.
528. Jiang Z, Sun L, Ding X, Zhang T, Li S, Ding X. Cytokine profile in aqueous humor of patients with ocular toxocariasis. Front Med (Lausanne). 2022;9:869976.
529. Marques A, Rodrigues A, Belo S, Guedes ME. Unusual panuveitis in a child: toxocariasis associated with ocular myiasis. BMJ Case Rep. 2014;2014:bcr2014204475.
530. Cai Y, Yang Y, Zhong X. A case report of intravitreal Dexamethasone implant with exudative retinal detachment for ocular toxocariasis treatment. Korean J Parasitol. 2022;60(2):133–7.
531. Frazier M, Anderson ML, Sophocleous S. Treatment of ocular toxocariasis with albendezole: a case report. Optometry. 2009;80(4):175–80.
532. Yoon DY, Woo SJ. Intravitreal administration of Ranibizumab and Bevacizumab for choroidal neovascularization secondary to ocular toxocariasis: a case report. Ocul Immunol Inflamm. 2018;26(4):639–41.
533. Sathiamoorthi S, Smith WM. The eye and tick-borne disease in the United States. Curr Opin Ophthalmol. 2016;27(6):530–7.
534. Radolf JD, Strle K, Lemieux JE, Strle F. Lyme disease in humans. Curr Issues Mol Biol. 2021;42:333–84.
535. Pritt BS, Mead PS, Johnson DKH, Neitzel DF, Respicio-Kingry LB, Davis JP, Schiffman E, Sloan LM, Schriefer ME, Replogle AJ, et al. Identification of a novel pathogenic Borrelia species causing Lyme borreliosis with unusually high spirochaetaemia: a descriptive study. Lancet Infect Dis. 2016;16(5):556–64.
536. Smith JL, Winward KE, Nicholson DF, Albert DW. Retinal vasculitis in Lyme borreliosis. J Clin Neuroophthalmol. 1991;11(1):7–15.
537. Shapiro ED. Borrelia burgdorferi (Lyme disease). Pediatr Rev. 2014;35(12):500–9.
538. Wan K-L. Current status and an outlook of Chinese Lyme disease. Chin J Vector Biol Control. 1998;9(6):401–5.
539. Niu Q-L, Yin H, Luo J-X. Progress on Lyme disease in China. Progr Vet Med. 2009;30(10):89–93.
540. Karma A, Seppala I, Mikkila H, Kaakkola S, Viljanen M, Tarkkanen A. Diagnosis and clinical characteristics of ocular Lyme borreliosis. Am J Ophthalmol. 1995;119(2):127–35.
541. Ross Russell AL, Dryden MS, Pinto AA, Lovett JK. Lyme disease: diagnosis and management. Pract Neurol. 2018;18(6):455–64.
542. Chomel B. Lyme disease. Rev Sci Tech. 2015;34(2):569–76.
543. Gerster JC, Peter O. Rheumatic manifestations related to acrodermatitis chronica atrophicans. A review of four cases. Rev Rhum Engl Ed. 1998;65(10):567–70.

544. Mikkila HO, Seppala IJ, Viljanen MK, Peltomaa MP, Karma A. The expanding clinical spectrum of ocular lyme borreliosis. Ophthalmology. 2000;107(3):581–7.
545. Steere AC, Bartenhagen NH, Craft JE, Hutchinson GJ, Newman JH, Rahn DW, Sigal LH, Spieler PN, Stenn KS, Malawista SE. The early clinical manifestations of Lyme disease. Ann Intern Med. 1983;99(1):76–82.
546. Morrison C, Seifter A, Aucott JN. Unusual presentation of Lyme disease: Horner syndrome with negative serology. J Am Board Fam Med. 2009;22(2):219–22.
547. Bergloff J, Gasser R, Feigl B. Ophthalmic manifestations in Lyme borreliosis. A review. J Neuroophthalmol. 1994;14(1):15–20.
548. Traisk F, Lindquist L. Optic nerve involvement in Lyme disease. Curr Opin Ophthalmol. 2012;23(6):485–90.
549. Rothermel H, Hedges TR 3rd, Steere AC. Optic neuropathy in children with Lyme disease. Pediatrics. 2001;108(2):477–81.
550. Raja H, Starr MR, Bakri SJ. Ocular manifestations of tick-borne diseases. Surv Ophthalmol. 2016a;61(6):726–44.
551. Sainz de la Maza M, Hemady RK, Foster CS. Infectious scleritis: report of four cases. Doc Ophthalmol. 1993;83(1):33–41.
552. Krist D, Wenkel H. Posterior scleritis associated with Borrelia burgdorferi (Lyme disease) infection. Ophthalmology. 2002;109(1):143–5.
553. Mikkila H, Karma A, Viljanen M, Seppala I. The laboratory diagnosis of ocular Lyme borreliosis. Graefes Arch Clin Exp Ophthalmol. 1999;237(3):225–30.
554. Seppala IJ, Kroneld R, Schauman K, Forsen KO, Lassenius R. Diagnosis of Lyme borreliosis: non-specific serological reactions with Borrelia burgdorferi sonicate antigen caused by IgG2 antibodies. J Med Microbiol. 1994;40(4):293–302.
555. Bernard A, Kodjikian L, Abukhashabh A, Roure-Sobas C, Boibieux A, Denis P, Broussolle C, Seve P. Diagnosis of Lyme-associated uveitis: value of serological testing in a tertiary centre. Br J Ophthalmol. 2018;102(3):369–72.
556. Magnarelli LA, Anderson JF, Johnson RC. Cross-reactivity in serological tests for Lyme disease and other spirochetal infections. J Infect Dis. 1987;156(1):183–8.
557. Steere AC. Lyme disease. N Engl J Med. 1989;321(9):586–96.
558. Steere AC, Duray PH, Kauffmann DJ, Wormser GP. Unilateral blindness caused by infection with the Lyme disease spirochete, Borrelia burgdorferi. Ann Intern Med. 1985;103(3):382–4.
559. Schubert HD, Greenebaum E, Neu HC. Cytologically proven seronegative Lyme choroiditis and vitritis. Retina. 1994;14(1):39–42.
560. Preac-Mursic V, Pfister HW, Spiegel H, Burk R, Wilske B, Reinhardt S, Bohmer R. First isolation of Borrelia burgdorferi from an iris biopsy. J Clin Neuroophthalmol. 1993;13(3):155–61; discussion 162.
561. Marques AR. Laboratory diagnosis of Lyme disease: advances and challenges. Infect Dis Clin North Am. 2015;29(2):295–307.
562. Picken MM, Picken RN, Han D, Cheng Y, Ruzic-Sabljic E, Cimperman J, Maraspin V, Lotric-Furlan S, Strle F. A two year prospective study to compare culture and polymerase chain reaction amplification for the detection and diagnosis of Lyme borreliosis. Mol Pathol. 1997;50(4):186–93.
563. Liveris D, Wang G, Girao G, Byrne DW, Nowakowski J, McKenna D, Nadelman R, Wormser GP, Schwartz I. Quantitative detection of Borrelia burgdorferi in 2-millimeter skin samples of erythema migrans lesions: correlation of results with clinical and laboratory findings. J Clin Microbiol. 2002;40(4):1249–53.
564. Liveris D, Schwartz I, McKenna D, Nowakowski J, Nadelman R, Demarco J, Iyer R, Bittker S, Cooper D, Holmgren D, et al. Comparison of five diagnostic modalities for direct detection of Borrelia burgdorferi in patients with early Lyme disease. Diagn Microbiol Infect Dis. 2012;73(3):243–5.

565. O'Rourke M, Traweger A, Lusa L, Stupica D, Maraspin V, Barrett PN, Strle F, Livey I. Quantitative detection of Borrelia burgdorferi sensu lato in erythema migrans skin lesions using internally controlled duplex real time PCR. PLoS One. 2013;8(5):e63968.
566. Karma A, Pirttila TA, Viljanen MK, Lahde YE, Raitta CM. Secondary retinitis pigmentosa and cerebral demyelination in Lyme borreliosis. Br J Ophthalmol. 1993;77(2):120–2.
567. Tilly K, Rosa PA, Stewart PE. Biology of infection with Borrelia burgdorferi. Infect Dis Clin North Am. 2008;22(2):217–34, v.
568. Karma A, Mikkila H. Ocular manifestations and treatment of Lyme disease. Curr Opin Ophthalmol. 1996;7(3):7–12.
569. Kullberg BJ, Vrijmoeth HD, van de Schoor F, Hovius JW. Lyme borreliosis: diagnosis and management. BMJ. 2020;369:m1041.
570. Bazzazi N, Yavarikia A, Keramat F. Ocular involvement of brucellosis. Middle East Afr J Ophthalmol. 2013;20(1):95–7.
571. Tabbara KF, Al-Kassimi H. Ocular brucellosis. Br J Ophthalmol. 1990;74(4):249–50.
572. Rajabi J, Hamidi-Farahani R, Mansouri F, Soleiman-Meigooni S. Incidence and risk factors of Brucellosis in Kermanshah Province, Iran during 2010-2014. Infect Disord Drug Targets. 2020;20(2):203–7.
573. Kaufmann AF, Fox MD, Boyce JM, Anderson DC, Potter ME, Martone WJ, Patton CM. Airborne spread of brucellosis. Ann N Y Acad Sci. 1980;353:105–14.
574. Walker J, Sharma OP, Rao NA. Brucellosis and uveitis. Am J Ophthalmol. 1992;114(3):374–5.
575. Al Dahouk S, Tomaso H, Nockler K, Neubauer H, Frangoulidis D. Laboratory-based diagnosis of brucellosis—a review of the literature. Part II: serological tests for brucellosis. Clin Lab. 2003;49(11-12):577–89.
576. Hasanjani Roushan MR, Ebrahimpour S. Human brucellosis: an overview. Caspian J Intern Med. 2015;6(1):46–7.
577. Pappas G, Akritidis N, Bosilkovski M, Tsianos E. Brucellosis. N Engl J Med. 2005;352(22):2325–36.
578. Rolando I, Olarte L, Vilchez G, Lluncor M, Otero L, Paris M, Carrillo C, Gotuzzo E. Ocular manifestations associated with brucellosis: a 26-year experience in Peru. Clin Infect Dis. 2008;46(9):1338–45.
579. Sungur GK, Hazirolan D, Gurbuz Y, Unlu N, Duran S, Duman S. Ocular involvement in brucellosis. Can J Ophthalmol. 2009;44(5):598–601.
580. Gungur K, Bekir NA, Namiduru M. Ocular complications associated with brucellosis in an endemic area. Eur J Ophthalmol. 2002;12(3):232–7.
581. Puig Solanes M, Heatley J, Arenas F, Guerrero Ibarra G. Ocular complications in brucellosis. Am J Ophthalmol. 1953;36(5):675–89.
582. Pacheco G, Veiga GP. Brucellosis as a medical and social problem; otolaringologica and ocular brucellosis. Rev Bras Med. 1946;3(7):574–7.
583. McCullough FE. Ocular brucellosis. Miss Doct. 1953;30(8):249–50.
584. Ghasemi Barghi R, Meraat H, Pahlevan AA. A review on ophthalmic manifestations of brucellosis and reporting a case of ophthalmic brucellosis. Iran Red Crescent Med J. 2011;13(5):352–3.
585. Rabinowitz R, Schneck M, Levy J, Lifshitz T. Bilateral multifocal choroiditis with serous retinal detachment in a patient with Brucella infection: case report and review of the literature. Arch Ophthalmol. 2005;123(1):116–8.
586. Rolando I, Vilchez G, Olarte L, Lluncor M, Carrillo C, Paris M, Guerra H, Gotuzzo E. Brucellar uveitis: intraocular fluids and biopsy studies. Int J Infect Dis. 2009;13(5):e206–11.
587. Corbel MJ. Brucellosis: an overview. Emerg Infect Dis. 1997;3(2):213–21.
588. Li YJ, Li XL, Liang S, Fang LQ, Cao WC. Epidemiological features and risk factors associated with the spatial and temporal distribution of human brucellosis in China. BMC Infect Dis. 2013;13:547.

589. Zheng R, Xie S, Lu X, Sun L, Zhou Y, Zhang Y, Wang K. A systematic review and meta-analysis of epidemiology and clinical manifestations of human brucellosis in China. Biomed Res Int. 2018;2018:5712920.
590. Abd Elrazak M. Brucella optic neuritis. Arch Intern Med. 1991;151(4):776–8.
591. Karakurum Goksel B, Yerdelen D, Karatas M, Pelit A, Demiroglu YZ, Kizilkilic O, Tan M, Toygar O. Abducens nerve palsy and optic neuritis as initial manifestation in brucellosis. Scand J Infect Dis. 2006;38(8):721–5.
592. Tunc M, Durukan H. Bilateral severe visual loss in brucellosis. Ocul Immunol Inflamm. 2004;12(3):233–6.
593. Al Faran MF. Brucella melitensis endogenous endophthalmitis. Ophthalmologica. 1990;201(1):19–22.
594. Chiu CY, Miller SA. Clinical metagenomics. Nat Rev Genet. 2019;20(6):341–55.
595. Xi H, Zhang L, Xu B, Liu H, Li S. Metagenomic next-generation sequencing to investigate infectious endophthalmitis of Brucella: a case report. Front Med (Lausanne). 2022;9:847143.
596. Shakir R. Brucellosis. J Neurol Sci. 2021;420:117280.
597. Ntirandekura JB, Matemba LE, Kimera SI, Muma JB, Karimuribo ED. Association of Brucellosis with abortion prevalence in humans and animals in africa: a review. Afr J Reprod Health. 2018;22(3):120–36.
598. Durand ML. Bacterial and fungal endophthalmitis. Clin Microbiol Rev. 2017;30(3):597–613.
599. Callegan MC, Booth MC, Jett BD, Gilmore MS. Pathogenesis of gram-positive bacterial endophthalmitis. Infect Immun. 1999;67(7):3348–56.
600. O'Callaghan RJ. The pathogenesis of Staphylococcus aureus eye infections. Pathogens. 2018;7(1):9.
601. Colas-Tomas T, Perez-Trigo S. Delayed-onset endophthalmitis following implantation of a XEN45 glaucoma device: a case report. J Glaucoma. 2018;27(10):936–8.
602. Muda R, Vayavari V, Subbiah D, Ishak H, Adnan A, Mohamed SO. Endogenous endophthalmitis: a 9-year retrospective study at a tertiary referral hospital in Malaysia. J Ophthalmic Inflamm Infect. 2018;8(1):14.
603. Michael NDB, Gunaseelan S, Tuan Jaffar TN, Noordin Z, Hussein A. Endogenous endophthalmitis: a five-year review of cases at the Raja Perempuan Zainab II Hospital, Kelantan, Malaysia. Cureus. 2018;10(7):e3066.
604. Harvey JP. Endogenous bacterial endophthalmitis and subretinal abscess complicating diabetic ketoacidosis. BMJ Case Rep. 2018;2018:bcr2018227025.
605. Joseph J, Sharma S, Narayanan R. Endogenous Cryptococcus neoformans endophthalmitis with subretinal abscess in a HIV-infected man. Indian J Ophthalmol. 2018;66(7):1015–7.
606. Rubin U, Benson MD, Kulkarni S, Greve MDJ. Endogenous endophthalmitis due to Klebsiella pneumoniae from an infected gallbladder. Can J Ophthalmol. 2018;53(6):e258–60.
607. Armesto E, Cubillas M, Anton S. Bacterial endogenous endophthalmitis after colonoscopy. Rev Esp Enferm Dig. 2018;110(9):601.
608. Lei B, Jiang R, Gu R, Xu G, Song F, Zhou M. Endogenous fungal endophthalmitis associated with genitourinary procedures. Ocul Immunol Inflamm. 2019;27(5):747–55.
609. AlQahtani GMS, AlSayed AAD, Gangadharan S, Adhi MI. Fungal endophthalmitis in a case of granulomatosis with polyangitis. Saudi J Ophthalmol. 2018;32(3):261–5.
610. Fernandez-Ruiz M, Vargas JC, Ruiz-Ruigomez M. Bilateral endophthalmitis as the initial presentation of pneumococcal endocarditis. Enferm Infecc Microbiol Clin (Engl Ed). 2019;37(7):488–90.
611. Schmid S, Martenet AC, Oelz O. Candida endophthalmitis: clinical presentation, treatment and outcome in 23 patients. Infection. 1991;19(1):21–4.
612. Jackson TL, Eykyn SJ, Graham EM, Stanford MR. Endogenous bacterial endophthalmitis: a 17-year prospective series and review of 267 reported cases. Surv Ophthalmol. 2003;48(4):403–23.

613. Lalwani GA, Flynn HW Jr, Scott IU, Quinn CM, Berrocal AM, Davis JL, Murray TG, Smiddy WE, Miller D. Acute-onset endophthalmitis after clear corneal cataract surgery (1996-2005). Clinical features, causative eorganisms, and visual acuity outcomes. Ophthalmology. 2008;115(3):473–6.
614. Taban M, Behrens A, Newcomb RL, Nobe MY, Saedi G, Sweet PM, McDonnell PJ. Acute endophthalmitis following cataract surgery: a systematic review of the literature. Arch Ophthalmol. 2005;123(5):613–20.
615. Zafar S, Siddiqui MAR. Sub-retinal abscess as presenting feature of endogenous Candida endophthalmitis. BMC Res Notes. 2018;11(1):598.
616. Mithal K, Pathengay A, Bawdekar A, Jindal A, Vira D, Relhan N, Choudhury H, Gupta N, Gupta V, Koday NK, et al. Filamentous fungal endophthalmitis: results of combination therapy with intravitreal amphotericin B and voriconazole. Clin Ophthalmol. 2015;9:649–55.
617. Mota SH. Pseudomonas aeruginosa-induced bilateral endophthalmitis after bilateral simultaneous cataract surgery: case report. Arq Bras Oftalmol. 2018;81(4):339–40.
618. Rashaed SA, Rushood A. Acute bacterial endophthalmitis after intravitreal bevacizumab injection: case report and literature review. Saudi J Ophthalmol. 2013;27(1):55–7.
619. Agarwal AK, Aggarwal K, Samanta R, Angrup A, Biswal M, Ray P, Dogra M, Katoch D, Bansal R, Singh R, et al. Cluster endophthalmitis due to Stenotrophomonas maltophilia following intravitreal bevacizumab: outcomes of patients from North India. Br J Ophthalmol. 2019c;103(9):1278–83.
620. Dave VP, Pathengay A, Sharma S, Naveen N, Basu S, Pappuru RR, Das T. Diagnosis, clinical presentations, and outcomes of nocardia endophthalmitis. Am J Ophthalmol. 2019;197:53–8.
621. Pongsachareonnont P, Honglertnapakul W, Chatsuwan T. Comparison of methods for identifying causative bacterial microorganisms in presumed acute endophthalmitis: conventional culture, blood culture, and PCR. BMC Infect Dis. 2017;17(1):165.
622. Bispo PJ, de Melo GB, Hofling-Lima AL, Pignatari AC. Detection and gram discrimination of bacterial pathogens from aqueous and vitreous humor using real-time PCR assays. Invest Ophthalmol Vis Sci. 2011;52(2):873–81.
623. Sowmya P, Madhavan HN. Diagnostic utility of polymerase chain reaction on intraocular specimens to establish the etiology of infectious endophthalmitis. Eur J Ophthalmol. 2009;19(5):812–7.
624. Seal D, Reischl U, Behr A, Ferrer C, Alio J, Koerner RJ, Barry P, Group EES. Laboratory diagnosis of endophthalmitis: comparison of microbiology and molecular methods in the European Society of Cataract & Refractive Surgeons multicenter study and susceptibility testing. J Cataract Refract Surg. 2008;34(9):1439–50.
625. Chiquet C, Lina G, Benito Y, Cornut PL, Etienne J, Romanet JP, Denis P, Vandenesch F. Polymerase chain reaction identification in aqueous humor of patients with postoperative endophthalmitis. J Cataract Refract Surg. 2007;33(4):635–41.
626. Anand AR, Madhavan HN, Therese KL. Use of polymerase chain reaction (PCR) and DNA probe hybridization to determine the Gram reaction of the infecting bacterium in the intraocular fluids of patients with endophthalmitis. J Infect. 2000;41(3):221–6.
627. Hykin PG, Tobal K, McIntyre G, Matheson MM, Towler HM, Lightman SL. The diagnosis of delayed post-operative endophthalmitis by polymerase chain reaction of bacterial DNA in vitreous samples. J Med Microbiol. 1994;40(6):408–15.
628. Mishra D, Satpathy G, Chawla R, Venkatesh P, Ahmed NH, Panda SK. Utility of broad-range 16S rRNA PCR assay versus conventional methods for laboratory diagnosis of bacterial endophthalmitis in a tertiary care hospital. Br J Ophthalmol. 2019;103(1):152–6.
629. Srinivasan R, Karaoz U, Volegova M, MacKichan J, Kato-Maeda M, Miller S, Nadarajan R, Brodie EL, Lynch SV. Use of 16S rRNA gene for identification of a broad range of clinically relevant bacterial pathogens. PLoS One. 2015;10(2):e0117617.
630. Ogawa M, Sugita S, Watanabe K, Shimizu N, Mochizuki M. Novel diagnosis of fungal endophthalmitis by broad-range real-time PCR detection of fungal 28S ribosomal DNA. Graefes Arch Clin Exp Ophthalmol. 2012;250(12):1877–83.

631. Budding AE, Hoogewerf M, Vandenbroucke-Grauls CM, Savelkoul PH. Automated broad-range molecular detection of bacteria in clinical samples. J Clin Microbiol. 2016;54(4):934–43.
632. Deshmukh D, Joseph J, Chakrabarti M, Sharma S, Jayasudha R, Sama KC, Sontam B, Tyagi M, Narayanan R, Shivaji S. New insights into culture negative endophthalmitis by unbiased next generation sequencing. Sci Rep. 2019;9(1):844.
633. Qian Z, Zhang Y, Wang L, Li Z, Wang H, Kang H, Feng J, Hu X, Tao Y. Application of metagenomic next-generation sequencing in suspected intraocular infections. Eur J Ophthalmol. 2022b;33:391.
634. Kolomeyer AM, Murphy KM, Traband A, Frank I, Kim BJ. Beta-D-Glucan testing in patients with fungal endophthalmitis. Retina. 2018;38(4):650–9.
635. Flynn HW Jr. The clinical challenge of endogenous endophthalmitis. Retina. 2001;21(6):572–4.
636. Slowik M, Biernat MM, Urbaniak-Kujda D, Kapelko-Slowik K, Misiuk-Hojlo M. Mycotic infections of the eye. Adv Clin Exp Med. 2015;24(6):1113–7.
637. Obayashi T, Yoshida M, Tamura H, Aketagawa J, Tanaka S, Kawai T. Determination of plasma (1-->3)-beta-D-glucan: a new diagnostic aid to deep mycosis. J Med Vet Mycol. 1992;30(4):275–80.
638. Yoshida K, Niki Y, Ohno M, Watanabe S, Hashiguchi K, Nakajima M, Matsushima T. Clinical significance of (1-->3)-beta-D-glucan in pleural effusion and liquor. Kansenshogaku Zasshi. 1997;71(12):1210–5.
639. Myint T, Chow FC, Bloch KC, Raymond-Guillen L, Davis TE, Wright PW, Woc-Colburn L, Khairy RN, Street AC, Yamamoto T, et al. Detection of (1,3)-beta-d-Glucan in cerebrospinal fluid in histoplasma meningitis. J Clin Microbiol. 2018;56(10):e00663.
640. Yasuoka A, Tachikawa N, Shimada K, Kimura S, Oka S. (1-->3) beta-D-glucan as a quantitative serological marker for Pneumocystis carinii pneumonia. Clin Diagn Lab Immunol. 1996;3(2):197–9.
641. Jeragh A, Ahmad S, Naseem J, Khan ZU. Candida lusitaniae arthritis in an intravenous drug user. Mycoses. 2007;50(5):430–2.
642. Chen L, Tao Y, Hu X. Utility of intraocular fluid beta-D-glucan testing in fungal endophthalmitis: a series of 5 cases. Am J Case Rep. 2020a;21:e921188.
643. Shimbo M, Ito N, Kadonosono K. Investigation of beta-D-glucan values in the vitreous. Nippon Ganka Gakkai Zasshi. 2002;106(9):579–82.
644. De Pauw B, Walsh TJ, Donnelly JP, Stevens DA, Edwards JE, Calandra T, Pappas PG, Maertens J, Lortholary O, Kauffman CA, et al. Revised definitions of invasive fungal disease from the European Organization for Research and Treatment of Cancer/Invasive Fungal Infections Cooperative Group and the National Institute of Allergy and Infectious Diseases Mycoses Study Group (EORTC/MSG) Consensus Group. Clin Infect Dis. 2008;46(12):1813–21.
645. Li XY, Wang C, Li JL, Cao J, Xing LH. The value of 1,3-beta-D-glucan assay for diagnosis of invasive fungal disease with automimmune disease. Chin J Respir Crit Care Med. 2017;16(3):237–40.
646. Haydour Q, Hage CA, Carmona EM, Epelbaum O, Evans SE, Gabe LM, Knox KS, Kolls JK, Wengenack NL, Prokop LJ, et al. Diagnosis of fungal infections. A systematic review and meta-analysis supporting American Thoracic Society Practice Guideline. Ann Am Thorac Soc. 2019;16(9):1179–88.
647. Pollreisz A, Rafferty B, Kozarov E, Lalla E. Klebsiella pneumoniae induces an inflammatory response in human retinal-pigmented epithelial cells. Biochem Biophys Res Commun. 2012;418(1):33–7.
648. Rossi EE, Pinheiro AL, Baltatu OC, Pacheco MT, Silveira L Jr. Differential diagnosis between experimental endophthalmitis and uveitis in vitreous with Raman spectroscopy and principal components analysis. J Photochem Photobiol B. 2012;107:73–8.

649. Chen L, Xu ZZ, Tao Y. Intraocular lipopolysaccharide examination for early diagnosis of Stenotrophomonas maltophilia endophthalmitis: a case report. J Int Med Res. 2020b;48(8):300060520929865.
650. Haynes RJ, Tighe PJ, Dua HS. Antimicrobial defensin peptides of the human ocular surface. Br J Ophthalmol. 1999;83(6):737–41.
651. Reviglio VE, Sambuelli RH, Olmedo A, Falco M, Echenique J, O'Brien TP, Kuo IC. Secretory leukocyte protease inhibitor is an inducible antimicrobial peptide expressed in Staphylococcus aureus endophthalmitis. Mediators Inflamm. 2007;2007:93857.
652. Giese MJ, Sumner HL, Berliner JA, Mondino BJ. Cytokine expression in a rat model of Staphylococcus aureus endophthalmitis. Invest Ophthalmol Vis Sci. 1998;39(13):2785–90.
653. Singh PK, Kumar A. Retinal photoreceptor expresses toll-like receptors (TLRs) and elicits innate responses following TLR ligand and bacterial challenge. PLoS One. 2015;10(3):e0119541.
654. Kumar A, Pandey RK, Miller LJ, Singh PK, Kanwar M. Muller glia in retinal innate immunity: a perspective on their roles in endophthalmitis. Crit Rev Immunol. 2013;33(2):119–35.
655. Talreja D, Singh PK, Kumar A. In vivo role of TLR2 and MyD88 signaling in eliciting innate immune responses in staphylococcal endophthalmitis. Invest Ophthalmol Vis Sci. 2015;56(3):1719–32.
656. Rajamani D, Singh PK, Rottmann BG, Singh N, Bhasin MK, Kumar A. Temporal retinal transcriptome and systems biology analysis identifies key pathways and hub genes in Staphylococcus aureus endophthalmitis. Sci Rep. 2016;6:21502.
657. Rosenzweig HL, Galster KT, Planck SR, Rosenbaum JT. NOD1 expression in the eye and functional contribution to IL-1beta-dependent ocular inflammation in mice. Invest Ophthalmol Vis Sci. 2009;50(4):1746–53.
658. Deshmukh D, Chakrabarti M, Jayasudha R, Hasnat Ali M, Tyagi M, Sharma S, Joseph J. Elevated cytokine levels in vitreous as biomarkers of disease severity in infectious endophthalmitis. PLoS One. 2018;13(10):e0205292.
659. Sandvig KU, Dannevig L. Postoperative endophthalmitis: establishment and results of a national registry. J Cataract Refract Surg. 2003;29(7):1273–80.
660. Ma WJ, Zhang H, Zhao SZ. Laboratory diagnosis of infectious endophthalmitis. Int J Ophthalmol. 2011;4(1):100–2.
661. Lingappan A, Wykoff CC, Albini TA, Miller D, Pathengay A, Davis JL, Flynn HW Jr. Endogenous fungal endophthalmitis: causative organisms, management strategies, and visual acuity outcomes. Am J Ophthalmol. 2012;153(1):162–166 e161.
662. Sridhar J, Flynn HW Jr, Kuriyan AE, Miller D, Albini T. Endogenous fungal endophthalmitis: risk factors, clinical features, and treatment outcomes in mold and yeast infections. J Ophthalmic Inflamm Infect. 2013;3(1):60.
663. Simonett JM, Igelman A, Taylor SC, Campbell JP, Hwang TS, Lin P, Lauer AK, Flaxel CJ. Culture-proven endophthalmitis after intravitreal injection: a 10-year analysis. Ophthalmic Surg Lasers Imaging Retina. 2019;50(1):33–8.
664. Ke Y. Domestic expert consensus of management for acute bacteria endophthalmitis after cataract surgery. Chin J Ophthalmol. 2010;46(8):764–6.
665. Ke Y. Domestic expert consensus of management for acute bacteria endophthalmitis after cataract surgery. Chin J Ophthalmol. 2017;53(11):810–3.
666. Ho IV, Fernandez-Sanz G, Levasseur S, Ting E, Liew G, Playfair J, Downie J, Gorbatov M, Hunyor AP, Chang AA. Early Pars Plana vitrectomy for treatment of acute infective endophthalmitis. Asia Pac J Ophthalmol (Phila). 2019;8(1):3–7.
667. Yoon YH, Lee SU, Sohn JH, Lee SE. Result of early vitrectomy for endogenous Klebsiella pneumoniae endophthalmitis. Retina. 2003;23(3):366–70.
668. Do T, Hon DN, Aung T, Hien ND, Cowan CL Jr. Bacterial endogenous endophthalmitis in Vietnam: a randomized controlled trial comparing vitrectomy with silicone oil versus vitrectomy alone. Clin Ophthalmol. 2014;8:1633–40.
669. Celiker H, Kazokoglu H. The role of pars plana vitrectomy in the management of fungal endogenous endophthalmitis. Eur J Ophthalmol. 2020;30(1):88–93.

670. Ghoraba HH, Ellakwa AF, Elgemai EM, Mansour HO, Heikal MA. Results of Pars Plana vitrectomy for the management of endogenous fungal endophthalmitis after urinary tract procedures. Retin Cases Brief Rep. 2017;11(2):171–4.
671. Lee S, Um T, Joe SG, Hwang JU, Kim JG, Yoon YH, Lee JY. Changes in the clinical features and prognostic factors of endogenous endophthalmitis: fifteen years of clinical experience in Korea. Retina. 2012;32(5):977–84.
672. Wykoff CC, Flynn HW Jr, Miller D, Scott IU, Alfonso EC. Exogenous fungal endophthalmitis: microbiology and clinical outcomes. Ophthalmology. 2008;115(9):1501–7, 1507 e1501-1502.
673. Tan TE, Wong TY. Diabetic retinopathy: Looking forward to 2030. Front Endocrinol (Lausanne). 2022;13:1077669.
674. Yau JW, Rogers SL, Kawasaki R, Lamoureux EL, Kowalski JW, Bek T, Chen SJ, Dekker JM, Fletcher A, Grauslund J, et al. Global prevalence and major risk factors of diabetic retinopathy. Diabetes Care. 2012;35(3):556–64.
675. Ruta LM, Magliano DJ, Lemesurier R, Taylor HR, Zimmet PZ, Shaw JE. Prevalence of diabetic retinopathy in Type 2 diabetes in developing and developed countries. Diabet Med. 2013;30(4):387–98.
676. Scott IU, Smiddy WE. Diabetes and ocular disease: past, present, and future therapies. In: Ophthalmology Monograph 14. 2nd ed. San Francisco: American Academy of Ophthalmology; 2009: Pooyan 66961526-66961527.
677. Collaborators GBDD. Global, regional, and national burden of diabetes from 1990 to 2021, with projections of prevalence to 2050: a systematic analysis for the Global Burden of Disease Study 2021. Lancet. 2023;402(10397):203–34.
678. Teo ZL, Tham YC, Yu M, Chee ML, Rim TH, Cheung N, Bikbov MM, Wang YX, Tang Y, Lu Y, et al. Global prevalence of diabetic retinopathy and projection of burden through 2045: systematic review and meta-analysis. Ophthalmology. 2021;128(11):1580–91.
679. Kohner EM, Aldington SJ, Stratton IM, Manley SE, Holman RR, Matthews DR, Turner RC. United Kingdom Prospective Diabetes Study, 30: diabetic retinopathy at diagnosis of non-insulin-dependent diabetes mellitus and associated risk factors. Arch Ophthalmol. 1998;116(3):297–303.
680. Klein R, Klein BE, Moss SE, Davis MD, DeMets DL. The Wisconsin Epidemiologic Study of Diabetic Retinopathy. IX. Four-year incidence and progression of diabetic retinopathy when age at diagnosis is less than 30 years. Arch Ophthalmol. 1989a;107(2):237–43.
681. Klein R, Klein BE, Moss SE, Davis MD, DeMets DL. The Wisconsin Epidemiologic Study of Diabetic Retinopathy. X. Four-year incidence and progression of diabetic retinopathy when age at diagnosis is 30 years or more. Arch Ophthalmol. 1989b;107(2):244–9.
682. Klein R, Klein BE, Moss SE, Cruickshanks KJ. The Wisconsin Epidemiologic Study of Diabetic Retinopathy. XV. The long-term incidence of macular edema. Ophthalmology. 1995;102(1):7–16.
683. Donaghue KC, Fairchild JM, Craig ME, Chan AK, Hing S, Cutler LR, Howard NJ, Silink M. Do all prepubertal years of diabetes duration contribute equally to diabetes complications? Diabetes Care. 2003;26(4):1224–9.
684. White NH, Sun W, Cleary PA, Danis RP, Davis MD, Hainsworth DP, Hubbard LD, Lachin JM, Nathan DM. Prolonged effect of intensive therapy on the risk of retinopathy complications in patients with type 1 diabetes mellitus: 10 years after the Diabetes Control and Complications Trial. Arch Ophthalmol. 2008;126(12):1707–15.
685. Hirsch IB, Brownlee M. Beyond hemoglobin A1c—need for additional markers of risk for diabetic microvascular complications. JAMA. 2010;303(22):2291–2.
686. Sadda SR. Assessing the severity of diabetic retinopathy: Early Treatment Diabetic Retinopathy Study Report Number 10. Ophthalmology. 2020;127(4S):S97–8.
687. Panel. AAoORV: preferred practice pattern guidelines. Diabetic retinopathy. San Francisco: American Academy of Ophthalmology; 2008. www.aao.org/ppp.
688. Davis MD, Fisher MR, Gangnon RE, Barton F, Aiello LM, Chew EY, Ferris FL 3rd, Knatterud GL. Risk factors for high-risk proliferative diabetic retinopathy and severe visual

loss: Early Treatment Diabetic Retinopathy Study Report #18. Invest Ophthalmol Vis Sci. 1998;39(2):233–52.
689. Kinyoun J, Barton F, Fisher M, Hubbard L, Aiello L, Ferris F. Detection of diabetic macular edema. Ophthalmoscopy versus photography—Early Treatment Diabetic Retinopathy Study Report Number 5. The ETDRS Research Group. Ophthalmology. 1989;96(6):746–50; discussion 750-741.
690. Ophthalmologists TRCo. Diabetic retinopathy guidelines. 2012.
691. Kanclerz P, Tuuminen R, Khoramnia R. Imaging modalities employed in diabetic retinopathy screening: a review and meta-analysis. Diagnostics (Basel). 2021;11(10):1802.
692. Sun JK, Lin MM, Lammer J, Prager S, Sarangi R, Silva PS, Aiello LP. Disorganization of the retinal inner layers as a predictor of visual acuity in eyes with center-involved diabetic macular edema. JAMA Ophthalmol. 2014b;132(11):1309–16.
693. Le D, Dadzie A, Son T, Lim JI, Yao X. Comparative analysis of OCT and OCT angiography characteristics in early diabetic retinopathy. Retina. 2023;43:992.
694. Aiello LP, Avery RL, Arrigg PG, Keyt BA, Jampel HD, Shah ST, Pasquale LR, Thieme H, Iwamoto MA, Park JE, et al. Vascular endothelial growth factor in ocular fluid of patients with diabetic retinopathy and other retinal disorders. N Engl J Med. 1994a;331(22):1480–7.
695. Adamis AP, Miller JW, Bernal MT, D'Amico DJ, Folkman J, Yeo TK, Yeo KT. Increased vascular endothelial growth factor levels in the vitreous of eyes with proliferative diabetic retinopathy. Am J Ophthalmol. 1994;118(4):445–50.
696. Funatsu H, Yamashita H, Ikeda T, Nakanishi Y, Kitano S, Hori S. Angiotensin II and vascular endothelial growth factor in the vitreous fluid of patients with diabetic macular edema and other retinal disorders. Am J Ophthalmol. 2002;133(4):537–43.
697. Watanabe D, Suzuma K, Suzuma I, Ohashi H, Ojima T, Kurimoto M, Murakami T, Kimura T, Takagi H. Vitreous levels of angiopoietin 2 and vascular endothelial growth factor in patients with proliferative diabetic retinopathy. Am J Ophthalmol. 2005a;139(3):476–81.
698. Hirase K, Ikeda T, Sotozono C, Nishida K, Sawa H, Kinoshita S. Transforming growth factor beta2 in the vitreous in proliferative diabetic retinopathy. Arch Ophthalmol. 1998;116(6):738–41.
699. Freyberger H, Brocker M, Yakut H, Hammer J, Effert R, Schifferdecker E, Schatz H, Derwahl M. Increased levels of platelet-derived growth factor in vitreous fluid of patients with proliferative diabetic retinopathy. Exp Clin Endocrinol Diabetes. 2000;108(2):106–9.
700. Watanabe D, Suzuma K, Matsui S, Kurimoto M, Kiryu J, Kita M, Suzuma I, Ohashi H, Ojima T, Murakami T, et al. Erythropoietin as a retinal angiogenic factor in proliferative diabetic retinopathy. N Engl J Med. 2005b;353(8):782–92.
701. Loukovaara S, Robciuc A, Holopainen JM, Lehti K, Pessi T, Liinamaa J, Kukkonen KT, Jauhiainen M, Koli K, Keski-Oja J, et al. Ang-2 upregulation correlates with increased levels of MMP-9, VEGF, EPO and TGFbeta1 in diabetic eyes undergoing vitrectomy. Acta Ophthalmol. 2013;91(6):531–9.
702. Abu El-Asrar AM, Mohammad G, Nawaz MI, Siddiquei MM, Van den Eynde K, Mousa A, De Hertogh G, Opdenakker G. Relationship between vitreous levels of matrix metalloproteinases and vascular endothelial growth factor in proliferative diabetic retinopathy. PLoS One. 2013;8(12):e85857.
703. McAuley AK, Sanfilippo PG, Hewitt AW, Liang H, Lamoureux E, Wang JJ, Connell PP. Vitreous biomarkers in diabetic retinopathy: a systematic review and meta-analysis. J Diabetes Complications. 2014;28(3):419–25.
704. Tao Y, Lu Q, Jiang YR, Qian J, Wang JY, Gao L, Jonas JB. Apelin in plasma and vitreous and in fibrovascular retinal membranes of patients with proliferative diabetic retinopathy. Invest Ophthalmol Vis Sci. 2010;51(8):4237–42.
705. Hillier RJ, Ojaimi E, Wong DT, Mak MYK, Berger AR, Kohly RP, Kertes PJ, Forooghian F, Boyd SR, Eng K, et al. Aqueous humor cytokine levels and anatomic response to intravitreal ranibizumab in diabetic macular edema. JAMA Ophthalmol. 2018;136(4):382–8.
706. Mastropasqua R, D'Aloisio R, Di Nicola M, Di Martino G, Lamolinara A, Di Antonio L, Tognetto D, Toto L. Relationship between aqueous humor cytokine level changes and

retinal vascular changes after intravitreal aflibercept for diabetic macular edema. Sci Rep. 2018;8(1):16548.

707. Sawada O, Kawamura H, Kakinoki M, Sawada T, Ohji M. Vascular endothelial growth factor in aqueous humor before and after intravitreal injection of bevacizumab in eyes with diabetic retinopathy. Arch Ophthalmol. 2007;125(10):1363–6.
708. Kwon JW, Jee D. Aqueous humor cytokine levels in patients with diabetic macular edema refractory to anti-VEGF treatment. PLoS One. 2018;13(9):e0203408.
709. Wang J, Chen S, Jiang F, You C, Mao C, Yu J, Han J, Zhang Z, Yan H. Vitreous and plasma VEGF levels as predictive factors in the progression of proliferative diabetic retinopathy after vitrectomy. PLoS One. 2014b;9(10):e110531.
710. Tang L, Xu GT, Zhang JF. Inflammation in diabetic retinopathy: possible roles in pathogenesis and potential implications for therapy. Neural Regen Res. 2023;18(5):976–82.
711. Kocabora MS, Telli ME, Fazil K, Erdur SK, Ozsutcu M, Cekic O, Ozbilen KT. Serum and aqueous concentrations of inflammatory markers in diabetic macular edema. Ocul Immunol Inflamm. 2016;24(5):549–54.
712. Costagliola C, Romano V, De Tollis M, Aceto F, dell'Omo R, Romano MR, Pedicino C, Semeraro F. TNF-alpha levels in tears: a novel biomarker to assess the degree of diabetic retinopathy. Mediators Inflamm. 2013;2013:629529.
713. Paine SK, Sen A, Choudhuri S, Mondal LK, Chowdhury IH, Basu A, Mukherjee A, Bhattacharya B. Association of tumor necrosis factor alpha, interleukin 6, and interleukin 10 promoter polymorphism with proliferative diabetic retinopathy in type 2 diabetic subjects. Retina. 2012;32(6):1197–203.
714. Marui N, Offermann MK, Swerlick R, Kunsch C, Rosen CA, Ahmad M, Alexander RW, Medford RM. Vascular cell adhesion molecule-1 (VCAM-1) gene transcription and expression are regulated through an antioxidant-sensitive mechanism in human vascular endothelial cells. J Clin Invest. 1993;92(4):1866–74.
715. Elner SG, Elner VM, Jaffe GJ, Stuart A, Kunkel SL, Strieter RM. Cytokines in proliferative diabetic retinopathy and proliferative vitreoretinopathy. Curr Eye Res. 1995;14(11):1045–53.
716. Feng S, Yu H, Yu Y, Geng Y, Li D, Yang C, Lv Q, Lu L, Liu T, Li G, et al. Levels of inflammatory cytokines IL-1beta, IL-6, IL-8, IL-17A, and TNF-alpha in aqueous humour of patients with diabetic retinopathy. J Diabetes Res. 2018a;2018:8546423.
717. Oh IK, Kim SW, Oh J, Lee TS, Huh K. Inflammatory and angiogenic factors in the aqueous humor and the relationship to diabetic retinopathy. Curr Eye Res. 2010;35(12):1116–27.
718. Chen H, Zhang X, Liao N, Wen F. Increased levels of IL-6, sIL-6R, and sgp130 in the aqueous humor and serum of patients with diabetic retinopathy. Mol Vis. 2016;22:1005–14.
719. Reddy S, Amutha A, Rajalakshmi R, Bhaskaran R, Monickaraj F, Rangasamy S, Anjana RM, Abhijit S, Gokulakrishnan K, Das A, et al. Association of increased levels of MCP-1 and cathepsin-D in young onset type 2 diabetes patients (T2DM-Y) with severity of diabetic retinopathy. J Diabetes Complications. 2017;31(5):804–9.
720. Hillier RJ, Ojaimi E, Wong DT, Mak MY, Berger AR, Kohly RP, Kertes PJ, Forooghian F, Boyd SR, Eng K, et al. Aqueous humor cytokine levels as biomarkers of disease severity in diabetic macular edema. Retina. 2017;37(4):761–9.
721. Figueras-Roca M, Sala-Puigdollers A, Alforja S, Torras J, Peraza-Nieves J, Zarranz-Ventura J, Adan Civera A, Molins B. Aqueous humour cytokine changes with intravitreal dexamethasone implant injection for diabetic macular edema. Ocul Immunol Inflamm. 2019a;27(8):1203–10.
722. Figueras-Roca M, Sala-Puigdollers A, Zarranz-Ventura J, Alba-Linero C, Alforja S, Esquinas C, Molins B, Adan A. Anatomic response to intravitreal dexamethasone implant and baseline aqueous humor cytokine levels in diabetic macular edema. Invest Ophthalmol Vis Sci. 2019b;60(5):1336–43.
723. UK Prospective Diabetes Study (UKPDS) Group. Intensive blood-glucose control with sulphonylureas or insulin compared with conventional treatment and risk of complications in patients with type 2 diabetes (UKPDS 33). Lancet. 1998;352(9131):837–53.

724. Sun JK, Glassman AR, Beaulieu WT, Stockdale CR, Bressler NM, Flaxel C, Gross JG, Shami M, Jampol LM, Diabetic Retinopathy Clinical Research N. Rationale and application of the protocol S anti-vascular endothelial growth factor algorithm for proliferative diabetic retinopathy. Ophthalmology. 2019;126(1):87–95.
725. Heier JS, Korobelnik JF, Brown DM, Schmidt-Erfurth U, Do DV, Midena E, Boyer DS, Terasaki H, Kaiser PK, Marcus DM, et al. Intravitreal Aflibercept for diabetic macular edema: 148-week results from the VISTA and VIVID studies. Ophthalmology. 2016;123(11):2376–85.
726. Garweg JG. A randomized, double-masked, multicenter, phase III study assessing the efficacy and safety of Brolucizumab versus Aflibercept in patients with visual impairment due to diabetic macular edema (KITE). Klin Monbl Augenheilkd. 2020;237(4):450–3.
727. Sahni J, Patel SS, Dugel PU, Khanani AM, Jhaveri CD, Wykoff CC, Hershberger VS, Pauly-Evers M, Sadikhov S, Szczesny P, et al. Simultaneous inhibition of angiopoietin-2 and vascular endothelial growth factor-A with Faricimab in diabetic macular edema: Boulevard phase 2 randomized trial. Ophthalmology. 2019;126(8):1155–70.
728. Verma LK, Vivek MB, Kumar A, Tewari HK, Venkatesh P. A prospective controlled trial to evaluate the adjunctive role of posterior subtenon triamcinolone in the treatment of diffuse diabetic macular edema. J Ocul Pharmacol Ther. 2004;20(4):277–84.
729. Mihalache A, Hatamnejad A, Patil NS, Popovic MM, Kertes PJ, Cruz-Pimentel M, Muni RH. Intravitreal triamcinolone acetonide for diabetic macular edema and macular edema secondary to retinal vein occlusion: a meta-analysis. Ophthalmologica. 2023;247:19.
730. Escobar-Barranco JJ, Pina-Marin B, Fernandez-Bonet M. Dexamethasone implants in patients with naive or refractory diffuse diabetic macular edema. Ophthalmologica. 2015;233(3-4):176–85.
731. Cunha-Vaz J, Ashton P, Iezzi R, Campochiaro P, Dugel PU, Holz FG, Weber M, Danis RP, Kuppermann BD, Bailey C, et al. Sustained delivery fluocinolone acetonide vitreous implants: long-term benefit in patients with chronic diabetic macular edema. Ophthalmology. 2014;121(10):1892–903.
732. Wei Q, Zhang T, Jiang R, Chang Q, Zhang Y, Huang X, Gao X, Jin H, Xu G. Vitreous fibronectin and fibrinogen expression increased in eyes with proliferative diabetic retinopathy after intravitreal anti-vegf therapy. Invest Ophthalmol Vis Sci. 2017;58(13):5783–91.
733. Feng J, Li B, Wen J, Jiang Y. Preoperative timing of intravitreal bevacizumab injection for proliferative diabetic retinopathy patients. Ophthalmic Res. 2018b;60(4):250–7.
734. Romano F, Lamanna F, Gabrielle PH, Teo KYC, Battaglia Parodi M, Iacono P, Fraser-Bell S, Cornish EE, Nassisi M, Viola F, et al. Update on retinal vein occlusion. Asia Pac J Ophthalmol (Phila). 2023;12(2):196–210.
735. Scott IU, Campochiaro PA, Newman NJ, Biousse V. Retinal vascular occlusions. Lancet. 2020;396(10266):1927–40.
736. Jonas J, Paques M, Mones J, Glacet-Bernard A. Retinal vein occlusions. Dev Ophthalmol. 2010;47:111–35.
737. Frangieh GT, Green WR, Barraquer-Somers E, Finkelstein D. Histopathologic study of nine branch retinal vein occlusions. Arch Ophthalmol. 1982;100(7):1132–40.
738. Coscas G, Loewenstein A, Augustin A, Bandello F, Battaglia Parodi M, Lanzetta P, Mones J, de Smet M, Soubrane G, Staurenghi G. Management of retinal vein occlusion—consensus document. Ophthalmologica. 2011;226(1):4–28.
739. Laouri M, Chen E, Looman M, Gallagher M. The burden of disease of retinal vein occlusion: review of the literature. Eye (Lond). 2011;25(8):981–8.
740. Rehak J, Rehak M. Branch retinal vein occlusion: pathogenesis, visual prognosis, and treatment modalities. Curr Eye Res. 2008;33(2):111–31.
741. Song P, Xu Y, Zha M, Zhang Y, Rudan I. Global epidemiology of retinal vein occlusion: a systematic review and meta-analysis of prevalence, incidence, and risk factors. J Glob Health. 2019;9(1):010427.
742. Klein R, Klein BE, Moss SE, Meuer SM. The epidemiology of retinal vein occlusion: the Beaver Dam Eye Study. Trans Am Ophthalmol Soc. 2000;98:133–41; discussion 141-133.

743. Mitchell P, Smith W, Chang A. Prevalence and associations of retinal vein occlusion in Australia. The Blue Mountains Eye Study. Arch Ophthalmol. 1996b;114(10):1243–7.
744. Kalva P, Akram R, Zuberi HZ, Kooner KS. Prevalence and risk factors of retinal vein occlusion in the United States: The National Health and Nutrition Examination Survey, 2005 to 2008. Proc (Bayl Univ Med Cent). 2023;36(3):335–40.
745. Hashimoto Y, Kaneko H, Aso S, Okada A, Matsui H, Yasunaga H, Aihara M, Obata R. Association between retinal vein occlusion and early-stage hypertension: a propensity score analysis using a large claims database. Eye (Lond). 2023;37(8):1741–7.
746. Kim HR, Lee NK, Lee CS, Byeon SH, Kim SS, Lee SW, Kim YJ. Retinal vascular occlusion risks in high blood pressure and the benefits of blood pressure control. Am J Ophthalmol. 2023;250:111–9.
747. The Central Vein Occlusion Study Group. Natural history and clinical management of central retinal vein occlusion. Arch Ophthalmol. 1997;115(4):486–91.
748. Rogers S, McIntosh RL, Cheung N, Lim L, Wang JJ, Mitchell P, Kowalski JW, Nguyen H, Wong TY, International Eye Disease C. The prevalence of retinal vein occlusion: pooled data from population studies from the United States, Europe, Asia, and Australia. Ophthalmology. 2010a;117(2):313–319e311.
749. Rath EZ, Frank RN, Shin DH, Kim C. Risk factors for retinal vein occlusions. A case-control study. Ophthalmology. 1992;99(4):509–14.
750. Nicholson L, Talks SJ, Amoaku W, Talks K, Sivaprasad S. Retinal vein occlusion (RVO) guideline: executive summary. Eye (Lond). 2022a;36(5):909–12.
751. McIntosh RL, Rogers SL, Lim L, Cheung N, Wang JJ, Mitchell P, Kowalski JW, Nguyen HP, Wong TY. Natural history of central retinal vein occlusion: an evidence-based systematic review. Ophthalmology. 2010;117(6):1113–1123e1115.
752. Pollack A, Leiba H, Oliver M. Progression of nonischemic central retinal vein occlusion. Ophthalmologica. 1997;211(1):13–20.
753. Rogers SL, McIntosh RL, Lim L, Mitchell P, Cheung N, Kowalski JW, Nguyen HP, Wang JJ, Wong TY. Natural history of branch retinal vein occlusion: an evidence-based systematic review. Ophthalmology. 2010b;117(6):1094–1101e1095.
754. Wong TY, Scott IU. Clinical practice. Retinal-vein occlusion. N Engl J Med. 2010;363(22):2135–44.
755. Hayreh SS, Klugman MR, Beri M, Kimura AE, Podhajsky P. Differentiation of ischemic from non-ischemic central retinal vein occlusion during the early acute phase. Graefes Arch Clin Exp Ophthalmol. 1990a;228(3):201–17.
756. Hayreh SS, Klugman MR, Podhajsky P, Servais GE, Perkins ES. Argon laser panretinal photocoagulation in ischemic central retinal vein occlusion. A 10-year prospective study. Graefes Arch Clin Exp Ophthalmol. 1990b;228(4):281–96.
757. Cochran MLMN, Czyz CN. Branch retinal vein occlusion. Treasure Island, FL: StatPearls; 2022.
758. The Central Vein Occlusion Study Group N Report. A randomized clinical trial of early panretinal photocoagulation for ischemic central vein occlusion. Ophthalmology. 1995;102(10):1434–44.
759. Hayreh SS. Photocoagulation for retinal vein occlusion. Prog Retin Eye Res. 2021;85:100964.
760. Schmidt-Erfurth U, Garcia-Arumi J, Gerendas BS, Midena E, Sivaprasad S, Tadayoni R, Wolf S, Loewenstein A. Guidelines for the management of retinal vein occlusion by the European Society of Retina Specialists (EURETINA). Ophthalmologica. 2019;242(3):123–62.
761. Ben Abdesslem N, Haddar S, Mahjoub A, Mahjoub A, Ghorbel M, Mahjoub H, Knani L, Krifa F. Retinal vein occlusions: an OCT-angiography analysis. Tunis Med. 2021;99(5):538–43.
762. Suzuki N, Hirano Y, Tomiyasu T, Esaki Y, Uemura A, Yasukawa T, Yoshida M, Ogura Y. Retinal hemodynamics seen on optical coherence tomography angiography before and after treatment of retinal vein occlusion. Invest Ophthalmol Vis Sci. 2016;57(13):5681–7.

763. Samara WA, Shahlaee A, Sridhar J, Khan MA, Ho AC, Hsu J. Quantitative optical coherence tomography angiography features and visual function in eyes with branch retinal vein occlusion. Am J Ophthalmol. 2016;166:76–83.
764. Martinet V, Guigui B, Glacet-Bernard A, Zourdani A, Coscas G, Soubrane G, Souied EH. Macular edema in central retinal vein occlusion: correlation between optical coherence tomography, angiography and visual acuity. Int Ophthalmol. 2012;32(4):369–77.
765. Glacet-Bernard A, Sellam A, Coscas F, Coscas G, Souied EH. Optical coherence tomography angiography in retinal vein occlusion treated with dexamethasone implant: a new test for follow-up evaluation. Eur J Ophthalmol. 2016;26(5):460–8.
766. Sivaprasad S, Amoaku WM, Hykin P, Group RVOG. The Royal College of Ophthalmologists Guidelines on retinal vein occlusions: executive summary. Eye (Lond). 2015;29(12):1633–8.
767. Flaxel CJ, Adelman RA, Bailey ST, Fawzi A, Lim JI, Vemulakonda GA, Ying GS. Retinal vein occlusions preferred practice pattern(R). Ophthalmology. 2020;127(2):P288–320.
768. Noma H, Funatsu H, Mimura T, Harino S, Hori S. Vitreous levels of interleukin-6 and vascular endothelial growth factor in macular edema with central retinal vein occlusion. Ophthalmology. 2009;116(1):87–93.
769. Noma H, Funatsu H, Yamasaki M, Tsukamoto H, Mimura T, Sone T, Hirayama T, Tamura H, Yamashita H, Minamoto A, et al. Aqueous humour levels of cytokines are correlated to vitreous levels and severity of macular oedema in branch retinal vein occlusion. Eye (Lond). 2008;22(1):42–8.
770. Noma H, Mimura T, Tatsugawa M, Shimada K. Aqueous flare and inflammatory factors in macular edema with central retinal vein occlusion: a case series. BMC Ophthalmol. 2013;13:78.
771. Yamada Y, Suzuma K, Matsumoto M, Tsuiki E, Fujikawa A, Harada T, Kitaoka T. Retinal blood flow correlates to aqueous vascular endothelial growth factor in central retinal vein occlusion. Retina. 2015;35(10):2037–42.
772. Ehlken C, Rennel ES, Michels D, Grundel B, Pielen A, Junker B, Stahl A, Hansen LL, Feltgen N, Agostini HT, et al. Levels of VEGF but not VEGF(165b) are increased in the vitreous of patients with retinal vein occlusion. Am J Ophthalmol. 2011;152(2):298–303 e291.
773. Yasuda S, Kachi S, Ueno S, Ushida H, Piao CH, Kondo M, Terasaki H. Electroretinograms and level of aqueous vascular endothelial growth factor in eyes with hemicentral retinal vein occlusion or branch retinal vein occlusion. Jpn J Ophthalmol. 2014;58(3):232–6.
774. Koss MJ, Pfister M, Rothweiler F, Michaelis M, Cinatl J, Schubert R, Koch FH. Comparison of cytokine levels from undiluted vitreous of untreated patients with retinal vein occlusion. Acta Ophthalmol. 2012;90(2):e98–e103.
775. Noma H, Funatsu H, Mimura T, Eguchi S, Shimada K, Hori S. Vitreous levels of pigment epithelium-derived factor and vascular endothelial growth factor in macular edema with central retinal vein occlusion. Curr Eye Res. 2011a;36(3):256–63.
776. Fonollosa A, Garcia-Arumi J, Santos E, Macia C, Fernandez P, Segura RM, Zapata MA, Rodriguez-Infante R, Boixadera A, Martinez-Castillo V. Vitreous levels of interleukine-8 and monocyte chemoattractant protein-1 in macular oedema with branch retinal vein occlusion. Eye (Lond). 2010;24(7):1284–90.
777. Pfister M, Rothweiler F, Michaelis M, Cinatl J Jr, Schubert R, Koch FH, Koss MJ. Correlation of inflammatory and proangiogenic cytokines from undiluted vitreous samples with spectral domain OCT scans, in untreated branch retinal vein occlusion. Clin Ophthalmol. 2013;7:1061–7.
778. Noma H, Funatsu H, Harino S, Mimura T, Eguchi S, Hori S. Vitreous inflammatory factors in macular edema with central retinal vein occlusion. Jpn J Ophthalmol. 2011b;55(3):248–55.
779. Noma H, Funatsu H, Mimura T, Shimada K. Increase of aqueous inflammatory factors in macular edema with branch retinal vein occlusion: a case control study. J Inflamm (Lond). 2010a;7:44.
780. Feng J, Zhao T, Zhang Y, Ma Y, Jiang Y. Differences in aqueous concentrations of cytokines in macular edema secondary to branch and central retinal vein occlusion. PLoS One. 2013;8(7):e68149.

781. Noma H, Funatsu H, Mimura T, Harino S, Eguchi S, Hori S. Pigment epithelium-derived factor and vascular endothelial growth factor in branch retinal vein occlusion with macular edema. Graefes Arch Clin Exp Ophthalmol. 2010b;248(11):1559–65.
782. Noma H, Funatsu H, Mimura T. Pigment epithelium-derived factor is related to macular microcirculation in patients with macular edema and branch retinal vein occlusion. Int Ophthalmol. 2012;32(5):485–9.
783. Wei P, He M, Teng H, Han G. Quantitative analysis of metabolites in glucose metabolism in the aqueous humor of patients with central retinal vein occlusion. Exp Eye Res. 2020;191:107919.
784. Yao J, Chen Z, Yang Q, Liu X, Chen X, Zhuang M, Liu Q. Proteomic analysis of aqueous humor from patients with branch retinal vein occlusion-induced macular edema. Int J Mol Med. 2013;32(6):1421–34.
785. Koban Y, Sahin S, Boy F, Kara F. Elevated lipocalin-2 level in aqueous humor of patients with central retinal vein occlusion. Int Ophthalmol. 2019;39(5):981–6.
786. Noma H, Funatsu H, Mimura T, Eguchi S, Shimada K. Visual prognosis and vitreous molecules after vitrectomy for macular edema with branch retinal vein occlusion. Clin Ophthalmol. 2011c;5:223–9.
787. Noma H, Funatsu H, Mimura T, Eguchi S, Shimada K. Influence of vitreous factors after vitrectomy for macular edema in patients with central retinal vein occlusion. Int Ophthalmol. 2011d;31(5):393–402.
788. Shimura M, Nakazawa T, Yasuda K, Kunikata H, Shiono T, Nishida K. Visual prognosis and vitreous cytokine levels after arteriovenous sheathotomy in branch retinal vein occlusion associated with macular oedema. Acta Ophthalmol. 2008;86(4):377–84.
789. Matsushima R, Noma H, Yasuda K, Goto H, Shimura M. Role of cytokines in ranibizumab therapy for macular edema in patients with central retinal vein occlusion. J Ocul Pharmacol Ther. 2019;35(7):407–12.
790. Noma H, Mimura T, Yasuda K, Shimura M. Functional-morphological parameters, aqueous flare and cytokines in macular oedema with branch retinal vein occlusion after ranibizumab. Br J Ophthalmol. 2017;101(2):180–5.
791. Noma H, Mimura T, Yasuda K, Nakagawa H, Motohashi R, Kotake O, Shimura M. Cytokines and recurrence of macular edema after intravitreal ranibizumab in patients with branch retinal vein occlusion. Ophthalmologica. 2016;236(4):228–34.
792. Park SP, Ahn JK. Changes of aqueous vascular endothelial growth factor and pigment epithelium-derived factor following intravitreal bevacizumab for macular oedema secondary to branch retinal vein occlusion. Clin Exp Ophthalmol. 2009;37(5):490–5.
793. Sohn HJ, Han DH, Lee DY, Nam DH. Changes in aqueous cytokines after intravitreal triamcinolone versus bevacizumab for macular oedema in branch retinal vein occlusion. Acta Ophthalmol. 2014;92(3):e217–24.
794. Kunikata H, Shimura M, Nakazawa T, Sonoda KH, Yoshimura T, Ishibashi T, Nishida K. Chemokines in aqueous humour before and after intravitreal triamcinolone acetonide in eyes with macular oedema associated with branch retinal vein occlusion. Acta Ophthalmol. 2012;90(2):162–7.
795. Park SP, Ahn JK. Changes of aqueous vascular endothelial growth factor and interleukin-6 after intravitreal triamcinolone for branch retinal vein occlusion. Clin Exp Ophthalmol. 2008;36(9):831–5.
796. Hayreh SS, Podhajsky PA, Zimmerman MB. Natural history of visual outcome in central retinal vein occlusion. Ophthalmology. 2011;118(1):119.
797. Hayreh SS, Zimmerman MB. Branch retinal vein occlusion: natural history of visual outcome. JAMA Ophthalmol. 2014;132(1):13–22.
798. Campochiaro PA, Sophie R, Pearlman J, Brown DM, Boyer DS, Heier JS, Marcus DM, Feiner L, Patel A, Group RS. Long-term outcomes in patients with retinal vein occlusion treated with ranibizumab: the RETAIN study. Ophthalmology. 2014;121(1):209–19.

799. Heier JS, Campochiaro PA, Yau L, Li Z, Saroj N, Rubio RG, Lai P. Ranibizumab for macular edema due to retinal vein occlusions: long-term follow-up in the HORIZON trial. Ophthalmology. 2012;119(4):802–9.
800. Clark WL, Boyer DS, Heier JS, Brown DM, Haller JA, Vitti R, Kazmi H, Berliner AJ, Erickson K, Chu KW, et al. Intravitreal Aflibercept for macular edema following branch retinal vein occlusion: 52-week results of the VIBRANT study. Ophthalmology. 2016;123(2):330–6.
801. Narayanan R, Panchal B, Das T, Chhablani J, Jalali S, Ali MH, Group MS. A randomised, double-masked, controlled study of the efficacy and safety of intravitreal bevacizumab versus ranibizumab in the treatment of macular oedema due to branch retinal vein occlusion: MARVEL Report No. 1. Br J Ophthalmol. 2015;99(7):954–9.
802. Davidorf FH, Mouser JG, Derick RJ. Rapid improvement of rubeosis iridis from a single bevacizumab (Avastin) injection. Retina. 2006;26(3):354–6.
803. Garweg JG, Zandi S. Retinal vein occlusion and the use of a dexamethasone intravitreal implant (Ozurdex(R)) in its treatment. Graefes Arch Clin Exp Ophthalmol. 2016;254(7):1257–65.
804. Chatziralli I, Nicholson L, Sivaprasad S, Hykin P. Intravitreal steroid and anti-vascular endothelial growth agents for the management of retinal vein occlusion: evidence from randomized trials. Expert Opin Biol Ther. 2015;15(12):1685–97.
805. Hou J, Tao Y, Jiang YR, Li XX, Gao L. Intravitreal bevacizumab versus triamcinolone acetonide for macular edema due to branch retinal vein occlusion: a matched study. Chin Med J (Engl). 2009;122(22):2695–9.
806. Lashay A, Riazi-Esfahani H, Mirghorbani M, Yaseri M. Intravitreal medications for retinal vein occlusion: systematic review and meta-analysis. J Ophthalmic Vis Res. 2019;14(3):336–66.
807. Jin ZY, Zhu D, Tao Y, Wong IY, Jonas JB. Meta-analysis of the effect of intravitreal bevacizumab versus intravitreal triamcinolone acetonide in central retinal vein occlusion. J Ocul Pharmacol Ther. 2013;29(9):826–31.
808. Nicholson L, Vazquez-Alfageme C, Sen P, Patrao NV, Peto T, Yang Y, Sivaprasad S, Hykin PG. The clinical relevance of ultra-widefield angiography findings in patients with central retinal vein occlusion and macular oedema receiving anti-VEGF therapy. Eye (Lond). 2022b;36(5):1086–93.
809. Lam HD, Blumenkranz MS. Treatment of central retinal vein occlusion by vitrectomy with lysis of vitreopapillary and epipapillary adhesions, subretinal peripapillary tissue plasminogen activator injection, and photocoagulation. Am J Ophthalmol. 2002;134(4):609–11.
810. Yeshaya A, Treister G. Pars plana vitrectomy for vitreous hemorrhage and retinal vein occlusion. Ann Ophthalmol. 1983;15(7):615–7.
811. Shields JA, Shields CL, Honavar SG, Demirci H, Cater J. Classification and management of Coats disease: the 2000 Proctor Lecture. Am J Ophthalmol. 2001a;131(5):572–83.
812. Yang X, Wang C, Su G. Recent advances in the diagnosis and treatment of Coats' disease. Int Ophthalmol. 2019;39(4):957–70.
813. Shields CL, Udyaver S, Dalvin LA, Lim LS, Atalay HT, Mazloumi M, Shields JA. Coats disease in 351 eyes: Analysis of features and outcomes over 45 years (by decade) at a single center. Indian J Ophthalmol. 2019;67(6):772–83.
814. Shields JA, Shields CL, Honavar SG, Demirci H. Clinical variations and complications of Coats disease in 150 cases: the 2000 Sanford Gifford Memorial Lecture. Am J Ophthalmol. 2001b;131(5):561–71.
815. Mandura RA, Alqahtani AS. Coats' disease diagnosed during adulthood. Cureus. 2021;13(7):e16303.
816. Smithen LM, Brown GC, Brucker AJ, Yannuzzi LA, Klais CM, Spaide RF. Coats' disease diagnosed in adulthood. Ophthalmology. 2005;112(6):1072–8.
817. Sen M, Shields CL, Honavar SG, Shields JA. Coats disease: an overview of classification, management and outcomes. Indian J Ophthalmol. 2019;67(6):763–71.

818. Dalvin LA, Udyaver S, Lim LS, Mazloumi M, Atalay HT, Khoo CTL, Shields CL. Coats disease: clinical features and outcomes by age category in 351 cases. J Pediatr Ophthalmol Strabismus. 2019;56(5):288–96.
819. Morris B, Foot B, Mulvihill A. A population-based study of Coats disease in the United Kingdom I: epidemiology and clinical features at diagnosis. Eye (Lond). 2010;24(12):1797–801.
820. Peng J, Zhang Q, Chen C, Huang Q, Li Y, Zhao P. Early onset Coats' disease initially treated as unilateral ROP at 39 weeks postmenstrual age: a case report. BMC Ophthalmol. 2017;17(1):145.
821. Lim Fat CP, Lee SY, Brundler MA, Scott CM, Parulekar MV. Coats disease in a 3-week-old boy. J AAPOS. 2014;18(1):86–8.
822. Al-Qahtani AA, Almasaud JM, Ghazi NG. Clinical characteristics and treatment outcomes of Coats disease in a saudi arabian population. Retina. 2015;35(10):2091–9.
823. Stanga PE, Romano F, Chwiejczak K, Tsamis E, Stringa F, Biswas S, Bento G, Arrigo A, Parodi MB, Bandello F. Swept-source optical coherence tomography angiography assessment of fellow eyes in Coats disease. Retina. 2019;39(3):608–13.
824. Ghorbanian S, Jaulim A, Chatziralli IP. Diagnosis and treatment of Coats' disease: a review of the literature. Ophthalmologica. 2012;227(4):175–82.
825. Grosso A, Pellegrini M, Cereda MG, Panico C, Staurenghi G, Sigler EJ. Pearls and pitfalls in diagnosis and management of Coats disease. Retina. 2015;35(4):614–23.
826. Helmi HA, Jammah A, Maktabi AM, AlMesfer S, Alkatan HM. Clinicopathological correlations in enucleated globes of late-stage Coats disease with a review of the literature. J Epidemiol Glob Health. 2022;12(4):496–503.
827. Shields JA, Shields CL. Review: Coats disease: the 2001 LuEsther T. Mertz lecture. Retina. 2002;22(1):80–91.
828. Daruich AL, Moulin AP, Tran HV, Matet A, Munier FL. Subfoveal nodule in Coats' disease: toward an updated classification predicting visual prognosis. Retina. 2017;37(8):1591–8.
829. Rabiolo A, Marchese A, Sacconi R, Cicinelli MV, Grosso A, Querques L, Querques G, Bandello F. Refining Coats' disease by ultra-widefield imaging and optical coherence tomography angiography. Graefes Arch Clin Exp Ophthalmol. 2017;255(10):1881–90.
830. Edward DP, Mafee MF, Garcia-Valenzuela E, Weiss RA. Coats' disease and persistent hyperplastic primary vitreous. Role of MR imaging and CT. Radiol Clin North Am. 1998;36(6):1119–31, x.
831. Ong SS, Mruthyunjaya P, Stinnett S, Vajzovic L, Toth CA. Macular features on spectral-domain optical coherence tomography imaging associated with visual acuity in Coats' disease. Invest Ophthalmol Vis Sci. 2018;59(7):3161–74.
832. Yonekawa Y, Todorich B, Trese MT. Optical coherence tomography angiography findings in Coats' disease. Ophthalmology. 2016;123(9):1964.
833. Cennamo G, Montorio D, Comune C, Laezza MP, Fallico M, Lionetti ME, Reibaldi M. Optical coherence tomography angiography findings after intravitreal ranibizumab in patients with Coats disease. Front Med (Lausanne). 2020;7:615015.
834. Dundar SO, Verdi F, Unsal AIA. Coats disease with retinal neovascularization under subfoveal nodule: optical coherence tomography-angiography findings before and after ranibizumab treatment. Arq Bras Oftalmol. 2021;84(4):383–6.
835. Hautz W, Golebiewska J, Kocyla-Karczmarewicz B. Optical coherence tomography and optical coherence tomography angiography in monitoring Coats' disease. J Ophthalmol. 2017;2017:7849243.
836. Eisenberg L, Castillo M, Kwock L, Mukherji SK, Wallace DK. Proton MR spectroscopy in Coats disease. AJNR Am J Neuroradiol. 1997;18(4):727–9.
837. Shields JSC. Intraocular tumors: an atlas and textbook. 3rd ed. Philadelphia, PA: Lippincott Williams & Wilkins; 2016. p. 1015–26.
838. Mafee MF, Goldberg MF, Cohen SB, Gotsis ED, Safran M, Chekuri L, Raofi B. Magnetic resonance imaging versus computed tomography of leukocoric eyes and use of in vitro proton

magnetic resonance spectroscopy of retinoblastoma. Ophthalmology. 1989;96(7):965–75; discussion 975-966.
839. Adam RS, Kertes PJ, Lam WC. Observations on the management of Coats' disease: less is more. Br J Ophthalmol. 2007;91(3):303–6.
840. Spitznas M, Joussen F, Wessing A, Meyer-Schwickerath Group Coats' disease. An epidemiologic and Fluorescein angiographic study. Albrecht Von Graefes Arch Klin Exp Ophthalmol 1975, 195(4):241-250.
841. Tarkkanen A, Laatikainen L. Coats' disease: clinical, angiographic, histopathological findings and clinical management. Br J Ophthalmol. 1983;67(11):766–76.
842. Egerer I, Tasman W, Tomer TT. Coats disease. Arch Ophthalmol. 1974;92(2):109–12.
843. Sun Y, Jain A, Moshfeghi DM. Elevated vascular endothelial growth factor levels in Coats disease: rapid response to pegaptanib sodium. Graefes Arch Clin Exp Ophthalmol. 2007;245(9):1387–8.
844. He YG, Wang H, Zhao B, Lee J, Bahl D, McCluskey J. Elevated vascular endothelial growth factor level in Coats' disease and possible therapeutic role of bevacizumab. Graefes Arch Clin Exp Ophthalmol. 2010;248(10):1519–21.
845. Zhao Q, Peng XY, Chen FH, Zhang YP, Wang L, You QS, Jonas JB. Vascular endothelial growth factor in Coats' disease. Acta Ophthalmol. 2014;92(3):e225–8.
846. Kase S, Rao NA, Yoshikawa H, Fukuhara J, Noda K, Kanda A, Ishida S. Expression of vascular endothelial growth factor in eyes with Coats' disease. Invest Ophthalmol Vis Sci. 2013b;54(1):57–62.
847. Feng J, Zheng X, Li B, Jiang Y. Differences in aqueous concentrations of cytokines in paediatric and adult patients with Coats' disease. Acta Ophthalmol. 2017;95(6):608–12.
848. Cackett P, Wong D, Cheung CM. Combined intravitreal bevacizumab and argon laser treatment for Coats' disease. Acta Ophthalmol. 2010;88(2):e48–9.
849. Kodama A, Sugioka K, Kusaka S, Matsumoto C, Shimomura Y. Combined treatment for Coats' disease: retinal laser photocoagulation combined with intravitreal bevacizumab injection was effective in two cases. BMC Ophthalmol. 2014;14:36.
850. Yang Q, Wei W, Shi X, Yang L. Successful use of intravitreal ranibizumab injection and combined treatment in the management of Coats' disease. Acta Ophthalmol. 2016;94(4):401–6.
851. Villegas VM, Gold AS, Berrocal AM, Murray TG. Advanced Coats' disease treated with intravitreal bevacizumab combined with laser vascular ablation. Clin Ophthalmol. 2014;8:973–6.
852. Liang T, Xu Y, Zhu X, Zhang X, Li J, Zhao P. Aqueous humour cytokines profiles in eyes with Coats disease and the association with the severity of the disease. BMC Ophthalmol. 2020;20(1):178.
853. Zhang J, Jiang C, Ruan L, Huang X. Associations of cytokine concentrations in aqueous humour with retinal vascular abnormalities and exudation in Coats' disease. Acta Ophthalmol. 2019;97(3):319–24.
854. Bergstrom CS, Hubbard GB 3rd. Combination intravitreal triamcinolone injection and cryotherapy for exudative retinal detachments in severe Coats disease. Retina. 2008;28(3 Suppl):S33–7.
855. Saatci AO, Doruk HC, Yaman A. Intravitreal dexamethasone implant (ozurdex) in Coats' disease. Case Rep Ophthalmol. 2013;4(3):122–8.
856. Martinez-Castillo S, Gallego-Pinazo R, Dolz-Marco R, Marin-Lambies C, Diaz-Llopis M. Adult Coats' disease successfully managed with the dexamethasone intravitreal implant (ozurdex(R)) combined with retinal photocoagulation. Case Rep Ophthalmol. 2012;3(1):123–7.
857. Wang Y, Fan H, Gao K, He W, Tao Y. Levels of cytokines in the aqueous humor guided treatment of refractory macular edema in adult-onset Coats' disease. BMC Ophthalmol. 2020;20(1):261.
858. Schefler AC, Berrocal AM, Murray TG. Advanced Coats' disease. Management with repetitive aggressive laser ablation therapy. Retina. 2008;28(3 Suppl):S38–41.

859. Haye C, Haut J, Aubry JP, Orsoni C. Treatment of a case of Coats' disease by photocoagulation. Bull Soc Ophtalmol Fr. 1968;68(9):711–4.
860. Spitznas M, Joussen F, Wessing A. Treatment of Coats' disease with photocoagulation. Albrecht Von Graefes Arch Klin Exp Ophthalmol. 1976;199(1):31–7.
861. Haut J, Van Effenterre G, Marre JM, Dureuil J, Moulin F. Treatment of Coats' disease with argon laser photocoagulation. Bull Soc Ophtalmol Fr. 1979;79(4-5):463–5.
862. Nucci P, Bandello F, Serafino M, Wilson ME. Selective photocoagulation in Coats disease: ten-year follow-up. Eur J Ophthalmol. 2002;12(6):501–5.
863. Haut J, Zeghal M, Limon S. Cryotherapy of Eales' disease and Coats' disease. Bull Soc Ophtalmol Fr. 1970;70(2):182–4.
864. Jarin RR, Teoh SC, Lim TH. Resolution of severe macular oedema in adult Coats' syndrome with high-dose intravitreal triamcinolone acetonide. Eye (Lond). 2006;20(2):163–5.
865. Jun JH, Kim YC, Kim KS. Resolution of severe macular edema in adult coats' disease with intravitreal triamcinolone and bevacizumab injection. Korean J Ophthalmol. 2008;22(3):190–3.
866. Bohm MR, Uhlig CE. Use of intravitreal triamcinolone and bevacizumab in Coats' disease with central macular edema. Graefes Arch Clin Exp Ophthalmol. 2011;249(7):1099–101.
867. Othman IS, Moussa M, Bouhaimed M. Management of lipid exudates in Coats disease by adjuvant intravitreal triamcinolone: effects and complications. Br J Ophthalmol. 2010;94(5):606–10.
868. Cakir M, Cekic O, Yilmaz OF. Combined intravitreal bevacizumab and triamcinolone injection in a child with Coats disease. J AAPOS. 2008;12(3):309–11.
869. Wang KY, Cheng CK. A combination of intravitreal bevacizumab injection with tunable argon yellow laser photocoagulation as a treatment for adult-onset Coats' disease. J Ocul Pharmacol Ther. 2011;27(5):525–30.
870. Goel N, Kumar V, Seth A, Raina UK, Ghosh B. Role of intravitreal bevacizumab in adult onset Coats' disease. Int Ophthalmol. 2011;31(3):183–90.
871. Venkatesh P, Mandal S, Garg S. Management of Coats disease with bevacizumab in 2 patients. Can J Ophthalmol. 2008;43(2):245–6.
872. Ramasubramanian A, Shields CL. Bevacizumab for Coats' disease with exudative retinal detachment and risk of vitreoretinal traction. Br J Ophthalmol. 2012;96(3):356–9.
873. Alvarez-Rivera LG, Abraham-Marin ML, Flores-Orta HJ, Mayorquin-Ruiz M, Cortes-Luna CF. Coats' disease treated with bevacizumab (Avastin). Arch Soc Esp Oftalmol. 2008;83(5):329–31.
874. Diago T, Valls B, Pulido JS. Coats' disease associated with muscular dystrophy treated with ranibizumab. Eye (Lond). 2010;24(7):1295–6.
875. Wells JR, Hubbard GB. The effect of intravitreal bevacizumab in the treatment of Coats disease in children. Retina. 2011;31(2):427–8; author reply 428.
876. Daruich A, Matet A, Munier FL. Younger age at presentation in children with coats disease is associated with more advanced stage and worse visual prognosis: a retrospective study. Retina. 2018;38(11):2239–46.
877. Smith W, Assink J, Klein R, Mitchell P, Klaver CC, Klein BE, Hofman A, Jensen S, Wang JJ, de Jong PT. Risk factors for age-related macular degeneration: pooled findings from three continents. Ophthalmology. 2001;108(4):697–704.
878. Thomas CJ, Mirza RG, Gill MK. Age-related macular degeneration. Med Clin North Am. 2021;105(3):473–91.
879. Yannuzzi LA, Sorenson J, Spaide RF, Lipson B. Idiopathic polypoidal choroidal vasculopathy (IPCV). Retina. 2012;32(Suppl 1):1–8.
880. Kwok AK, Lai TY, Chan CW, Neoh EL, Lam DS. Polypoidal choroidal vasculopathy in Chinese patients. Br J Ophthalmol. 2002;86(8):892–7.
881. Wen F, Chen C, Wu D, Li H. Polypoidal choroidal vasculopathy in elderly Chinese patients. Graefes Arch Clin Exp Ophthalmol. 2004;242(8):625–9.
882. Khetan V, Shanmugam MP, Bhende MP, Shetty NS. Polypoidal choroidal vasculopathy. Surv Ophthalmol. 2004;49(6):620–1; author reply 621.

883. Lim TH, Laude A, Tan CS. Polypoidal choroidal vasculopathy: an angiographic discussion. Eye (Lond). 2010;24(3):483–90.
884. Escano MF, Fujii S, Ishibashi K, Matsuo H, Yamamoto M. Indocyanine green videoangiography in macular variant of idiopathic polypoidal choroidal vasculopathy. Jpn J Ophthalmol. 2000;44(3):313–6.
885. Chan WM, Lam DS, Lai TY, Liu DT, Li KK, Yao Y, Wong TH. Photodynamic therapy with verteporfin for symptomatic polypoidal choroidal vasculopathy: one-year results of a prospective case series. Ophthalmology. 2004;111(8):1576–84.
886. Hajar S, Al Hazmi A, Wasli M, Mousa A, Rabiu M. Prevalence and causes of blindness and diabetic retinopathy in Southern Saudi Arabia. Saudi Med J. 2015;36(4):449–55.
887. Chou R, Bougatsos C, Jungbauer R, Grusing S, Blazina I, Selph S, Jonas DE, Tehrani S. Screening for impaired visual acuity in older adults: updated evidence report and systematic review for the US Preventive Services Task Force. JAMA. 2022;327(21):2129–40.
888. Deng Y, Qiao L, Du M, Qu C, Wan L, Li J, Huang L. Age-related macular degeneration: epidemiology, genetics, pathophysiology, diagnosis, and targeted therapy. Genes Dis. 2022;9(1):62–79.
889. Chakravarthy U, Wong TY, Fletcher A, Piault E, Evans C, Zlateva G, Buggage R, Pleil A, Mitchell P. Clinical risk factors for age-related macular degeneration: a systematic review and meta-analysis. BMC Ophthalmol. 2010;10:31.
890. Rastogi N, Smith RT. Association of age-related macular degeneration and reticular macular disease with cardiovascular disease. Surv Ophthalmol. 2016;61(4):422–33.
891. Choudhury F, Varma R, McKean-Cowdin R, Klein R, Azen SP, Los Angeles Latino Eye Study Group. Risk factors for four-year incidence and progression of age-related macular degeneration: the Los Angeles Latino Eye Study. Am J Ophthalmol. 2011;152(3):385–95.
892. Fischer T. The age-related macular degeneration as a vascular disease/part of systemic vasculopathy: contributions to its pathogenesis. Orv Hetil. 2015;156(9):358–65.
893. Srinivasan S, Swaminathan G, Kulothungan V, Ganesan S, Sharma T, Raman R. Age-related macular degeneration in a South Indian population, with and without diabetes. Eye (Lond). 2017;31(8):1176–83.
894. Choi JK, Lym YL, Moon JW, Shin HJ, Cho B. Diabetes mellitus and early age-related macular degeneration. Arch Ophthalmol. 2011;129(2):196–9.
895. Houston T. Smoking and age-related macular degeneration. Am Fam Physician. 2001;63(2):225.
896. Humphries JM, Khachik F. Distribution of lutein, zeaxanthin, and related geometrical isomers in fruit, vegetables, wheat, and pasta products. J Agric Food Chem. 2003;51(5):1322–7.
897. Merle BMJ, Silver RE, Rosner B, Seddon JM. Associations between Vitamin D intake and progression to incident advanced age-related macular degeneration. Invest Ophthalmol Vis Sci. 2017;58(11):4569–78.
898. Fritsche LG, Fariss RN, Stambolian D, Abecasis GR, Curcio CA, Swaroop A. Age-related macular degeneration: genetics and biology coming together. Annu Rev Genomics Hum Genet. 2014;15:151–71.
899. Barondes M, Pauleikhoff D, Chisholm IC, Minassian D, Bird AC. Bilaterality of drusen. Br J Ophthalmol. 1990;74(3):180–2.
900. Zweifel SA, Imamura Y, Spaide TC, Fujiwara T, Spaide RF. Prevalence and significance of subretinal drusenoid deposits (reticular pseudodrusen) in age-related macular degeneration. Ophthalmology. 2010;117(9):1775–81.
901. Klein R, Meuer SM, Knudtson MD, Iyengar SK, Klein BE. The epidemiology of retinal reticular drusen. Am J Ophthalmol. 2008;145(2):317–26.
902. Zhou Q, Daniel E, Maguire MG, Grunwald JE, Martin ER, Martin DF, Ying GS, Comparison of Age-Related Macular Degeneration Treatments Trials Research Group. Pseudodrusen and incidence of late age-related macular degeneration in fellow eyes in the comparison of age-related macular degeneration treatments trials. Ophthalmology. 2016;123(7):1530–40.

903. Shijo T, Sakurada Y, Yoneyama S, Sugiyama A, Kikushima W, Tanabe N, Iijima H. Prevalence and characteristics of pseudodrusen subtypes in advanced age-related macular degeneration. Graefes Arch Clin Exp Ophthalmol. 2017;255(6):1125–31.
904. Green WR, McDonnell PJ, Yeo JH. Pathologic features of senile macular degeneration. Retina. 2005;25(5 Suppl):615–27.
905. Klein R, Klein BE, Tomany SC, Meuer SM, Huang GH. Ten-year incidence and progression of age-related maculopathy: The Beaver Dam Eye Study. Ophthalmology. 2002;109(10):1767–79.
906. Gehrs KM, Anderson DH, Johnson LV, Hageman GS. Age-related macular degeneration--emerging pathogenetic and therapeutic concepts. Ann Med. 2006;38(7):450–71.
907. Grunwald JE, Pistilli M, Daniel E, Ying GS, Pan W, Jaffe GJ, Toth CA, Hagstrom SA, Maguire MG, Martin DF, et al. Incidence and growth of geographic atrophy during 5 years of comparison of age-related macular degeneration treatments trials. Ophthalmology. 2017;124(1):97–104.
908. Stahl A. The diagnosis and treatment of age-related macular degeneration. Dtsch Arztebl Int. 2020;117(29-30):513–20.
909. Friedman D, Parker JS, Kimble JA, Delori FC, McGwin G Jr, Curcio CA. Quantification of fluorescein-stained drusen associated with age-related macular degeneration. Retina. 2012;32(1):19–24.
910. Manjunath V, Goren J, Fujimoto JG, Duker JS. Analysis of choroidal thickness in age-related macular degeneration using spectral-domain optical coherence tomography. Am J Ophthalmol. 2011;152(4):663–8.
911. Cheung CMG, Yanagi Y, Akiba M, Tan A, Mathur R, Chan CM, Yeo I, Wong TY. Improved detection and diagnosis of polypoidal choroidal vasculopathy using a combination of optical coherence tomography and optical coherence tomography angiography. Retina. 2019;39(9):1655–63.
912. Ma J, Desai R, Nesper P, Gill M, Fawzi A, Skondra D. Optical coherence tomographic angiography imaging in age-related macular degeneration. Ophthalmol Eye Dis. 2017;9:1179172116686075.
913. Kermany DS, Goldbaum M, Cai W, Valentim CCS, Liang H, Baxter SL, McKeown A, Yang G, Wu X, Yan F, et al. Identifying medical diagnoses and treatable diseases by image-based deep learning. Cell. 2018;172(5):1122–1131e1129.
914. Treder M, Lauermann JL, Eter N. Automated detection of exudative age-related macular degeneration in spectral domain optical coherence tomography using deep learning. Graefes Arch Clin Exp Ophthalmol. 2018;256(2):259–65.
915. Muether PS, Hermann MM, Viebahn U, Kirchhof B, Fauser S. Vascular endothelial growth factor in patients with exudative age-related macular degeneration treated with ranibizumab. Ophthalmology. 2012;119(10):2082–6.
916. Hsu MY, Hung YC, Hwang DK, Lin SC, Lin KH, Wang CY, Choi HY, Wang YP, Cheng CM. Detection of aqueous VEGF concentrations before and after intravitreal injection of anti-VEGF antibody using low-volume sampling paper-based ELISA. Sci Rep. 2016;6:34631.
917. Mimura T, Funatsu H, Noma H, Shimura M, Kamei Y, Yoshida M, Kondo A, Watanabe E, Mizota A. Aqueous humor levels of cytokines in patients with age-related macular degeneration. Ophthalmologica. 2019;241(2):81–9.
918. Neuhaus T, Stier S, Totzke G, Gruenewald E, Fronhoffs S, Sachinidis A, Vetter H, Ko YD. Stromal cell-derived factor 1alpha (SDF-1alpha) induces gene-expression of early growth response-1 (Egr-1) and VEGF in human arterial endothelial cells and enhances VEGF induced cell proliferation. Cell Prolif. 2003;36(2):75–86.
919. Keles A, Erol YO, Ayyildiz SN, Karaman SK, Ogus E. Aqueous humor levels of vascular endothelial growth factor and stromal cell-derived factor-1alpha in age-related macular degeneration. Beyoglu Eye J. 2021;6(4):298–303.
920. Sakamoto S, Takahashi H, Tan X, Inoue Y, Nomura Y, Arai Y, Fujino Y, Kawashima H, Yanagi Y. Changes in multiple cytokine concentrations in the aqueous humour of neo-

vascular age-related macular degeneration after 2 months of ranibizumab therapy. Br J Ophthalmol. 2018;102(4):448–54.
921. Jonas JB, Tao Y, Neumaier M, Findeisen P. Cytokine concentration in aqueous humour of eyes with exudative age-related macular degeneration. Acta Ophthalmol. 2012;90(5):e381–8.
922. Liu F, Ding X, Yang Y, Li J, Tang M, Yuan M, Hu A, Zhan Z, Li Z, Lu L. Aqueous humor cytokine profiling in patients with wet AMD. Mol Vis. 2016b;22:352–61.
923. Chappelow AV, Kaiser PK. Neovascular age-related macular degeneration: potential therapies. Drugs. 2008;68(8):1029–36.
924. Wong TY, Liew G, Mitchell P. Clinical update: new treatments for age-related macular degeneration. Lancet. 2007;370(9583):204–6.
925. Cheung N, Wong TY. Changing trends of blindness: the initial harvest from translational public health and clinical research in ophthalmology. Am J Ophthalmol. 2012;153(2):193–5.
926. Hikichi T, Agarie M. Reduced vessel density of the choriocapillaris during anti-vascular endothelial growth factor therapy for neovascular age-related macular degeneration. Invest Ophthalmol Vis Sci. 2019;60(4):1088–95.
927. Mantel I. Optimizing the anti-VEGF treatment strategy for neovascular age-related macular degeneration: from clinical trials to real-life requirements. Transl Vis Sci Technol. 2015;4(3):6.
928. Macular Photocoagulation Study Group. Persistent and recurrent neovascularization after laser photocoagulation for subfoveal choroidal neovascularization of age-related macular degeneration. Arch Ophthalmol. 1994;112(4):489–99.
929. Macular Photocoagulation Study Group. Laser photocoagulation of subfoveal neovascular lesions of age-related macular degeneration. Updated findings from two clinical trials. Arch Ophthalmol. 1993;111(9):1200–9.
930. Chen YX, Ge J, Yan M, Jin CJ, Zhang MX, Dong FT, Lu F, Zhang CF, Zhao JL. Clinical trial of verteporfin photodynamic therapy in Chinese age-related macular degeneration with subfoveal predominant choroidal neovascularization patients. Zhonghua Yan Ke Za Zhi. 2007;43(3):198–205.
931. Incorvaia C, Campa C, Parmeggiani F, Menzione M, D'Angelo S, Della Corte M, Rinaldi M, Romano M, Dell'omo R, Costagliola C. 12-month retrospective study and review of photodynamic therapy with verteporfin for subfoveal choroidal neovascularization in age-related macular degeneration. Retina. 2008;28(2):289–97.
932. Chen FK, Patel PJ, Uppal GS, Tufail A, Coffey PJ, Da Cruz L. Long-term outcomes following full macular translocation surgery in neovascular age-related macular degeneration. Br J Ophthalmol. 2010;94(10):1337–43.
933. Schwartz SD, Hubschman JP, Heilwell G, Franco-Cardenas V, Pan CK, Ostrick RM, Mickunas E, Gay R, Klimanskaya I, Lanza R. Embryonic stem cell trials for macular degeneration: a preliminary report. Lancet. 2012;379(9817):713–20.
934. Khanani AM, Thomas MJ, Aziz AA, Weng CY, Danzig CJ, Yiu G, Kiss S, Waheed NK, Kaiser PK. Review of gene therapies for age-related macular degeneration. Eye (Lond). 2022;36(2):303–11.
935. Gelfman CM, Grishanin R, Bender KO, Nguyen A, Greengard J, Sharma P, Nieves J, Kiss S, Gasmi M. Comprehensive preclinical assessment of ADVM-022, an intravitreal anti-VEGF gene therapy for the treatment of neovascular AMD and diabetic macular edema. J Ocul Pharmacol Ther. 2021;37(3):181–90.
936. Huisingh C, McGwin G Jr. Aqueous humor levels of vascular endothelial growth factor before and after intravitreal bevacizumab in type 3 versus type 1 and 2 neovascularization: a prospective, case-control study. Am J Ophthalmol. 2012;153(5):1009–10; author reply 1010-1001.
937. Krohne TU, Eter N, Holz FG, Meyer CH. Intraocular pharmacokinetics of bevacizumab after a single intravitreal injection in humans. Am J Ophthalmol. 2008;146(4):508–12.
938. Mitchell P, Korobelnik JF, Lanzetta P, Holz FG, Prunte C, Schmidt-Erfurth U, Tano Y, Wolf S. Ranibizumab (Lucentis) in neovascular age-related macular degeneration: evidence from clinical trials. Br J Ophthalmol. 2010;94(1):2–13.

939. Stewart MW, Rosenfeld PJ, Penha FM, Wang F, Yehoshua Z, Bueno-Lopez E, Lopez PF. Pharmacokinetic rationale for dosing every 2 weeks versus 4 weeks with intravitreal ranibizumab, bevacizumab, and aflibercept (vascular endothelial growth factor Trap-eye). Retina. 2012;32(3):434–57.
940. Brown DM, Nguyen QD, Marcus DM, Boyer DS, Patel S, Feiner L, Schlottmann PG, Rundle AC, Zhang J, Rubio RG, et al. Long-term outcomes of ranibizumab therapy for diabetic macular edema: the 36-month results from two phase III trials: RISE and RIDE. Ophthalmology. 2013;120(10):2013–22.
941. Fauser S, Schwabecker V, Muether PS. Suppression of intraocular vascular endothelial growth factor during aflibercept treatment of age-related macular degeneration. Am J Ophthalmol. 2014;158(3):532–6.
942. Nigam N, Hedaya J, Freeman WR. Non-responders to bevacizumab (Avastin) therapy of choroidal neovascular lesions. Br J Ophthalmol. 2008;92(6):864–5; author reply 865-866.
943. Schmidt-Erfurth U, Eldem B, Guymer R, Korobelnik JF, Schlingemann RO, Axer-Siegel R, Wiedemann P, Simader C, Gekkieva M, Weichselberger A, et al. Efficacy and safety of monthly versus quarterly ranibizumab treatment in neovascular age-related macular degeneration: the EXCITE study. Ophthalmology. 2011;118(5):831–9.
944. Rali A, Xu LT, Craven C, Cohen JB, Yeh S, Grossniklaus HE, O'Keefe GD. Diagnostic retinal biopsy in the management of secondary non-CNS vitreoretinal lymphoma masquerading as viral retinitis: a case report. Int J Retina Vitreous. 2021;7(1):58.
945. Reddy V, Winslow R, Cao JH, Robertson ZM, Chen B, Ufret-Vincenty RL. Vitreoretinal lymphoma, secondary to non-CNS systemic lymphoma, masquerading as an infectious retinitis. Am J Ophthalmol Case Rep. 2019;16:100545.
946. Ryan ME, Shantha JG, Grossniklaus HE, Yeh S. Secondary vitreoretinal lymphoma masquerading as acute retinal necrosis. Ophthalmic Surg Lasers Imaging Retina. 2015;46(10):1048–50.
947. Say EA, Knupp CL, Gertsch KR, Chavala SH. Metastatic B-cell lymphoma masquerading as infectious retinitis and vasculitis. Oncol Lett. 2012;3(6):1245–8.
948. Lee KE, Kim YJ. Bilateral multiple retinal detachments associated with diffuse large B-cell lymphoma: Masquerading as Vogt-Koyanagi-Harada disease. Ocul Immunol Inflamm. 2021;31:7–10.
949. Moussa K, Begaj T, Ma K, Barrantes PC, Eliott D, Sobrin L. Systemic lymphoma masquerading as Vogt-Koyanagi-Harada syndrome: report of a case with multimodal imaging and histopathology. Am J Ophthalmol Case Rep. 2022;27:101643.
950. Touhami S, Audo I, Terrada C, Gaudric A, LeHoang P, Touitou V, Bodaghi B. Neoplasia and intraocular inflammation: from masquerade syndromes to immunotherapy-induced uveitis. Prog Retin Eye Res. 2019;72:100761.
951. Cooper EL, Riker JL. Malignant lymphoma of the uveal tract. Am J Ophthalmol. 1951;34(8):1153–8.
952. Givner I. Malignant lymphoma with ocular involvement; a clinico-pathologic report. Am J Ophthalmol. 1955;39(1):29–32.
953. Raval V, Binkley E, Aronow ME, Valenzuela J, Peereboom DM, Singh AD. Primary central nervous system lymphoma - ocular variant: an interdisciplinary review on management. Surv Ophthalmol. 2021;66(6):1009–20.
954. Tang LJ, Gu CL, Zhang P. Intraocular lymphoma. Int J Ophthalmol. 2017;10(8):1301–7.
955. Chan CC, Buggage RR, Nussenblatt RB. Intraocular lymphoma. Curr Opin Ophthalmol. 2002;13(6):411–8.
956. Buggage RR, Chan CC, Nussenblatt RB. Ocular manifestations of central nervous system lymphoma. Curr Opin Oncol. 2001;13(3):137–42.
957. Sagoo MS, Mehta H, Swampillai AJ, Cohen VM, Amin SZ, Plowman PN, Lightman S. Primary intraocular lymphoma. Surv Ophthalmol. 2014;59(5):503–16.
958. Karakawa A, Taoka K, Kaburaki T, Tanaka R, Shinozaki-Ushiku A, Hayashi H, Miyagi-Maeshima A, Nishimura Y, Uekusa T, Kojima Y, et al. Clinical features and outcomes of secondary intraocular lymphoma. Br J Haematol. 2018;183(4):668–71.

959. Fredrick DR, Char DH, Ljung BM, Brinton DA. Solitary intraocular lymphoma as an initial presentation of widespread disease. Arch Ophthalmol. 1989;107(3):395–7.
960. Cunningham ET, Miserocchi E, Smith JR, Gonzales JA, Zierhut M. Intraocular lymphoma. Ocul Immunol Inflamm. 2021;29(3):425–9.
961. Coupland SE, Damato B. Understanding intraocular lymphomas. Clin Exp Ophthalmol. 2008;36(6):564–78.
962. Chan CC, Wallace DJ. Intraocular lymphoma: update on diagnosis and management. Cancer Control. 2004;11(5):285–95.
963. Barr CC, Green WR, Payne JW, Knox DL, Jensen AD, Thompson RL. Intraocular reticulum-cell sarcoma: clinico-pathologic study of four cases and review of the literature. Surv Ophthalmol. 1975;19(4):224–39.
964. Kaplan HJ, Meredith TA, Aaberg TM, Keller RH. Reclassification of intraocular reticulum cell sarcoma (histiocytic lymphoma). Immunologic characterization of vitreous cells. Arch Ophthalmol. 1980;98(4):707–10.
965. Freeman LN, Schachat AP, Knox DL, Michels RG, Green WR. Clinical features, laboratory investigations, and survival in ocular reticulum cell sarcoma. Ophthalmology. 1987;94(12):1631–9.
966. Sen HN, Bodaghi B, Hoang PL, Nussenblatt R. Primary intraocular lymphoma: diagnosis and differential diagnosis. Ocul Immunol Inflamm. 2009;17(3):133–41.
967. Wang Z, Liu Y, Mo J, Cao X, Xu X, Shen L, Wang H, Wei W. Mucosal associated lymphoid tissue lymphoma of the uvea: an analysis of 3 cases. BMC Ophthalmol. 2022;22(1):371.
968. Gaucher D, Bodaghi B, Charlotte F, Schneider C, Cassoux N, Lemaitre C, Leblond V, Rao N, LeHoang P. MALT-type B-cell lymphoma masquerading as scleritis or posterior uveitis. J Fr Ophtalmol. 2005;28(1):31–8.
969. Soussain C, Malaise D, Cassoux N. Primary vitreoretinal lymphoma: a diagnostic and management challenge. Blood. 2021;138(17):1519–34.
970. Raja H, Snyder MR, Johnston PB, O'Neill BP, Caraballo JN, Balsanek JG, Peters BE, Decker PA, Pulido JS. Effect of intravitreal methotrexate and rituximab on interleukin-10 levels in aqueous humor of treated eyes with vitreoretinal lymphoma. PLoS One. 2013;8(6):e65627.
971. Levasseur SD, Wittenberg LA, White VA. Vitreoretinal lymphoma: a 20-year review of incidence, clinical and cytologic features, treatment, and outcomes. JAMA Ophthalmol. 2013;131(1):50–5.
972. Venkatesh R, Bavaharan B, Mahendradas P, Yadav NK. Primary vitreoretinal lymphoma: prevalence, impact, and management challenges. Clin Ophthalmol. 2019;13:353–64.
973. Hoffman PM, McKelvie P, Hall AJ, Stawell RJ, Santamaria JD. Intraocular lymphoma: a series of 14 patients with clinicopathological features and treatment outcomes. Eye (Lond). 2003;17(4):513–21.
974. Cassoux N, Merle-Beral H, Leblond V, Bodaghi B, Milea D, Gerber S, Fardeau C, Reux I, Xuan KH, Chan CC, et al. Ocular and central nervous system lymphoma: clinical features and diagnosis. Ocul Immunol Inflamm. 2000;8(4):243–50.
975. Wender A, Adar A, Maor E, Yassur Y. Primary B-cell lymphoma of the eyes and brain in a 3-year-old boy. Arch Ophthalmol. 1994;112(4):450–1.
976. Sobrin L, Dubovy SR, Davis JL, Murray TG. Isolated, bilateral intraocular lymphoma in a 15-year-old girl. Retina. 2005;25(3):370–3.
977. Berenbom A, Davila RM, Lin HS, Harbour JW. Treatment outcomes for primary intraocular lymphoma: implications for external beam radiotherapy. Eye (Lond). 2007;21(9):1198–201.
978. Buettner H, Bolling JP. Intravitreal large-cell lymphoma. Mayo Clin Proc. 1993;68(10):1011–5.
979. Peterson K, Gordon KB, Heinemann MH, DeAngelis LM. The clinical spectrum of ocular lymphoma. Cancer. 1993;72(3):843–9.
980. Qualman SJ, Mendelsohn G, Mann RB, Green WR. Intraocular lymphomas. Natural history based on a clinicopathologic study of eight cases and review of the literature. Cancer. 1983;52(5):878–86.

981. Zhao XY, Cheng TT, Meng LH, Zhang WF, Chen YX. Clinical features, diagnosis, management and prognosis of primary intraocular lymphoma. Front Oncol. 2022;12:808511.
982. Hochberg FH, Miller DC. Primary central nervous system lymphoma. J Neurosurg. 1988;68(6):835–53.
983. Cho BJ, Yu HG. Risk factors for intraocular involvement in patients with primary central nervous system lymphoma. J Neurooncol. 2014;120(3):523–9.
984. Char DH, Ljung BM, Miller T, Phillips T. Primary intraocular lymphoma (ocular reticulum cell sarcoma) diagnosis and management. Ophthalmology. 1988;95(5):625–30.
985. Chan CC, Rubenstein JL, Coupland SE, Davis JL, Harbour JW, Johnston PB, Cassoux N, Touitou V, Smith JR, Batchelor TT, et al. Primary vitreoretinal lymphoma: a report from an International Primary Central Nervous System Lymphoma Collaborative Group symposium. Oncologist. 2011;16(11):1589–99.
986. Kalogeropoulos D, Vartholomatos G, Mitra A, Elaraoud I, Ch'ng SW, Zikou A, Papoudou-Bai A, Moschos MM, Kanavaros P, Kalogeropoulos C. Primary vitreoretinal lymphoma. Saudi J Ophthalmol. 2019;33(1):66–80.
987. Velez G, de Smet MD, Whitcup SM, Robinson M, Nussenblatt RB, Chan CC. Iris involvement in primary intraocular lymphoma: report of two cases and review of the literature. Surv Ophthalmol. 2000;44(6):518–26.
988. Chan SM, Hutnik CM, Heathcote JG, Orton RB, Banerjee D. Iris lymphoma in a pediatric cardiac transplant recipient: clinicopathologic findings. Ophthalmology. 2000;107(8):1479–82.
989. Lobo A, Larkin G, Clark BJ, Towler HM, Lightman S. Pseudo-hypopyon as the presenting feature in B-cell and T-cell intraocular lymphoma. Clin Exp Ophthalmol. 2003;31(2):155–8.
990. Corriveau C, Easterbrook M, Payne D. Lymphoma simulating uveitis (masquerade syndrome). Can J Ophthalmol. 1986;21(4):144–9.
991. Zhou M, Xu G. Recent progress in the diagnosis and treatment of primary vitreoretinal lymphoma. Taiwan J Ophthalmol. 2016;6(4):170–6.
992. Augsburger JJ, Greatrex KV. Intraocular lymphoma: clinical presentations, differential diagnosis and treatment. Trans PA Acad Ophthalmol Otolaryngol. 1989;41:796–808.
993. Akpek EK, Ahmed I, Hochberg FH, Soheilian M, Dryja TP, Jakobiec FA, Foster CS. Intraocular-central nervous system lymphoma: clinical features, diagnosis, and outcomes. Ophthalmology. 1999;106(9):1805–10.
994. Gass JD, Sever RJ, Grizzard WS, Clarkson JG, Blumenkranz M, Wind CA, Shugarman R. Multifocal pigment epithelial detachments by reticulum cell sarcoma. A characteristic funduscopic picture. Retina. 1984;4(3):135–43.
995. Tsai T, O'Brien JM. Masquerade syndromes: malignancies mimicking inflammation in the eye. Int Ophthalmol Clin. 2002;42(1):115–31.
996. Hedayatfar A, Phaik Chee S. Presumptive primary intraocular lymphoma presented as an intraocular mass involving the optic nerve head. J Ophthalmic Inflamm Infect. 2012;2(1):49–51.
997. Gill MK, Jampol LM. Variations in the presentation of primary intraocular lymphoma: case reports and a review. Surv Ophthalmol. 2001;45(6):463–71.
998. Egawa M, Mitamura Y, Hayashi Y, Semba K, Naito T. Changes of fundus autofluorescence and spectral-domain optical coherence tomographic findings after treatment of primary intraocular lymphoma. J Ophthalmic Inflamm Infect. 2014;4(1):7.
999. Fardeau C, Lee CP, Merle-Beral H, Cassoux N, Bodaghi B, Davi F, Lehoang P. Retinal fluorescein, indocyanine green angiography, and optic coherence tomography in non-Hodgkin primary intraocular lymphoma. Am J Ophthalmol. 2009;147(5):886–94, 894 e881.
1000. Xiao Z. Precise dignosis and treatment of myelodysplastic syndromes: current state and problems. J Clin Hematol (China). 2017;30(5):339–41.
1001. Ursea R, Heinemann MH, Silverman RH, Deangelis LM, Daly SW, Coleman DJ. Ophthalmic, ultrasonographic findings in primary central nervous system lymphoma with ocular involvement. Retina. 1997;17(2):118–23.

1002. Chaput F, Amer R, Baglivo E, Touitou V, Kozyreff A, Bron D, Bodaghi B, LeHoang P, Bergstrom C, Grossniklaus HE, et al. Intraocular T-cell lymphoma: clinical presentation, diagnosis, treatment, and outcome. Ocul Immunol Inflamm. 2017;25(5):639–48.
1003. Brown SM, Jampol LM, Cantrill HL. Intraocular lymphoma presenting as retinal vasculitis. Surv Ophthalmol. 1994;39(2):133–40.
1004. Abedi F, Borovik AM, Waring D, Hariz S, Francis IC. Primary intraocular natural killer/T-cell lymphoma unmasked with infective endophthalmitis after an intravitreal injection of bevacizumab. Clin Exp Ophthalmol. 2019;47(8):1088–9.
1005. Gao S, Zhou Y, Jin X, Lin Z, Zhong Y, Shen X. Primary vitreoretinal natural killer/T-cell lymphoma with breast involvement: a case report and review of the literature. Surv Ophthalmol. 2019;64(2):225–32.
1006. Matsuo T, Shimizu T, Tanaka T, Yamamoto A, Takasuka H. Pathologically proven intraocular infiltration with adult T-cell leukemia/lymphoma: two new cases with either vitreous opacity or aqueous hypopyon and literature review of 16 cases. J Investig Med High Impact Case Rep. 2020;8:2324709620966843.
1007. Araujo I, Coupland SE. Primary vitreoretinal lymphoma—a review. Asia Pac J Ophthalmol (Phila). 2017;6(3):283–9.
1008. Fend F, Ferreri AJ, Coupland SE. How we diagnose and treat vitreoretinal lymphoma. Br J Haematol. 2016;173(5):680–92.
1009. Dalal M, Casady M, Moriarty E, Faia L, Nussenblatt R, Chan CC, Sen HN. Diagnostic procedures in vitreoretinal lymphoma. Ocul Immunol Inflamm. 2014;22(4):270–6.
1010. Takase H, Arai A, Iwasaki Y, Imai A, Nagao T, Kawagishi M, Ishida T, Mochizuki M. Challenges in the diagnosis and management of vitreoretinal lymphoma—clinical and basic approaches. Prog Retin Eye Res. 2022;90:101053.
1011. Davis JL. Intraocular lymphoma: a clinical perspective. Eye (Lond). 2013;27(2):153–62.
1012. Bonzheim I, Giese S, Deuter C, Susskind D, Zierhut M, Waizel M, Szurman P, Federmann B, Schmidt J, Quintanilla-Martinez L, et al. High frequency of MYD88 mutations in vitreoretinal B-cell lymphoma: a valuable tool to improve diagnostic yield of vitreous aspirates. Blood. 2015;126(1):76–9.
1013. Gorochov G, Parizot C, Bodaghi B, Raphael D, Cassoux N, Merle-Beral H, Debre P, LeHoang P. Characterization of vitreous B-cell infiltrates in patients with primary ocular lymphoma, using CDR3 size polymorphism analysis of antibody transcripts. Invest Ophthalmol Vis Sci. 2003;44(12):5235–41.
1014. Wang Y, Shen D, Wang VM, Sen HN, Chan CC. Molecular biomarkers for the diagnosis of primary vitreoretinal lymphoma. Int J Mol Sci. 2011;12(9):5684–97.
1015. Heiferman MJ, Yu MD, Mruthyunjaya P. Update in molecular testing for intraocular lymphoma. Cancers (Basel). 2022;14(19):4546.
1016. Miserocchi E, Ferreri AJM, Giuffre C, Cangi MG, Francaviglia I, Calimeri T, Ponzoni M, Pecciarini L, Bandello FM, Modorati GM. Myd88 L265p mutation detection in the aqueous humor of patients with vitreoretinal lymphoma. Retina. 2019;39(4):679–84.
1017. Dunn JP. Interleukins in the diagnosis of intraocular lymphoma: do we still need histologic confirmation? Retina. 2018;38(4):647–9.
1018. Nussenblatt RB, Chan CC, Wilson WH, Hochman J, Gottesman M, Cns, Ocular Lymphoma Workshop Group. International Central Nervous System and Ocular Lymphoma Workshop: recommendations for the future. Ocul Immunol Inflamm. 2006;14(3):139–44.
1019. Davis JL, Miller DM, Ruiz P. Diagnostic testing of vitrectomy specimens. Am J Ophthalmol. 2005;140(5):822–9.
1020. Davis JL, Viciana AL, Ruiz P. Diagnosis of intraocular lymphoma by flow cytometry. Am J Ophthalmol. 1997;124(3):362–72.
1021. Finger PT, Papp C, Latkany P, Kurli M, Iacob CE. Anterior chamber paracentesis cytology (cytospin technique) for the diagnosis of intraocular lymphoma. Br J Ophthalmol. 2006;90(6):690–2.

1022. Cassoux N, Giron A, Bodaghi B, Tran TH, Baudet S, Davy F, Chan CC, Lehoang P, Merle-Beral H. IL-10 measurement in aqueous humor for screening patients with suspicion of primary intraocular lymphoma. Invest Ophthalmol Vis Sci. 2007;48(7):3253–9.
1023. Banchereau J, Briere F, Liu YJ, Rousset F. Molecular control of B lymphocyte growth and differentiation. Stem Cells. 1994;12(3):278–88.
1024. Chan CC, Whitcup SM, Solomon D, Nussenblatt RB. Interleukin-10 in the vitreous of patients with primary intraocular lymphoma. Am J Ophthalmol. 1995;120(5):671–3.
1025. Buggage RR, Whitcup SM, Nussenblatt RB, Chan CC. Using interleukin 10 to interleukin 6 ratio to distinguish primary intraocular lymphoma and uveitis. Invest Ophthalmol Vis Sci. 1999;40(10):2462–3.
1026. Ohta K, Sano K, Imai H, Kikuchi T. Cytokine and molecular analyses of intraocular lymphoma. Ocul Immunol Inflamm. 2009;17(3):142–7.
1027. Merle-Beral H, Davi F, Cassoux N, Baudet S, Colin C, Gourdet T, Bodaghi B, LeHoang P. Biological diagnosis of primary intraocular lymphoma. Br J Haematol. 2004;124(4):469–73.
1028. Hiemcke-Jiwa LS, Ten Dam-van Loon NH, Leguit RJ, Nierkens S, Ossewaarde-van Norel J, de Boer JH, Roholl FF, de Weger RA, Huibers MMH, de Groot-Mijnes JDF, et al. Potential diagnosis of vitreoretinal lymphoma by detection of MYD88 mutation in aqueous humor with ultrasensitive droplet digital polymerase chain reaction. JAMA Ophthalmol. 2018;136(10):1098–104.
1029. Chen K, Li X, Wang D, Ma Y, Chen B, Wang Q, Ma J, Guan M. The diagnostic value of IL-10 and IL-6 level in vitreous fluid and aqueous humor for vitreoretinal lymphoma. Clin Chim Acta. 2021b;515:21–6.
1030. Costopoulos M, Touitou V, Golmard JL, Darugar A, Fisson S, Bonnemye P, Le Lez ML, Soussain C, Cassoux N, Lamy T, et al. ISOLD: a new highly sensitive interleukin score for intraocular lymphoma diagnosis. Ophthalmology. 2016;123(7):1626–8.
1031. Sugita S, Takase H, Sugamoto Y, Arai A, Miura O, Mochizuki M. Diagnosis of intraocular lymphoma by polymerase chain reaction analysis and cytokine profiling of the vitreous fluid. Jpn J Ophthalmol. 2009;53(3):209–14.
1032. Tanaka R, Kaburaki T, Taoka K, Karakawa A, Tsuji H, Nishikawa M, Yatomi Y, Shinozaki-Ushiku A, Ushiku T, Araki F. More accurate diagnosis of vitreoretinal lymphoma using a combination of diagnostic test results: a prospective observational study. Ocul Immunol Inflamm. 2022;30(6):1354–60.
1033. Kase S, Namba K, Iwata D, Mizuuchi K, Suzuki K, Ito T, Hase K, Kitaichi N, Ishida S. Diagnostic accuracy of cell block preparations and clinical features affecting it in vitreoretinal lymphoma. J Clin Med. 2022;11(5):1391.
1034. Whitcup SM, Stark-Vancs V, Wittes RE, Solomon D, Podgor MJ, Nussenblatt RB, Chan CC. Association of interleukin 10 in the vitreous and cerebrospinal fluid and primary central nervous system lymphoma. Arch Ophthalmol. 1997;115(9):1157–60.
1035. Wolf LA, Reed GF, Buggage RR, Nussenblatt RB, Chan CC. Vitreous cytokine levels. Ophthalmology. 2003;110(8):1671–2.
1036. Castellino A, Pulido JS, Johnston PB, Ristow KM, Nora Bennani N, Inwards DJ, Macon WR, Micallef INM, King RL, Salomao DR, et al. Role of systemic high-dose methotrexate and combined approaches in the management of vitreoretinal lymphoma: a single center experience 1990-2018. Am J Hematol. 2019;94(3):291–8.
1037. Kuo DE, Wei MM, Armbrust KR, Knickelbein JE, Yeung IYL, Nussenblatt RB, Chan CC, Sen HN. Gradient boosted decision tree classification of endophthalmitis versus uveitis and lymphoma from aqueous and vitreous IL-6 and IL-10 levels. J Ocul Pharmacol Ther. 2017;33(4):319–24.
1038. Fisson S, Ouakrim H, Touitou V, Baudet S, Ben Abdelwahed R, Donnou S, Miloudi A, Galand C, Bodaghi B, Lehoang P, et al. Cytokine profile in human eyes: contribution of a new cytokine combination for differential diagnosis between intraocular lymphoma or uveitis. PLoS One. 2013;8(2):e52385.

1039. Ranty ML, Laurent C, Aziza J, Mahieu L, Olle P, Quintyn JC, Garnier L, Bienvenu J, Collin L, Delisle MB, et al. Improving the cytological diagnosis of intraocular lymphoma from vitreous fluid. Histopathology. 2015;67(1):48–61.
1040. White VA, Gascoyne RD, Paton KE. Use of the polymerase chain reaction to detect B- and T-cell gene rearrangements in vitreous specimens from patients with intraocular lymphoma. Arch Ophthalmol. 1999;117(6):761–5.
1041. Shen DF, Zhuang Z, LeHoang P, Boni R, Zheng S, Nussenblatt RB, Chan CC. Utility of microdissection and polymerase chain reaction for the detection of immunoglobulin gene rearrangement and translocation in primary intraocular lymphoma. Ophthalmology. 1998;105(9):1664–9.
1042. Kimura K, Usui Y, Goto H, Japanese Intraocular Lymphoma Study Group. Clinical features and diagnostic significance of the intraocular fluid of 217 patients with intraocular lymphoma. Jpn J Ophthalmol. 2012;56(4):383–9.
1043. Bruno A, Boisselier B, Labreche K, Marie Y, Polivka M, Jouvet A, Adam C, Figarella-Branger D, Miquel C, Eimer S, et al. Mutational analysis of primary central nervous system lymphoma. Oncotarget. 2014;5(13):5065–75.
1044. Gonzalez-Aguilar A, Idbaih A, Boisselier B, Habbita N, Rossetto M, Laurenge A, Bruno A, Jouvet A, Polivka M, Adam C, et al. Recurrent mutations of MYD88 and TBL1XR1 in primary central nervous system lymphomas. Clin Cancer Res. 2012;18(19):5203–11.
1045. Montesinos-Rongen M, Godlewska E, Brunn A, Wiestler OD, Siebert R, Deckert M. Activating L265P mutations of the MYD88 gene are common in primary central nervous system lymphoma. Acta Neuropathol. 2011;122(6):791–2.
1046. Raja H, Salomao DR, Viswanatha DS, Pulido JS. Prevalence of Myd88 L265p mutation in histologically proven, diffuse large B-cell vitreoretinal lymphoma. Retina. 2016b;36(3):624–8.
1047. Pulido JS, Raja H, Vile RG, Salomao DR, Viswanatha DS. Mighty MyD88 in health and disease. Retina. 2016;36(3):429–31.
1048. Coupland SE. Molecular pathology of lymphoma. Eye (Lond). 2013;27(2):180–9.
1049. Gametchu B. Glucocorticoid receptor-like antigen in lymphoma cell membranes: correlation to cell lysis. Science. 1987;236(4800):456–61.
1050. Fernandez-Rodriguez C, Bellosillo B, Garcia-Garcia M, Sanchez-Gonzalez B, Gimeno E, Vela MC, Serrano S, Besses C, Salar A. MYD88 (L265P) mutation is an independent prognostic factor for outcome in patients with diffuse large B-cell lymphoma. Leukemia. 2014;28(10):2104–6.
1051. Liu S, Gu J, Zhang T, Ping B, Zhou M, Huang X, Jiang R, Xu G, Chang Q. Clinical features, diagnostic significance, and prognosis of vitreoretinal lymphoma in young patients. Retina. 2021;41(12):2596–604.
1052. Yonese I, Takase H, Yoshimori M, Onozawa E, Tsuzura A, Miki T, Mochizuki M, Miura O, Arai A. CD79B mutations in primary vitreoretinal lymphoma: diagnostic and prognostic potential. Eur J Haematol. 2019;102(2):191–6.
1053. Takhar J, Doan T, Gonzales JA. Vitreoretinal lymphoma: a literature review and introduction of a new diagnostic method. Asia Pac J Ophthalmol (Phila). 2021;10(1):93–8.
1054. Coupland SE, Bechrakis NE, Anastassiou G, Foerster AM, Heiligenhaus A, Pleyer U, Hummel M, Stein H. Evaluation of vitrectomy specimens and chorioretinal biopsies in the diagnosis of primary intraocular lymphoma in patients with Masquerade syndrome. Graefes Arch Clin Exp Ophthalmol. 2003;241(10):860–70.
1055. Zaldivar RA, Martin DF, Holden JT, Grossniklaus HE. Primary intraocular lymphoma: clinical, cytologic, and flow cytometric analysis. Ophthalmology. 2004;111(9):1762–7.
1056. Yeh S, Weichel ED, Faia LJ, Albini TA, Wroblewski KK, Stetler-Stevenson M, Ruiz P, Sen HN, Chan CC, Nussenblatt RB. 25-Gauge transconjunctival sutureless vitrectomy for the diagnosis of intraocular lymphoma. Br J Ophthalmol. 2010b;94(5):633–8.
1057. Kanavi MR, Soheilian M, Hosseini SB, Azari AA. 25-gauge transconjunctival diagnostic vitrectomy in suspected cases of intraocular lymphoma: a case series and review of the literature. Int J Ophthalmol. 2014;7(3):577–81.

1058. Hoang-Xuan K, Bessell E, Bromberg J, Hottinger AF, Preusser M, Ruda R, Schlegel U, Siegal T, Soussain C, Abacioglu U, et al. Diagnosis and treatment of primary CNS lymphoma in immunocompetent patients: guidelines from the European Association for Neuro-Oncology. Lancet Oncol. 2015;16(7):e322–32.
1059. Pui CH, Robison LL, Look AT. Acute lymphoblastic leukaemia. Lancet. 2008;371(9617):1030–43.
1060. de Smet MD, Vancs VS, Kohler D, Solomon D, Chan CC. Intravitreal chemotherapy for the treatment of recurrent intraocular lymphoma. Br J Ophthalmol. 1999;83(4):448–51.
1061. de Smet MD, Stark-Vancs V, Kohler DR, Smith J, Wittes R, Nussenblatt RB. Intraocular levels of methotrexate after intravenous administration. Am J Ophthalmol. 1996;121(4):442–4.
1062. Wang JK, Yang CM, Lin CP, Shan YD, Lo AY, Tien HF. An Asian patient with intraocular lymphoma treated by intravitreal methotrexate. Jpn J Ophthalmol. 2006;50(5):474–8.
1063. Frenkel S, Hendler K, Siegal T, Shalom E, Pe'er J. Intravitreal methotrexate for treating vitreoretinal lymphoma: 10 years of experience. Br J Ophthalmol. 2008;92(3):383–8.
1064. Smith JR, Rosenbaum JT, Wilson DJ, Doolittle ND, Siegal T, Neuwelt EA, Pe'er J. Role of intravitreal methotrexate in the management of primary central nervous system lymphoma with ocular involvement. Ophthalmology. 2002;109(9):1709–16.
1065. Klimova A, Heissigerova J, Rihova E, Brichova M, Pytlik R, Spicka I, Mrazova K, Karolova J, Svozilkova P. Combined treatment of primary vitreoretinal lymphomas significantly prolongs the time to first relapse. Br J Ophthalmol. 2018;102(11):1579–85.
1066. Zhou X, Zhou X, Shi H, Lai J, Wang Q, Li Y, Chen K, Li Q, Zhou Q, Cao X, et al. Reduced frequency of intravitreal methotrexate injection lowers the risk of Keratopathy in vitreoretinal lymphoma patients. BMC Ophthalmol. 2020;20(1):189.
1067. Pulido JS, Johnston PB, Nowakowski GS, Castellino A, Raja H. The diagnosis and treatment of primary vitreoretinal lymphoma: a review. Int J Retina Vitreous. 2018;4:18.
1068. Seregard S. Posterior uveal melanoma. The Swedish perspective. Acta Ophthalmol Scand. 1996;74(4):315–29.
1069. Chang AE, Karnell LH, Menck HR. The National Cancer Data Base report on cutaneous and noncutaneous melanoma: a summary of 84,836 cases from the past decade. The American College of Surgeons Commission on Cancer and the American Cancer Society. Cancer. 1998;83(8):1664–78.
1070. Mooy CM, De Jong PT. Prognostic parameters in uveal melanoma: a review. Surv Ophthalmol. 1996;41(3):215–28.
1071. Gragoudas ES, Egan KM, Seddon JM, Walsh SM, Munzenrider JE. Intraocular recurrence of uveal melanoma after proton beam irradiation. Ophthalmology. 1992;99(5):760–6.
1072. Shields CL, Shields JA, Milite J, De Potter P, Sabbagh R, Menduke H. Uveal melanoma in teenagers and children. A report of 40 cases. Ophthalmology. 1991;98(11):1662–6.
1073. Journée-de Korver JG, Keunen JE. Thermotherapy in the management of choroidal melanoma. Prog Retin Eye Res. 2002;21(3):303–17.
1074. Grossniklaus HE, Albert DM, Green WR, Conway BP, Hovland KR. Clear cell differentiation in choroidal melanoma. COMS report no. 8. Collaborative Ocular Melanoma Study Group. Arch Ophthalmol. 1997;115(7):894–8.
1075. Grisanti S, Ranjbar M, Tura A, Heindl LM, Kakkassery V. Uveal melanoma: early detection as the key to successful personalized medicine. Ophthalmologe. 2020;117(6):508–20.
1076. Damato EM, Damato BE. Detection and time to treatment of uveal melanoma in the United Kingdom: an evaluation of 2,384 patients. Ophthalmology. 2012;119(8):1582–9.
1077. Andreoli MT, Mieler WF, Leiderman YI. Epidemiological trends in uveal melanoma. Br J Ophthalmol. 2015;99(11):1550–3.
1078. Virgili G, Gatta G, Ciccolallo L, Capocaccia R, Biggeri A, Crocetti E, Lutz JM, Paci E. Incidence of uveal melanoma in Europe. Ophthalmology. 2007;114(12):2309–15.
1079. Vajdic CM, Kricker A, Giblin M, McKenzie J, Aitken J, Giles GG, Armstrong BK. Incidence of ocular melanoma in Australia from 1990 to 1998. Int J Cancer. 2003;105(1):117–22.
1080. Margo CE, Mulla Z, Billiris K. Incidence of surgically treated uveal melanoma by race and ethnicity. Ophthalmology. 1998;105(6):1087–90.

1081. Gupta MP, Lane AM, DeAngelis MM, Mayne K, Crabtree M, Gragoudas ES, Kim IK. Clinical characteristics of uveal melanoma in patients with germline BAP1 mutations. JAMA Ophthalmol. 2015;133(8):881–7.
1082. Singh P, Singh A. Choroidal melanoma. Oman J Ophthalmol. 2012;5(1):3–9.
1083. Branisteanu DC, Bogdanici CM, Branisteanu DE, Maranduca MA, Zemba M, Balta F, Branisteanu CI, Moraru AD. Uveal melanoma diagnosis and current treatment options (Review). Exp Ther Med. 2021;22(6):1428.
1084. Bedi DG, Gombos DS, Ng CS, Singh S. Sonography of the eye. AJR Am J Roentgenol. 2006;187(4):1061–72.
1085. Chattopadhyay C, Kim DW, Gombos DS, Oba J, Qin Y, Williams MD, Esmaeli B, Grimm EA, Wargo JA, Woodman SE, et al. Uveal melanoma: from diagnosis to treatment and the science in between. Cancer. 2016;122(15):2299–312.
1086. Kivela T. Diagnosis of uveal melanoma. Dev Ophthalmol. 2012;49:1–15.
1087. Accuracy of diagnosis of choroidal melanomas in the Collaborative Ocular Melanoma Study. COMS report no. 1. Arch Ophthalmol. 1990;108(9):1268–73.
1088. Char DH, Miller T. Accuracy of presumed uveal melanoma diagnosis before alternative therapy. Br J Ophthalmol. 1995;79(7):692–6.
1089. Damato B, Eleuteri A, Taktak AF, Coupland SE. Estimating prognosis for survival after treatment of choroidal melanoma. Prog Retin Eye Res. 2011;30(5):285–95.
1090. Vader MJC, Madigan MC, Versluis M, Suleiman HM, Gezgin G, Gruis NA, Out-Luiting JJ, Bergman W, Verdijk RM, Jager MJ, et al. GNAQ and GNA11 mutations and downstream YAP activation in choroidal nevi. Br J Cancer. 2017;117(6):884–7.
1091. Van Raamsdonk CD, Griewank KG, Crosby MB, Garrido MC, Vemula S, Wiesner T, Obenauf AC, Wackernagel W, Green G, Bouvier N, et al. Mutations in GNA11 in uveal melanoma. N Engl J Med. 2010;363(23):2191–9.
1092. Damato B. Ocular treatment of choroidal melanoma in relation to the prevention of metastatic death—a personal view. Prog Retin Eye Res. 2018;66:187–99.
1093. Nagarkatti-Gude N, Bronkhorst IH, van Duinen SG, Luyten GP, Jager MJ. Cytokines and chemokines in the vitreous fluid of eyes with uveal melanoma. Invest Ophthalmol Vis Sci. 2012;53(11):6748–55.
1094. Lattanzio L, Tonissi F, Torta I, Gianello L, Russi E, Milano G, Merlano M, Lo Nigro C. Role of IL-8 induced angiogenesis in uveal melanoma. Invest New Drugs. 2013;31(5):1107–14.
1095. Oliva M, Rullan AJ, Piulats JM. Uveal melanoma as a target for immune-therapy. Ann Transl Med. 2016;4(9):172.
1096. Bronkhorst IH, Jager MJ. Uveal melanoma: the inflammatory microenvironment. J Innate Immun. 2012;4(5-6):454–62.
1097. Jager MJ, Ly LV, El Filali M, Madigan MC. Macrophages in uveal melanoma and in experimental ocular tumor models: friends or foes? Prog Retin Eye Res. 2011;30(2):129–46.
1098. Ly LV, Bronkhorst IH, van Beelen E, Vrolijk J, Taylor AW, Versluis M, Luyten GP, Jager MJ. Inflammatory cytokines in eyes with uveal melanoma and relation with macrophage infiltration. Invest Ophthalmol Vis Sci. 2010;51(11):5445–51.
1099. Koga M, Kai H, Egami K, Murohara T, Ikeda A, Yasuoka S, Egashira K, Matsuishi T, Kai M, Kataoka Y, et al. Mutant MCP-1 therapy inhibits tumor angiogenesis and growth of malignant melanoma in mice. Biochem Biophys Res Commun. 2008;365(2):279–84.
1100. Amaro A, Mirisola V, Angelini G, Musso A, Tosetti F, Esposito AI, Perri P, Lanza F, Nasciuti F, Mosci C, et al. Evidence of epidermal growth factor receptor expression in uveal melanoma: inhibition of epidermal growth factor-mediated signalling by Gefitinib and Cetuximab triggered antibody-dependent cellular cytotoxicity. Eur J Cancer. 2013;49(15):3353–65.
1101. Topcu-Yilmaz P, Kiratli H, Saglam A, Söylemezoglu F, Hascelik G. Correlation of clinicopathological parameters with HGF, c-Met, EGFR, and IGF-1R expression in uveal melanoma. Melanoma Res. 2010;20(2):126–32.
1102. Bröcker EB, Magiera H, Herlyn M. Nerve growth and expression of receptors for nerve growth factor in tumors of melanocyte origin. J Invest Dermatol. 1991;96(5):662–5.

1103. Li B, Cai S, Zhao Y, He Q, Yu X, Cheng L, Zhang Y, Hu X, Ke M, Chen S, et al. Nerve growth factor modulates the tumor cells migration in ovarian cancer through the WNT/β-catenin pathway. Oncotarget. 2016;7(49):81026–48.
1104. Manni L, Lundeberg T, Fiorito S, Bonini S, Vigneti E, Aloe L. Nerve growth factor release by human synovial fibroblasts prior to and following exposure to tumor necrosis factor-alpha, interleukin-1 beta and cholecystokinin-8: the possible role of NGF in the inflammatory response. Clin Exp Rheumatol. 2003;21(5):617–24.
1105. Yue XJ, Xu LB, Zhu MS, Zhang R, Liu C. Over-expression of nerve growth factor-β in human cholangiocarcinoma QBC939 cells promote tumor progression. PLoS One. 2013;8(4):e62024.
1106. Missotten GS, Notting IC, Schlingemann RO, Zijlmans HJ, Lau C, Eilers PH, Keunen JE, Jager MJ. Vascular endothelial growth factor a in eyes with uveal melanoma. Arch Ophthalmol. 2006;124(10):1428–34.
1107. Boyd SR, Tan D, Bunce C, Gittos A, Neale MH, Hungerford JL, Charnock-Jones S, Cree IA. Vascular endothelial growth factor is elevated in ocular fluids of eyes harbouring uveal melanoma: identification of a potential therapeutic window. Br J Ophthalmol. 2002a;86(4):448–52.
1108. Boyd SR, Tan DS, de Souza L, Neale MH, Myatt NE, Alexander RA, Robb M, Hungerford JL, Cree IA. Uveal melanomas express vascular endothelial growth factor and basic fibroblast growth factor and support endothelial cell growth. Br J Ophthalmol. 2002b;86(4):440–7.
1109. Wierenga APA, Gezgin G, van Beelen E, Eikmans M, Spruyt-Gerritse M, Brouwer NJ, Versluis M, Verdijk RM, van Duinen SG, Marinkovic M, et al. Soluble HLA in the aqueous humour of uveal melanoma is associated with unfavourable tumour characteristics. Cancers (Basel). 2019;11(8):1202.
1110. Ragusa M, Barbagallo C, Statello L, Caltabiano R, Russo A, Puzzo L, Avitabile T, Longo A, Toro MD, Barbagallo D, et al. miRNA profiling in vitreous humor, vitreal exosomes and serum from uveal melanoma patients: pathological and diagnostic implications. Cancer Biol Ther. 2015;16(9):1387–96.
1111. Cochran AJ, Holland GN, Saxton RE, Damato BE, Foulds WR, Herschman HR, Foos RY, Straatsma BR, Lee WR. Detection and quantification of S-100 protein in ocular tissues and fluids from patients with intraocular melanoma. Br J Ophthalmol. 1988;72(11):874–9.
1112. Shields CL, Shields JA, Perez N, Singh AD, Cater J. Primary transpupillary thermotherapy for small choroidal melanoma in 256 consecutive cases: outcomes and limitations. Ophthalmology. 2002;109(2):225–34.
1113. Takiar V, Gombos DS, Mourtada F, Rechner LA, Lawyer AA, Morrison WH, Garden AS, Beadle BM. Disease control and toxicity outcomes using ruthenium eye plaque brachytherapy in the treatment of uveal melanoma. Pract Radiat Oncol. 2014;4(4):e189–94.
1114. Egger E, Zografos L, Schalenbourg A, Beati D, Böhringer T, Chamot L, Goitein G. Eye retention after proton beam radiotherapy for uveal melanoma. Int J Radiat Oncol Biol Phys. 2003;55(4):867–80.
1115. Damato BE, Foulds WS. Chapter 40. Surgical resection of choroidal melanoma. In: Ryan SJ, Hinton DR, Schachat AP, Wilkinson CP, editors. Retina. 4th ed. Edinburgh: Mosby; 2006. p. 769–78.
1116. Folberg R, Rummelt V, Parys-Van Ginderdeuren R, Hwang T, Woolson RF, Pe'er J, Gruman LM. The prognostic value of tumor blood vessel morphology in primary uveal melanoma. Ophthalmology. 1993;100(9):1389–98.
1117. Jager MJ, Shields CL, Cebulla CM, Abdel-Rahman MH, Grossniklaus HE, Stern MH, Carvajal RD, Belfort RN, Jia R, Shields JA, et al. Uveal melanoma. Nat Rev Dis Primers. 2020;6(1):24.
1118. Kaliki S, Shields CL, Shields JA. Uveal melanoma: estimating prognosis. Indian J Ophthalmol. 2015;63(2):93–102.
1119. Damato B, Dopierala JA, Coupland SE. Genotypic profiling of 452 choroidal melanomas with multiplex ligation-dependent probe amplification. Clin Cancer Res. 2010;16(24):6083–92.

1120. Parrella P, Sidransky D, Merbs SL. Allelotype of posterior uveal melanoma: implications for a bifurcated tumor progression pathway. Cancer Res. 1999;59(13):3032–7.
1121. Onken MD, Worley LA, Harbour JW. A metastasis modifier locus on human chromosome 8p in uveal melanoma identified by integrative genomic analysis. Clin Cancer Res. 2008;14(12):3737–45.
1122. Broaddus E, Topham A, Singh AD. Incidence of retinoblastoma in the USA: 1975-2004. Br J Ophthalmol. 2009;93(1):21–3.
1123. Friend SH, Bernards R, Rogelj S, Weinberg RA, Rapaport JM, Albert DM, Dryja TP. A human DNA segment with properties of the gene that predisposes to retinoblastoma and osteosarcoma. Nature. 1986;323(6089):643–6.
1124. Grossniklaus HE. Retinoblastoma. Fifty years of progress. The LXXI Edward Jackson Memorial Lecture. Am J Ophthalmol. 2014;158(5):875–91.
1125. Knudson AG Jr. Mutation and cancer: statistical study of retinoblastoma. Proc Natl Acad Sci U S A. 1971;68(4):820–3.
1126. McEvoy JD, Dyer MA. Genetic and epigenetic discoveries in human retinoblastoma. Crit Rev Oncog. 2015;20(3-4):217–25.
1127. Moin M, Malik TG, Siddiq L. Clinical patterns and outcomes of retinoblastoma in a tertiary care centre of a developing country. J Pak Med Assoc. 2023;73(9):1881–3.
1128. Roy SR, Kaliki S. Retinoblastoma: a major review. Mymensingh Med J. 2021;30(3):881–95.
1129. Parkin DM, Stiller CA, Draper GJ, Bieber CA. The international incidence of childhood cancer. Int J Cancer. 1988;42(4):511–20.
1130. Lohmann DR, Gallie BL. Retinoblastoma. In: Adam MP, Mirzaa GM, Pagon RA, Wallace SE, LJH B, Gripp KW, Amemiya A, editors. GeneReviews(®). Seattle, WA: University of Washington; 1993. Copyright © 1993-2023, University of Washington, Seattle. GeneReviews is a registered trademark of the University of Washington, Seattle. All rights reserved.
1131. Bilbeisi T, Almasry R, Obeidat M, Mohammad M, Jaradat I, Halalsheh H, Alni'mat A, Ahmad DK, Alsaket N, Mehyar M, et al. Causes of death and survival analysis for patients with retinoblastoma in Jordan. Front Med (Lausanne). 2023;10:1244308.
1132. Dimaras H, Kimani K, Dimba EA, Gronsdahl P, White A, Chan HS, Gallie BL. Retinoblastoma. Lancet. 2012;379(9824):1436–46.
1133. Kanukollu VM, Tripathy K. Leukocoria. In: Disclosure: Koushik Tripathy declares no relevant financial relationships with ineligible companies. Treasure Island, FL: StatPearls; 2023.
1134. Gu H, Wang Y, Huang D. Clinical features and imaging manifestations of retinoblastoma with hepatic metastasis. Pediatr Blood Cancer. 2021;68(10):e28959.
1135. Fang X, Wang H, Ma X, Guo Y. Clinical features of children with retinoblastoma and neuroblastoma. J Ophthalmol. 2020;2020:9315784.
1136. Lindahl S. Computed tomography of retinoblastoma. Acta Radiol Diagn (Stockh). 1986;27(5):513–8.
1137. de Jong MC, Kors WA, de Graaf P, Castelijns JA, Kivelä T, Moll AC. Trilateral retinoblastoma: a systematic review and meta-analysis. Lancet Oncol. 2014a;15(10):1157–67.
1138. Fabian ID, Abdallah E, Abdullahi SU, Abdulqader RA, Adamou Boubacar S, Ademola-Popoola DS, Adio A, Afshar AR, Aggarwal P, Aghaji AE, et al. Global retinoblastoma presentation and analysis by National Income Level. JAMA Oncol. 2020;6(5):685–95.
1139. de Jong MC, de Graaf P, Noij DP, Göricke S, Maeder P, Galluzzi P, Brisse HJ, Moll AC, Castelijns JA. Diagnostic performance of magnetic resonance imaging and computed tomography for advanced retinoblastoma: a systematic review and meta-analysis. Ophthalmology. 2014b;121(5):1109–18.
1140. Karcioglu ZA. Fine needle aspiration biopsy (FNAB) for retinoblastoma. Retina. 2002;22(6):707–10.
1141. Berry JL, Xu L, Murphree AL, Krishnan S, Stachelek K, Zolfaghari E, McGovern K, Lee TC, Carlsson A, Kuhn P, et al. Potential of aqueous humor as a surrogate tumor biopsy for retinoblastoma. JAMA Ophthalmol. 2017;135(11):1221–30.

1142. Kim ME, Xu L, Prabakar RK, Shen L, Peng CC, Kuhn P, Gai X, Hicks J, Berry JL. Aqueous humor as a liquid biopsy for retinoblastoma: clear corneal paracentesis and genomic analysis. J Vis Exp. 2021;(175).

1143. Rushlow DE, Mol BM, Kennett JY, Yee S, Pajovic S, Thériault BL, Prigoda-Lee NL, Spencer C, Dimaras H, Corson TW, et al. Characterisation of retinoblastomas without RB1 mutations: genomic, gene expression, and clinical studies. Lancet Oncol. 2013;14(4):327–34.

1144. Dias PL, Shanmuganathan SS, Rajaratnam M. Lactic dehydrogenase activity of aqueous humour in retinoblastoma. Br J Ophthalmol. 1971;55(2):130–2.

1145. Shehata HH, Abou Ghalia AH, Elsayed EK, Ziko OO, Mohamed SS. Detection of survivin protein in aqueous humor and serum of retinoblastoma patients and its clinical significance. Clin Biochem. 2010;43(4-5):362–6.

1146. Shehata HH, Abou Ghalia AH, Elsayed EK, Ahmed Said AM, Mahmoud SS. Clinical significance of high levels of survivin and transforming growth factor beta-1 proteins in aqueous humor and serum of retinoblastoma patients. J AAPOS. 2016;20(5):444e441–9.

1147. Comoy E, Roussat B, Henry I, Bloch-Michel E. Neuron-specific enolase in the aqueous humor. Its significance in the differential diagnosis of retinoblastoma. Ophtalmologie. 1990;4(3):233–5.

1148. Hervas Benito I, Ruiz Rodriguez JC, Saura Quiles A, Borghol Kassar R, Harto MA, Bello Arques P, Sancho Gaspar A, Perez Pastor JL, Mateo Navarro A. Radioimmunometric assay of neuron specific enolase in aqueous humor and serum in patients with retinoblastoma. Rev Esp Med Nucl. 2000;19(7):472–8.

1149. Hadjistilianou T, Giglioni S, Micheli L, Vannoni D, Brogi E, Cevenini G, Cortelazzo A, De Francesco S, Menicacci F, Leoncini R. Analysis of aqueous humour proteins in patients with retinoblastoma. Clin Exp Ophthalmol. 2012;40(1):e8–e15.

1150. Szeto W, Jiang W, Tice DA, Rubinfeld B, Hollingshead PG, Fong SE, Dugger DL, Pham T, Yansura DG, Wong TA, et al. Overexpression of the retinoic acid-responsive gene Stra6 in human cancers and its synergistic induction by Wnt-1 and retinoic acid. Cancer Res. 2001;61(10):4197–205.

1151. Berry JL, Xu L, Kooi I, Murphree AL, Prabakar RK, Reid M, Stachelek K, Le BHA, Welter L, Reiser BJ, et al. Genomic cfDNA analysis of aqueous humor in retinoblastoma predicts eye salvage: the surrogate tumor biopsy for retinoblastoma. Mol Cancer Res. 2018;16(11):1701–12.

1152. Ancona-Lezama D, Dalvin LA, Shields CL. Modern treatment of retinoblastoma: a 2020 review. Indian J Ophthalmol. 2020;68(11):2356–65.

1153. Schaiquevich P, Francis JH, Cancela MB, Carcaboso AM, Chantada GL, Abramson DH. Treatment of retinoblastoma: what is the latest and what is the future. Front Oncol. 2022;12:822330.

1154. Leclerc R, Olin J. An overview of retinoblastoma and enucleation in pediatric patients. AORN J. 2020;111(1):69–79.

1155. Munier FL, Soliman S, Moulin AP, Gaillard MC, Balmer A, Beck-Popovic M. Profiling safety of intravitreal injections for retinoblastoma using an anti-reflux procedure and sterilisation of the needle track. Br J Ophthalmol. 2012;96(8):1084–7.

1156. Ueda M, Tanabe J, Inomata M, Kaneko A, Kimura T. Study on conservative treatment of retinoblastoma—effect of intravitreal injection of melphalan on the rabbit retina. Nippon Ganka Gakkai Zasshi. 1995;99(11):1230–5.

1157. Brodie SE, Munier FL, Francis JH, Marr B, Gobin YP, Abramson DH. Persistence of retinal function after intravitreal melphalan injection for retinoblastoma. Doc Ophthalmol. 2013;126(1):79–84.

1158. Sun YB, Hui P, Punyara K, Bi MC, Li SH, Teng SY, Song E. Intravitreal injection of melphalan in the treatment of retinoblastoma with vitreous cavity seeding. Chin Med J (Engl). 2013;126(8):1587.

1159. Suzuki S, Aihara Y, Fujiwara M, Sano S, Kaneko A. Intravitreal injection of melphalan for intraocular retinoblastoma. Jpn J Ophthalmol. 2015;59(3):164–72.

1160. Wong FL, Boice JD Jr, Abramson DH, Tarone RE, Kleinerman RA, Stovall M, Goldman MB, Seddon JM, Tarbell N, Fraumeni JF Jr, et al. Cancer incidence after retinoblastoma. Radiation dose and sarcoma risk. JAMA. 1997;278(15):1262–7.
1161. Dalvin LA, Bas Z, Tadepalli S, Rao R, Vaidya S, Pacheco R, Shields CL. Risk factors for tumor recurrence following primary intravenous chemotherapy (chemoreduction) for retinoblastoma in 869 eyes of 551 patients. J Pediatr Ophthalmol Strabismus. 2020;57(4):224–34.
1162. Kletke SN, Mallipatna A, Mireskandari K, Gallie BL, Ali A. Pediatric cataract surgery following treatment for retinoblastoma: a case series and systematic review. Am J Ophthalmol. 2022;239:130–41.
1163. Kohe SE, Bennett CD, Gill SK, Wilson M, McConville C, Peet AC. Metabolic profiling of the three neural derived embryonal pediatric tumors retinoblastoma, neuroblastoma and medulloblastoma, identifies distinct metabolic profiles. Oncotarget. 2018;9(13):11336–51.
1164. Gomatou G, Trontzas I, Ioannou S, Drizou M, Syrigos N, Kotteas E. Mechanisms of resistance to cyclin-dependent kinase 4/6 inhibitors. Mol Biol Rep. 2021;48(1):915–25.
1165. Togashi K, Okada M, Suzuki S, Sanomachi T, Seino S, Yamamoto M, Yamashita H, Kitanaka C. Inhibition of retinoblastoma cell growth by CEP1347 through activation of the P53 pathway. Anticancer Res. 2020;40(9):4961–8.
1166. Russo E, Spallarossa A. Nanotechnology for pediatric retinoblastoma therapy. Pharmaceuticals. 2022;15:1087.
1167. Hubens WHG, Mohren RJC, Liesenborghs I, Eijssen LMT, Ramdas WD, Webers CAB, Gorgels T. The aqueous humor proteome of primary open angle glaucoma: an extensive review. Exp Eye Res. 2020;197:108077.
1168. Guo T, Guo L, Fan Y, Fang L, Wei J, Tan Y, Chen Y, Fan X. Aqueous humor levels of TGFbeta2 and SFRP1 in different types of glaucoma. BMC Ophthalmol. 2019;19(1):170.
1169. Wang Y, Chen S, Liu Y, Huang W, Li X, Zhang X. Inflammatory cytokine profiles in eyes with primary angle-closure glaucoma. Biosci Rep. 2018;38(6):BSR20181411.
1170. Oribio-Quinto C, Burgos-Blasco B, Perez-Garcia P, Espino-Paisan L, Sarria B, Fernandez-Vigo JI, Garcia-Feijoo J. Aqueous humor cytokine profile in primary congenital glaucoma. J Clin Med. 2023;12(9):3142.
1171. Junemann AGM, Michalke B, Lucio M, Chaudhri A, Schlotzer-Schrehardt U, Rejdak R, Rekas M, Hohberger B. Aqueous humor selenium level and open-angle glaucoma. J Trace Elem Med Biol. 2018;50:67–72.
1172. Yin Z, Gao Y, Tang Y, Tian X, Zheng Y, Han Q. Aqueous humor cytokine levels are associated with the severity of visual field defects in patients with primary open-angle glaucoma. BMC Ophthalmol. 2023;23(1):141.
1173. Picht G, Welge-Luessen U, Grehn F, Lutjen-Drecoll E. Transforming growth factor beta 2 levels in the aqueous humor in different types of glaucoma and the relation to filtering bleb development. Graefes Arch Clin Exp Ophthalmol. 2001;239(3):199–207.
1174. Cvenkel B, Kopitar AN, Ihan A. Inflammatory molecules in aqueous humour and on ocular surface and glaucoma surgery outcome. Mediators Inflamm. 2010;2010:939602.
1175. Aketa N, Yamaguchi T, Asato T, Yagi-Yaguchi Y, Suzuki T, Higa K, Kurihara T, Satake Y, Tsubota K, Shimazaki J. Elevated aqueous cytokine levels in eyes with ocular surface diseases. Am J Ophthalmol. 2017;184:42–51.
1176. Wang L, Zhang Z, Koch DD, Jia Y, Cao W, Zhang S. Anterior chamber interleukin 1beta, interleukin 6 and prostaglandin E2 in patients undergoing femtosecond laser-assisted cataract surgery. Br J Ophthalmol. 2016b;100(4):579–82.
1177. Ji Y, Rong X, Lu Y. Metabolic characterization of human aqueous humor in the cataract progression after pars plana vitrectomy. BMC Ophthalmol. 2018;18(1):63.

MIX
Papier aus verantwortungsvollen Quellen
Paper from responsible sources
FSC® C105338

If you have any concerns about our products,
you can contact us on
ProductSafety@springernature.com

In case Publisher is established outside the EU,
the EU authorized representative is:
Springer Nature Customer Service Center GmbH
Europaplatz 3, 69115 Heidelberg, Germany

Printed by Libri Plureos GmbH
in Hamburg, Germany